Elementary School Health

EDUCATION AND SERVICE

Ronald L. Rhodes
Brent Q. Hafen
Keith J. Karren
L. McKay Rollins
Brigham Young University

ALLYN AND BACON, INC.
Boston   London   Sydney   Toronto

Library of Congress Cataloging in Publication Data

Main entry under title:

Elementary school health.

  Earlier ed. (c1977) published under title: Health and the elementary teacher.
  Bibliography: p.
  Includes index.
  1. School hygiene. 2. School children—Health and hygiene. I. Rhodes, Ronald L. II. Health and the elementary teacher.
LB3405.E43   372.17   80-17511
ISBN 0-205-06979-7

Series Editor: Hiram G. Howard

Printed in the United States of America

Contents

Preface

The elementary school can and should actively look after the health and welfare of its students. Although the school is adjunctive to the home, an alert, sensitive faculty and staff who can deal with existing health threats or problems and impart to children knowledge, attitudes, and skills that will enhance the quality and continuity of their lives render an invaluable service.

We had two purposes for writing this book. First, we wanted to acquaint prospective school personnel with common health problems of elementary schoolchildren and to provide a guide for the prompt detection and follow-up essential to the satisfactory resolution of those problems. Second, we agreed that teachers need a brief overview of the educational elements of health care and guidelines for presenting instructional programs that will effectively foster early acquisition of health habits and skills necessary to maintain optimum health throughout life.

We hope that this text will be a resource for concerned school personnel who are aware of children's health needs, perceive the potential for effective school involvement, and desire to help children develop healthful behaviors and life-styles. Certainly parents and teachers should practice the principles presented in the book and create an atmosphere that will encourage children to emulate their healthful behaviors. Equally important is the attitude that adults convey in their practice and teaching of health habits. Not even skilled teachers can give children a positive attitude about something they themselves care little about.

CHAPTER 1
The Concept of Health

One of the most popular words of our time is "health." This word generates some confusion, much frustration, and a lot of money, and it is the focus of all types of fads and fallacies. Certainly, if we have good health, we have the most precious of all gifts. Hundreds of organizations, including the government, support health programs. Health seems to have a direct relationship to the quality of life. Good health is prerequisite for a full, rich life. Teachers who do not appreciate or understand health give up the opportunity to influence the health of their students.

There are many definitions of health. Benjamin Disraeli, a former British prime minister, stated, "The health of the people is really the foundation upon which all their happiness and all their powers as a State depend."[1] The World Health Organization tried to be more explicit. In 1947, it asserted, "health is a state of complete physical, mental, and social well-being and not merely the absence of disease or infirmity." This definition, though not complete, added a new dimension to the concept of health. Many tend to regard themselves as healthy unless they are sick or injured. A much more positive concept strives for optimal, personal fitness.

Dr. Howard S. Hoyman describes health as "optimal, personal fitness for full, fruitful, creative living."[2] Using Hoyman's levels

FIGURE 1-1. *A continuum of well-being.*

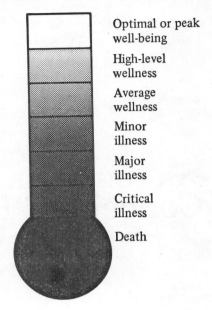

Optimal or peak
well-being

High-level
wellness

Average
wellness

Minor
illness

Major
illness

Critical
illness

Death

of well-being, we can think of health as a continuum (see Figure
1-1).

Cornacchia and Staton describe health through a set of concepts:

Health is personal—it is individual in nature and variability.
Health is complex—it relates to physical, psychologic, social, and spiritual
aspects.
Health is constantly changing—it is a phenomenon that is the result of the
interaction of the growing and developing human organism with the
environment.
Health is dependent upon self-actualization—it necessitates internalization
and action by the individual.
Health is the result of intelligent decisions—it demands selection from the
positive and negative alternatives and their consequences.
Health is necessary for effective learning and living—it is a means to an
end.[3]

Health is greatly influenced by heredity, environment, and behavior. Genetic defects and weaknesses can have a serious effect on
personal health. The environment, or surroundings, can assault tissue
and cause disease. In addition, it can seriously affect emotional
health. Behavior bears directly on our health-related decisions in
the sense that if health values are not well defined and the concept

of health is shallow, we will be easily susceptible to quackery and will make poor health decisions. It is essential, therefore, to prepare students to seek high quality and quantity of life by helping them to understand health and to make good health-related decisions.

The concept of health has evolved from the mysticism and sorcery of day-to-day survival to today's search for well-being and continuing youthfulness. Throughout history the search for survival and longevity has opened new frontiers of health. Each culture and each generation has had its own health problems. New concerns have generated new concepts of health.

The first concept of health was survival in the face of communicable disease, pestilence and famine, ignorance, and war. In the early 1800s the Industrial Revolution gave rise to adverse living conditions, including overcrowding, poor sanitation, overwork and poor nutrition. People became concerned with their quality of living. Health and freedom from disease became synonymous. By 1900 full-scale public sanitation measures had reduced the threat of disease substantially, so health attention shifted to personal hygiene. By the early 1950s, two world wars had revealed that many Americans were in poor physical shape, and the national health emphasis turned to physical fitness. The sixties stressed overall well-being. Today we seek a consensus on health values and the resolution of value conflicts that result from "future shock." Higher-level needs (such as the needs for knowledge, belonging, positive self-concept, and self-actualization) are taking precedence over biological needs. This generation is making more complicated health-related decisions than ever.

Sorochan characterizes health as a style of living. Accepting Metchnikoff's concept of *orthobiosis,* which means a right or proper style of living, he believes that the daily interaction of people and their social and physical environment affects the quality and quantity of their lives.[4] Thus Sorochan's definition of health is an extension of Hoyman's levels of well-being. Though well-being is an abstract concept, a continuum makes it easier to comprehend. Sorochan and Bender identified the levels of well-being labeled on Figure 1–1.[5]

Health is a dynamic, ever-changing process. Whether we move upward or downward on the continuum depends on the effectiveness of health-related decision making and behavior.

Sorochan and Bender delineate fitness components of well-being. The five components are implicated as *unidimensions* of fitness— that is, factors of "wellness" considered separately but functioning together as a whole.[6] Figure 1–2 is a graphic representation of the components of fitness.

There is no way to measure well-being or fitness, but the con-

FIGURE 1-2. *Sorochan and Bender's components of fitness.*

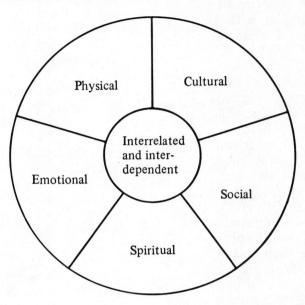

tinuum concept combined with the subjective concept of health can give us a reasonably accurate description. You need not be a diagnostician to recognize that some characteristics distinguish healthy from unhealthy children. For example, healthy children

1. Display the energy and normal development of their age group and participate regularly in physical education.
2. Have the ability to carry out normal school and home responsibilities without undue emotional upset or fatigue.
3. Experience progressive, normal gains in weight and height.
4. Have clear, smooth skin unmarked by eruptions, discoloration, or unusual dryness or oiliness.
5. Experience normal spells of illness and accidents for their age.
6. Have enthusiasm or zest for life.
7. Experience good social (peer) health and are honest and truthful.
8. Have emotional control.

In 1969 the Metropolitan Life Insurance Company released a film designed to "foster greater understanding about the teacher's role as health observer."[7] Called *Looking at Children,* the film provides information about typical health problems of school-age children. A supplement to the film suggests that teachers should become familiar with each child's normal and healthy physical and emotional characteristics. They should also learn to use the other class members as a frame of reference for each child so that they can detect clues to developing chronic conditions, such as vision, hearing, and postural problems. Alert teachers can recognize the signs and symptoms of respiratory infections and other communicable diseases; skin abnormalities; dental problems; poor nutrition; vision, hearing, and other perceptual impairments; speech problems, and other emotional, physical, and intellectual handicaps. In addition, our environment presents special health hazards, such as drug abuse and increased emotional difficulties, which we will discuss in subsequent chapters. Suspected health problems warrant a report to parents and to the school health service.

It is good to remember that elementary teachers who most effectively teach health epitomize an optimal level of well-being. Students learn from their example. Develop your educational program to reinforce opportunities for optimal well-being.

The potential for optimal well-being comes from various sources. A gene pool from parents and, to a less extent, grandparents, contains the blueprint for the body. This blueprint or framework may predispose an individual to diabetes, hemophilia, epilepsy, obesity, and heart disease. Conversely, genetics may ordain a strong, well-coordinated body that experiences little disease.

The environment also contributes to our potential well-being. The physical, cultural, and social environments can enhance or detract from our well-being and developing personalities. The cultural and social environments develop *values,* the standards that guide our behavior and decision making. Our cultural traditions and the society in which we live teach us about people and social interaction and prepare us to get along in the world. People continuously interact with the environment for the purpose of achieving a harmonious balance that is compatible with optimal wellness. In fact, the way in which individuals react to their surroundings determines whether they will be successful in adapting to them. Successful adaptation is necessary for wellness. One type of adaptive mechanism is *coping behavior,* such as means of handling anger or peer pressure. Teachers should teach the students coping behaviors.

Teachers have some control over their students' environment. To a great measure, elementary teachers can influence behavior, create positive health-related attitudes, teach the recognition of alternatives in any decision-making situation, and help students to make good decisions regarding their own health, thereby helping them to achieve positive health and well-being.

NOTES

1. Harold J. Cornacchia and Wesley M. Staton, *Health in Elementary Schools* (St. Louis: C.V. Mosby Co., 1974), p. 3.
2. Quoted in ibid., p. 14.
3. Ibid.
4. Walter D. Sorochan, "Health Concepts as a Basis for Orthobiosis," *Journal of School Health,* December 1968, pp. 673–82.
5. Walter Sorochan and Stephen Bender, *Teaching Elementary Health Science* (Reading, Mass.: Addison-Wesley Publishing Co., 1975), p. 8.
6. Ibid., p. 9.
7. Metropolitan Life Insurance Company, *Looking for Health,* 1969, p. 1.

CHAPTER 2
The School Health Program

To understand the teacher's role in the total elementary-school health program it is essential to know the functions and goals of the program. Promoting the health of elementary students involves school programs and activities that extend beyond the traditional classroom. The comprehensive school health program includes health services, health instruction, and healthful school living. Table 2–1 shows a more detailed breakdown. These components are mutually supportive, not mutually exclusive, and have a strong interrelationship.

Health services refer to the methods used by teachers, school nurses, psychologists, physicians, dentists, counselors, and others to appraise, protect, promote, and maintain the health of the students. Generally, the health services program strives to:

1. Appraise the health status of students and school personnel.
2. Counsel students and their parents and school personnel relative to the appraisal findings.
3. Assist and encourage the remediation of defects.
4. Identify and assist in the educational program for handicapped students.
5. Observe students for any correctable health problems.
6. Refer specific health problems to proper specialists.
7. Follow up to see that students receive the help they need.

TABLE 2–1.   The School Health Program

Health Services	Health Instruction	Healthful Living

Appraisal aspects
  health examination
  dental examination
  teacher health assess-
    ment
  vision testing
  height and weight
    measurement
  cleanliness inspection
  guidance and supervi-
    sion
  teacher health
Preventive aspects
  Communicable disease
    control
  safety
  first aid to prevent
    injury
Remedial aspects
  Follow-up services
  correction of remedi-
    able defects
  practitioner services
  school functions
	Planned instruction
	  practice
	  attitudes
	  knowledge
	Correlated instruction
	  arts
	  social studies
	  sciences
	Integrated learning
	  personal experiences
	  pupil-teacher relation-
	    ships
	  classroom experiences
	  school experiences
	Incidental instruction
	  personal experiences
	  classroom experiences
	  school activity
	  community events
		Physical environment
		  site
		  plant plan
		  heating
		  ventilation
		  lighting
		  water
		  lunch room facilities
		  sewage disposal
		Mentally healthy en-
		  vironment
		  pupil status
		  pupil-teacher rela-
		    tionships
		  provision for indi-
		    vidual differences
		  curriculum adapta-
		    tion
		  atmosphere of mu-
		    tual respect
		Practices
		  schedules
		  time allotments
		  activity and rest
		  fire protection/safety
		  inspection
		  housekeeping

8. Assist in the prevention and control of communicable disease.
9. Provide or obtain emergency care for any member of the school
   community who becomes sick or injured.

The major role of elementary teachers in health services is observation and referral. It is their responsibility to report health problems to proper authorities. Teachers need to know their limitations—what they can safely and wisely handle themselves and what to refer to someone else. Serious health problems require referral and follow-up to make sure students receive proper treatment. Stay clear of legal entanglements by following prescribed procedures. Successful teachers maintain good rapport and public relations with others who have an effect on student health, such as the principal, janitor, parents, school cafeteria personnel, and social workers.

The second component of the school health program, *health in-*

struction, is not the highly structured, didactic, teacher-centered process it once was. Today we understand that knowing is not enough (i.e., knowing that cigarette smoking is a health hazard does not prevent people from smoking). Today health instruction involves a broad range of sequential learning activities whose purpose is to positively influence students' health knowledge, attitudes, and practices. These activities include formal classroom teaching; correlated, integrated, and incidental instruction; and planned learning experiences outside the classroom. Essential cognitive (knowledge) input emphasizes "such skills as knowing, analyzing, evaluating, synthesizing, comprehending, and applying gained insight."[1]

The affective (emotional) domain is also an essential focus of health education. This domain has a potential effect upon attitudes and practices. Since the goal of the teacher is to positively influence the health and well-being of the student, it is necessary to deal with health attitudes and practices.

Health education units should help students develop positive, scientifically oriented attitudes that will effect positive health behavior. In some areas the development of positive attitudes may even be more important than the acquisition of facts. Concepts within the units should influence how students interpret health information, how they evaluate it, and whether or not they apply it to change their behavior. Concepts can influence and direct behavior.

Teachers must actively involve students in health instruction. The action domain of education, or active involvement of students with concepts and knowledge, may have a very positive effect on observable, nonobservable, and delayed-onset health behaviors.

In many schools very little health education takes place because their teachers have not received any health education. The major reason is that most states do not require health education for teacher certification. Therefore your exposure to health education may equip you as a health education resource person in your school. Don't back away from the challenge. It can be a very exciting one.

Health education training for elementary school faculties may be available through teacher in-service education. Many states will provide funds to bring in health education specialists. Where teachers understand how to integrate health education into other subject areas in the curriculum, the students will benefit greatly.

The third interrelated phase of the school health program is *healthful school living.* To fulfill its obligation to the community the school must provide an environment that fosters positive physical, social, and emotional health. The physical plant itself should be on a healthy site with safe playgrounds, adequate sewage, water supply and refuse disposal, safe building construction and pleasant decoration, adequate lighting, temperature control and ventilation, and a healthy food-service program. With administrative support, teachers are largely responsible for the emotional climate in their classrooms. Healthy interpersonal relationships and respect between the teacher and students is essential for good health.

Usually teachers have the freedom to decorate their classroom. The attention they give to the physical characteristics of the classroom in part determines their students' learning environment. A bright, cheery room has a definite effect on student behavior. Emphasis in the classroom on healthful living will have a very positive effect on those whose homes do not stress good health habits. The room temperature should be conducive to learning, for example. Because elementary students generate more body heat, they need a cooler room than adults. If the temperature is comfortable for the students, the teacher will probably have to wear a sweater. Ideally the temperature should be between 66°F and 71°F with a humidity of approximately 50 percent. A classroom that is too warm will cause students to experience drowsiness, headaches, depression, and a lack of motivation or general loss of vigor.

The social mood or environment of the classroom depends to a large extent on the teacher and to a smaller extent on the students. The students will mirror or model the warmth, acceptance, love, and respect of the teacher. By becoming involved in the affective domain or level teachers can effect a positive emotional climate. As Glasser explains in *Schools Without Failure*,[2] when responsible teachers interact with students at an affective level they learn to make responsible choices and behave constructively. Involvement on an affective level means being personal, warm, sincerely interested, and much more. It is a life-style that cannot be turned on and off. The use of students' first names is essential, as are decreased threat levels and increased trust levels. The successful "affective" teacher shows background and out-of-school interests as much as possible. A lot of this information comes from being a good listener. In Glasser's view, emotion directs behavior. Successful behavior results in pleasant emotions, and unsuccessful behavior brings unpleasant emotions. Therefore, the role of the teacher is to create as many opportunities for successful behavior as possible. Glasser's approach is unique and deserves thorough examination by pre-professional and professional teachers.

THE ELEMENTARY TEACHER'S ROLE

With the exception of parents, peers, and, in some cases, television, no one has more potential influence on the health of children than the elementary school teacher. The elementary years are very sensitive ones when children acquire health attitudes, practices, and values. Sorochan states that "much of the learned behavior and attitudes of a health nature that will prevail throughout a lifetime are established during the elementary years."[3] If the attitudes and habits developed in childhood are positive, they will most likely continue into adult life. It is the goal of the school health program to foster such attitudes and habits. Parents retain the primary responsibility for the health and safety of their children, but elementary teachers have more hours of communication with them. Although the school's role is generally a supplementary one, in many instances it assumes primary importance for children who receive no direct health education at home. Failure of a child for untreated health problems is inexcusable.

Elementary teachers naturally take part in health education, but they can have a very positive effect on health services and healthful school living if they choose to play an active role in integrating these concerns with other school activities. Few other professional educators develop such a wide variety of competencies. As health educators, psychologists, mathematicians, English teachers, historians, chemists, geographers, anthropologists, and nutritionists combined, elementary teachers, above all, are facilitators of learning for inquisitive, developing young minds.

Teachers' health attitudes, practices, and knowledge determine their effectiveness as health educators. It is also in the area of health education that elementary teachers can have some of the greatest teaching experiences. Because it is such a personal subject, health education enlarges individual student differences. In addition, some aspects of the subject are controversial.

On some health-related subjects, such as tobacco smoking, teachers may run into student apathy. The reasons for this attitude vary, depending on parental example and background, but overconcern will not eliminate apathy because it is too direct. The subtle process of teaching decision-making and healthful values will be much more effective. No other area of learning in the elementary school depends so heavily on teacher participation. Through experience and understanding students may develop positive attitudes that will lead to positive behavior, even if they approach the subject with false notions, poor attitudes, and harmful health and safety habits nurtured in the family and community.

Health science is dynamic, or constantly changing. There are some areas which are consistently black and white, but many are gray. Thus elementary teachers not only must stay abreast of current scientific information but also must help students understand the scientific process and teach them to recognize alternatives, to cope with peer and cultural pressure, and to make health-related decisions. Health is a participant subject, not a spectator one, and requires active involvement for successful results.

Some subject areas within health education may be very controversial and emotional and so demand preparation. Examples are fluoridation, sex education, venereal disease, nutrition, socialized medicine, and unscientific healing professions (quackery). All of these subjects are intimately related to the cultural patterns of any community. For this reason, objections to your instruction may arise. Don't be intimidated. Hold firm to your value system and your beliefs. In addition, you will be on safe ground if you:

1. Follow the prescribed unit outlines of your school board.
2. Welcome student input to the course and incorporate their needs and interests.
3. Select a text that is scientifically sound, up-to-date, and acceptable to the school board.
4. Use materials developed by reputable organizations, such as the American Medical Association, the American Dental Association, the National Education Association, the American Public Health Association, and the American Association of Health Education.
5. Take advantage of local resources, including people and organizations who prepare and present health education (e.g., voluntary health agencies, public health agencies, PTA, and religious leaders).
6. Maintain a scientific, unbiased approach.
7. Keep up-to-date records of student health needs, interests, and activities.

Stay abreast of current information:

1. Review current periodicals, such as *Health Education, Family Health,* and *American Journal of Public Health.*
2. Read medical sections of *Time* and *Newsweek,* and other reputable magazines. (Check with your local medical professionals for additional suggestions.)
3. Scan newspaper articles on health-related subjects (be careful of their credibility).
4. Write to publishers for information on current elementary health texts and readers.
5. Get one or two good college health texts for reference.
6. Obtain up-to-date government publications on health. Voluntary health agencies, including the American Lung Association, American Heart Association, and National Dairy Council, also furnish excellent information and teacher kits.
7. Enroll in college health education courses to renew teacher certification.
8. Know your state's health-related policies.
9. Get to know and use state health professionals and the consulting services provided by most states.
10. Conduct surveys and experiments in the area of health.

11. Retain membership in national and state educational associations. Professional organizations in health education include the Association for the Advancement of Health Education, American School Health Association, American Public Health Association (school health section), and National Safety Council (for reference).
12. Know the attitudes of school administrators and school board members toward health education.

As important as these suggestions are, the key to a good health education program is accommodating student differences. Therefore teachers should include the following practices in their teaching:

1. Maintain and know the health record of each child. Know the child's health status and learning problems.
2. Know each child's name and background. Children's goals, attitudes, and values will be closely aligned with those of their parents.
3. Keep in mind that children mature at different rates. Some are more socially or academically adept than others at the same age. Children's development follows a general pattern, but each individual has a unique schedule.

An important curriculum problem seems to be how much time and emphasis to give to specific health and safety topics. Make these decisions with student and community involvement. Find out the health needs and interests of your students through checklists, essays, brainstorming, panels, health histories, and talks with teaching colleagues. Assess the community's health needs and problems and balance the curriculum accordingly.

Teachers not only teach but also serve as health counselors to the students. They are part of a coordinated team that includes the school nurse; administrators; dentists and dental hygienists; physicians; vision, hearing, and speech specialists; and parents. Perhaps the best vehicle for coordinating the efforts of the team is the school health council.

A GLOSSARY OF TERMS

The following definitions help to characterize school health programs.

Daily health inspection is a daily nondiagnostic survey of pupils by the teacher or nurse to detect physical defects and symptoms of health disorders and to monitor the practice or avoidance of health habits. The daily inspection of all students is idealistic and probably does not occur in many classrooms. However, teachers should continually be alert for evidence of health disorders among students.

Only those habits that allow objective evaluation should be part of a regular inspection. These include cleanliness of hands and fingernails, face, ears, neck, teeth, handkerchief, and clothing; neatly combed hair; condition of shoes; removal of overshoes and wraps while in the classroom; and so on.

The purposes of daily health inspection are (1) to motivate and establish health habits and (2) to note early symptoms of illness among children and refer them to the proper health authorities (these signs include fatigue, worry, and maladjustment).

Dental examination is an appraisal of the structure, hygiene and condition of the mouth by a dentist, a dental hygienist, and perhaps an orthodontist.

Dental hygienist is a member of the school staff who aids in dental examinations, cleans teeth when advisable, teaches toothbrush drill technique, gives instruction in nutrition for healthy development of teeth, and encourages pupils in the proper care of their teeth. He or she is really an assistant to the dentist.

Functional examination is a test and/or examination to determine the physiological condition of the whole body or any of its parts. In this category are the Snellen Vision Test, the Spirometer Test, Foster's Test, Brace's Motor Ability Test, Roger's Strength Test, Cozen's Athletic Ability Test, McCurdy's Physical Fitness Test, and the Schneider Cardiovascular Examination.

Health appraisal is the assessment of the physical, mental, emotional, and social health status of individual pupils and school personnel by means of health histories, teachers' and nurses' observations, screening tests, and medical, dental, and psychological examinations.

Health coordination is the process of developing relationships within the school health program and between school and community health programs that will facilitate the harmonious solution of problems relating to pupil health.

Health examination is revealed in the operation of health service. The health examination is inclusive of all other phases of the examination.

Health history is a written record of a student's hereditary history; previous illnesses (diseases), immunizations or protective and preventive treatments and innoculations, operations, and accidents; and previous and present method of life management, regime, and environment. Usually this information comes from a questionnaire circulated to the parents.

Healthful school living is a term that describes a safe and healthful environment, the organization of a healthful school day, and the establishment of interpersonal relationships favorable to the best emotional, social, and physical health of pupils.

Physical examination is a nondiagnostic study by a nonmedical examiner of the appearance, structure, and functional condition of the body by means of some generally acceptable objective test that does not require interpretation. It includes items that might appear under "Physical Measurement and Observation." (For example, an investigation of the heart sounds is a judgment or interpretation that requires medical training and is diagnostic in the sense that a description of the condition is not sufficient without a statement of the cause. On the other hand, blood pressure and pulse rate may be recorded as seen or measured. They may be observed, described, and measured objectively without a statement of cause and thus might be items in a physical examination.)

A physically handicapped child is one who, by reason of one or more defects that are either congenital in nature, or were sustained through accident or disease, is totally or partially incapacitated.

Prevention and protection is the phase of health services that encourages the child's cooperation in health protection and maintenance, improved habits of living, health control through protection from acute and chronic infectious diseases by inoculation and vaccination, and prevention of the spread of contagious diseases by isolation and exclusion.

The school health council is an ad hoc advisory committee that coordinates the health education efforts of the school and the community. An organized effort aimed at improving the school health program, the committee should include representatives from the school administration (e.g., principal), students, teachers, parents, dental and medical societies, county health department, voluntary health agencies, town council, food service and custodial staffs, and school nurses and physicians. The council has three objectives:

1. To discover health and safety interests and needs of students and school personnel.
2. To study health and safety interests and needs of students and school personnel.
3. To make recommendations concerning health interests and needs to the school administration.

The elementary teacher can be a real asset to the school by participating in the school health council and working closely with the school health coordinator.

The school health coordinator in the elementary school is usually one of the teaching faculty who has had at least one course in health education. Ideally the health coordinator is a specialist in school health and health education, but in reality this is seldom the case. The duties of the health coordinator include curriculum development, research and problem solving in health care, individual guidance, resources, and communication. More specifically, the health coordinator helps the elementary faculty:

1. Interpret philosophy.
2. Determine objectives.
3. Set curriculum and unit content.
4. Evaluate new methods and techniques in health teaching.
5. Obtain health texts, readers, and so on.
6. Obtain community resources and personnel.
7. Strengthen the school's health program.
8. Gain information and ideas.

The successful coordinator sends out a weekly or bimonthly news-letter which summarizes new information on texts, articles, resources, films, community programs, ongoing research, and so on. Having an energetic health coordinator in the school or district can lift the level of health knowledge, attitudes, and practices of elementary students.

School health counseling is the procedure by which nurses, teachers, physicians, guidance personnel, and others interpret to pupils and parents the nature and significance of a health problem and aid them in formulating a plan to solve the problem.

School health educator is a person specially qualified to serve as a teacher, consultant, coordinator, or supervisor of health education in an individual school or school system.

School health instruction (from the point of view of the school program) is the provision of learning experiences for the purpose of imparting knowledge and attitudes and influencing conduct in the area of individual and group health.

The school health program is the school's contribution to the understanding, maintenance, and improvement of the health of pupils and school personnel through health services, health education, and healthful school living.

A sign is any evidence of a health characteristic or condition that emerges during objective measurement.

A symptom is any evidence of a health characteristic or condition that is not sensitive to objective measurement. Unable to see or measure symptoms, the examiner learns of the symptom from an examinee. It is subjective in nature. For example, the student "feels" a symptom.

NOTES

1. Walter D. Sorochan and Stephen J. Bender, *Teaching Elementary Health Science* (Reading, Mass.: Addison-Wesley Publishing Co., 1975). p. 29.
2. William Glasser, *Schools Without Failure* (New York: Harper and Row, Publishers, 1969).
3. Sorochan and Bender, p. 28.

RESOURCES

America's Children 1976: A Bicentennial Assessment. National Council of Organizations for Children and Youth, 1910 K. St., Washington, D.C. 20006.

Child Health in America. U.S. Department of Health, Education, and Welfare, Bureau of Community Health Services, 5600 Fishers Lane, Rockville, Md. 20852.

Harold J. Cornacchia and Wesley M. Staton. *Health in Elementary Schools.* St. Louis: C.V. Mosby Co., 1974.

Gere B. Fulton and William V. Fassbender. *Health Education in the Elementary School.* Pacific Palisades, Calif.: Goodyear Publishing Co., 1972.

Health and Safety Education Materials (catalog). Available free of charge from the Health and Welfare Division, Metropolitan Life Insurance Company, 1 Madison Avenue, New York, N.Y. 10010.

The Health of Children (1970). Selected data from the National Center for Health Statistics, U.S. Department of Health, Education, and Welfare, Rockville, Md.

Joint Committee on Health Problems. *School Health Services.* National Education Association and the American Medical Association, 1964.

Alma Nemir and Warren Schaller. *The School Health Program.* Philadelphia: W.B. Saunders Co., 1975.

School Health Education Study. 3M Center, Building 220-10W, St. Paul, Minn. 55101.

Walter D. Sorochan and Stephen J. Bender. *Teaching Elementary Health Science,* Reading, Mass.: Addison-Wesley Publishing Co., 1975.

George M. Wheatley and Grace T. Hallock. *Health Observations of School Children* (textbook). New York: McGraw-Hill Book Co., 1965. Guide to observing and understanding the school child in health and illness.

CHAPTER 3
Child Growth and Development

GROWING UP NORMALLY[1]

Growth patterns in childhood and the ultimate stature of an individual are influenced by heredity, the hormones and nutrients required for growth, acute and chronic health disorders, and even the emotional environment of the home. In the final analysis, however, ultimate height depends on (1) the yearly growth in height and (2) the number of years in which growth occurs.

The yearly growth in height, or *height velocity,* which is measured in inches or centimeters per year, is subject to many hereditary and environmental factors. The rate of growth is not consistent over the twelve months of the year, and periods of rapid growth may follow periods of slow growth and vice versa. The duration, or number of years during which growth occurs, is largely a function of the age at which puberty occurs, for the hormones that initiate the processes of puberty also terminate the process of physical growth.

Before puberty, most children of the same age grow at approximately the same rate. This is an important principle to remember, for children who seem "too short" or "too tall" may actually have a normal growth velocity for their age. Exceptionally short or tall children, in other words, may simply represent one extreme or the other of the normal range of sizes. The normal height range for each age of childhood has been well established and is the basis for the growth curves that are familiar to all physicians and many parents (see Figures 3-1–3-4). Physicians use growth curves to determine whether a particular child has a normal growth pattern—that is, a normal progression of growth over a period of time.[2]

Only 5 percent of normal children are taller at each age than

FIGURE 3–1. *Growth curves for girls aged birth to eighteen showing height by percentile, or rank relative to 100 children. Thus an eight-year-old girl at the 10th percentile by height is shorter than 90 out of every 100 girls her age in the United States. (National Center for Health Statistics, U.S. Department of Health, Education and Welfare.)*

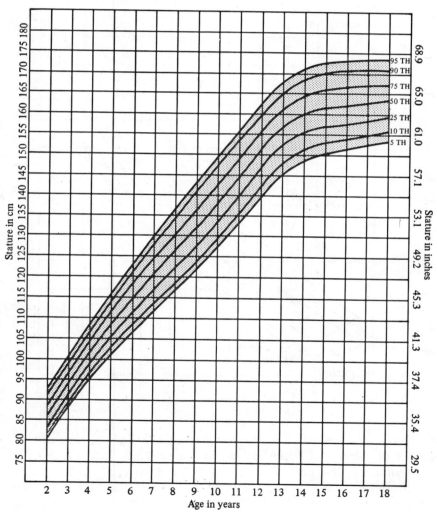

FIGURE 3-2. *Girls' weight by stature percentiles. To compare a girl with her peers, find where her weight and height intersect; judge the distance from the 5th, 50th, and 95th curves for a more exact percentile. If she is near or outside the top or bottom percentile, this fact should be called to the attention of her physician. (National Center for Health Statistics, U.S. Department of Health, Education and Welfare.)*

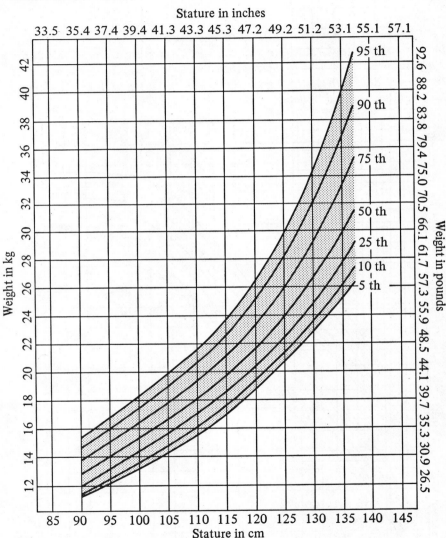

the height represented by the top line in the figures, and only 5 percent of normal children are shorter at each age than the heights represented by the bottom line. Thus the 95th and 5th percentile growth patterns are equally "normal," and neither is better or worse than the other. The 50th percentile line represents the growth

FIGURE 3-3. *Growth curve for boys aged birth to eighteen showing height by percentile, or rank relative to 100 children. Thus an eleven-year-old boy at the 50th percentile by height is taller than 50 out of every 100 boys his age in the United States and shorter than the other 50. (National Center for Health Statistics, U.S. Department of Health, Education and Welfare.)*

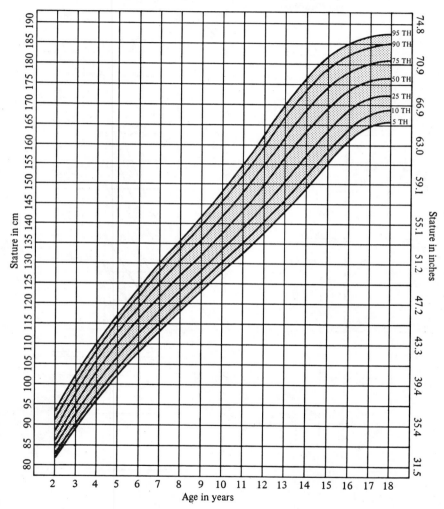

pattern of the average child: 50 percent of normal children will be taller and 50 percent will be shorter than children who grow at such a rate. Normal growth is defined as any pattern that lies between or just outside the 95th and 5th percentile limits and runs parallel to the normal growth curves. In general, growth curves that cross these lines or move progressively away from them are not normal and warrant investigation to determine if some treatable condition is the cause.

FIGURE 3-4. *Boys' weight by stature percentiles. To compare a boy with his peers, find where his weight and height intersect; judge the distance from the 5th, 50th, and 95th curves for a more exact percentile. If he is near or outside the top or bottom percentile, this fact should be called to the attention of his physician. (National Center for Health Statistics, U.S. Department of Health, Education and Welfare.)*

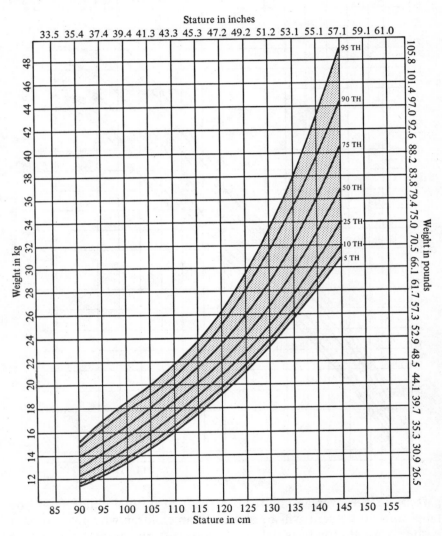

The following example gives some idea of how these normal growth curves work. The average length of a two-year-old boy is about 35 inches, but most boys that age will be 32–37 inches tall. And from the third year of life until puberty, normal growth velocity for most children is 2–2.5 inches per year.

Growth in height stops only after pubertal changes are complete. By the time of the first menstrual period (usually at the age of 12 to 13 years), the growth velocity of girls is already slowing down. Puberty starts and finishes about two years later in boys than in girls. If puberty occurs at an unusually early age, growth will cease earlier than in other children of the same age. In the same way, if puberty is delayed, growth will continue for a longer period of time than is the case with other youngsters of the same age. The chronologic age at which puberty will occur and the number of years of growth potential remaining in a particular child, may often be estimated by the maturity of the skeleton, or *bone age,* determined by an X-ray of the hand and wrist.

FACTORS INFLUENCING GROWTH

Heredity is probably the most important single factor that determines childhood growth and adult height. A child's growth pattern is often similar to those of other members of the family who are of the same sex. Generally children enter into and complete puberty at ages that are appropriate for their family.

Constitutional factors that are usually unidentifiable cause some children to be unusually tall or short during childhood, although their bone age is appropriate for their height. Among these children puberty compensates to some extent for their unusual stature by terminating growth earlier or later than expected for the child's chronologic age. Many can anticipate normal adult height.

Primordial factors that also are usually unidentifiable cause some children to be small at birth and to remain short during childhood, although their bone age is appropriate for their chronologic age. These children enter puberty at the appropriate age and most of them become short adults.

Five hormones greatly influence the growth pattern: growth hormone (secreted by the pituitary gland), thyroxin (secreted by the thyroid gland), androgens (secreted by the testes and adrenal glands), estrogens (secreted by the ovary and adrenal gland), and insulin (secreted by the pancreas). With the exception of insulin, all are directly or indirectly under the control of the pituitary gland and are essential for normal growth. In excessive amounts they may result in excess growth. Likewise, a deficiency will slow down growth velocity. Estrogens and androgens accelerate growth velocity and signs of puberty. They are the agents that terminate skeletal growth and, thus, prevent a further increase in height.

A wide variety of illnesses may cause abnormal growth patterns. Abnormally slow growth (falling progressively below the original growth curve) may result from reduced secretion of any of the hormones required for normal growth, malnutrition, or either congenital or acquired disorders of the skeletal system, liver, kidneys, and most other organ systems. Following correction of the causal disorder growth velocity usually increases for a time and the child shows some degree of "catch-up" growth. Abnormally rapid growth may be attributable to excess amounts of growth hormones or to the unusually early appearance of hormones responsible for the changes of puberty. As with growth failure, correction of the causal disorder, if it is possible, should adjust growth velocity.

Evidently, emotional as well as nutritional starvation can retard normal growth. The short stature of some children has been traced to a family environment troubled by unemployment, alcoholism, marital breakup, and the like. Fortunately, catch-up growth may follow correction of the adverse emotional environment.

Growth failure may accompany prolonged therapy with adrenal glucocorticoid hormones (e.g., cortisone), which are sometimes used in treating asthma, arthritis, and other disorders.

Disturbances during prenatal life may result in permanent growth problems. Often, low-birthweight babies who were born prematurely or were part of a multiple birth reach normal size during the first year or two after birth. Babies who are unusually small for their gestational age at birth (such as a four-pound infant born after a full-term pregnancy) have limited ability to catch up.

DETECTION OF GROWTH PROBLEMS

In measuring a child's growth, the examiner ideally should compare the individual to a growth standard derived from a group of children of the same racial and socioeconomic background. For practical purposes, however, the standardized growth curves shown in Figures 3-1-3-4 seem appropriate for most children. Records of previous heights and weights obtained from school records or family physicians make it possible to determine the trend of growth over a period of time and to use the growth curve as a diagnostic method. Without such records, it may be necessary to obtain additional growth measurements over a six-month to twelve-month period in order to establish whether a "problem" of growth velocity actually exists. As mentioned before, a child whose growth curve parallels the normal percentile lines, even if it is slightly above the 95th percentile or slightly below the 5th percentile, probably does not have a treatable growth problem. But any growth curve that is significantly or progressively outside these limits or one that crosses several percentile lines should increase the suspicion that a child may have a significant growth disorder.

TREATMENT OF GROWTH PROBLEMS

Most suspected growth problems turn out to be either a variation of normal growth or a disorder causing the onset of puberty to be early or late. These problems usually are self-correcting. Significant growth failures caused by some underlying health problem are generally reversible if the condition has been recognized early. In the same way, treatment of an imbalance in the production and release of a hormone required for normal growth and development should trigger a more normal pattern of growth. Thyroid hormone deficiency is a relatively common endocrinologic cause of significant growth failure. Fortunately, replacement of thyroid hormone is easy and inexpensive. In the last decade small supplies of human growth hormone have become available to treat childhood deficiencies. Proof of a deficiency of growth hormone may enable a physician or a consultant to obtain a supply of the hormone for experimental purposes. For children of short stature who have no proven hormonal deficiency, there is no evidence that provision of growth hormone, thyroid hormone, or any other hormone will increase the growth rate.

Delayed puberty is common in boys and is usually self-correcting. Primary treatment of this condition should be based on reassurance and understanding of the social problems that often accompany it. If delayed puberty is due to the permanent lack of testicular function, testosterone treatment will generate most of the normal virilizing changes of puberty. In rare situations of extreme pubertal delay, hormones similar to the testicular hormones may accelerate development and speed up skeletal maturation to the point at which a spontaneous puberty will occur. Unfortunately, such treatment may also reduce adult height potential by preventing further skeletal growth. This risk must be balanced against the possible psychological benefits of accelerating maturation. The same considerations apply to the use of estrogens to accelerate pubertal development in girls.

Rarely is excessive growth in girls treated by inducing puberty, a procedure that accelerates bone maturation and terminates growth at an earlier than expected age. Although the question of adverse effects from the hormones used is still open and few physicians would consider such treatment unless the predicted adult height is greater than six feet, hormonal therapy may produce a moderate reduction in the final height of still-growing girls whose present height is interfering with their home, school, or social life.

Unusual stature in childhood has many possible causes. Fortunately, the majority of them are simply variations of normal growth, normal puberty, or both. In addition, the processes of growth and development are well understood, and parents and children need not suffer unnecessary anxiety over present or potential growth patterns. A review of a child's past and present growth processes, combined with a thorough history and physical examination and supplemented, if necessary, by appropriate laboratory and X-ray procedures, will usually resolve the most growth-related questions.

Most epidemiological studies have shown that children from low socioeconomic classes mature more slowly and are somewhat shorter and lighter than children of the same age from more privileged socioeconomic groups. Although the causes for these differences are not entirely clear, they probably reflect the net effect of the many nutritional, health, and environmental advantages that accompany affluence. Probably because of generally improved nutrition, health care and sanitation and other environmental benefits, over the last one hundred years each new generation has been a little taller at a given age than the previous one.[3]

However, whether you measure them in inches or centimeters, tomorrow's American children are likely to stand no taller than today's, the National Center for Health Statistics reports. The national genetic destiny—in which each successive generation has been taller than the one before—has apparently been fulfilled. Thus we may have seen a fulfillment of those factors that have been increasing the size of American children.[4] All we can say with certainty is that whatever factors have been responsible for the trend to increasing size, their effects seem to have ceased across almost all socioeconomic levels of the American population.

PERSONAL GROWTH FROM SIX TO TWELVE YEARS[5]

Think about the differences between the first-grader and the high school youth. They are worlds apart in emotional maturity, ability to do things for themselves, and social relations with friends of the same and different sex, interests, and skills. The six-year-old is just learning to read; the twelve-year-old may be able to read everything that an adult does. The six-year-old depends on his or her parents and may brag about how great father and mother are. The twelve-year-old may insist on being independent and may often look for ways of showing parents' limitations. Changes in thinking, understanding, feeling, and social relations between the ages of six and twelve is the result of development during the school years. Other terms for this process are "maturation" and "personal growth."

Children in six-to-twelve age range are so different that it is useful to separate them for discussion. As shown in Table 3–1, we can divide children by age, educational level, or general emotional and social development.

Middle childhood covers the period between five or six and eleven

TABLE 3–1. Groups of Children in Similar Phases of Development

Age Range	Education Range	Development Range	
6–8	Grades K–3	Early elementary school period	Middle Childhood
8–11/12	Grades 4–7	Late elementary period	
12–13/14	Junior high school	Preadolescence or early adolescence	

or twelve years of age. Compared to infancy and the preschool years, childhood is more leisurely with respect to both physical and mental growth. In a way, middle childhood is a period of consolidation and adjustment to past gains in preparation for the increased pace of change and transformation that adolescence brings.

Slow growth is typical of the period of middle childhood. In both size and proportions, these children change relatively little from year to year. The period of slow growth ends several months before menarche in girls and a corresponding point of sexual maturity in boys.[6] The average boy is slightly taller than the average girl until the girl's adolescent spurt begins. Between the ages of about eleven and thirteen the average girl is taller than the average boy. Moreover, she is also heavier, in most respects she is equally strong, and sexually she is much more mature. Only when the boy's spurt begins does he surge toward his adult status of being the larger and physically more powerful sex. This leapfrog effect is one cause of problems in the organization of school activities.[7]

The middle years are healthier than the preschool period. Because growth needs and the burdens of illness claim less energy than they did in an earlier stage of life, the schoolchild has more energy to invest in relationships, problem solving, and acquisition of skills and knowledge.

Sometimes you will hear middle childhood called the *latency period*. According to one developmental theory, a child's aggressive and sexual urges are relatively less powerful, in other words, are more latent, during this stage than they were earlier in life or will be during adolescence. This theory may not be completely accurate, but children during middle childhood do tend to show less emotional upheaval than before or afterward and usually put more effort into work and hobbies. Consequently, some professionals call this stage a *period of industry*.

Some children develop more rapidly than most. In effect, they enter adolescence while they are in elementary school, when other children are still developmentally in middle childhood. Other children are slower and may not reach adolescence until late in high school. Similarly, some children progress faster than others educationally but develop at the usual speed emotionally. Such children may be capable of high-school-level work at age eleven, although emotionally and socially they act like preadolescent children.

Teachers must understand a child's educational and developmental needs. Children develop at different paces based on genetic endowment, experience, family background, physical constitution, social and cultural expectations, and other factors. Just knowing a child's age does not enable you to know that child's needs. In the next sections, we will describe typical behavior of children in different developmental stages. The major questions that we will address are "What helps a child develop and how can a classroom teacher provide necessary guidance?"

DEVELOPMENT OF THE ELEMENTARY-SCHOOL-AGE CHILD[8]

School entry can be quite a shock to children who are making their first separation from home. For children who have been in nursery school, day care, or kindergarten, going to regular school may not be a big change in life. Nevertheless school provides all children with new opportunities and makes new demands.

Typically, preschoolers at home or in a nursery program receive a great deal of individual attention and have a lot of freedom. In a day-care or preschool program, children usually may move around a lot during the day, participate in activities that interest them, express themselves emotionally, and make themselves physically comfortable by sitting on the floor or lounging about. At home they generally are masters of their own schedules and can nap, eat, and play as they wish without interference from their caregivers.

The situation differs in school. In school, children must sit in one place for longer periods of time, engage in activities assigned by the teacher, and restrain their emotions and "act like big boys and girls." Instead of doing what they think is fun, they are expected to apply themselves to learning. Finding themselves in a classroom filled with many children who are strangers and in a school with so many hallways, rooms, and people, they may feel bewildered.

School Readiness

Most children are capable of dealing with the new tasks that school presents. Early in the elementary school years children show rapid improvement in their ability to think, speak, and remember details. They begin to do more for themselves, and eat, dress, wash, and go to the toilet more or less independently. At this age children become increasingly able to sit still and concentrate.

The beginning schoolchild's social interests broaden, too. Younger children may show interest in playmates and their opinions, but for children in the early grades of elementary school, peers of the same sex become important behavior influences. In addition, these children sometimes see their teachers as ideal people. Little by little they begin to separate themselves from their families. Forming a separate identity as an individual is a normal process, and it is always interesting to watch the way a child reacts to meeting a teacher in a store, especially if the teacher is with his or her own family. Elementary school children typically become quite bashful and yet excited. They are relatively surprised that their teacher has a personal life outside the classroom.

Imaginary Friends

During the process of taking emotional steps away from the family, children sometimes create an imaginary friend. Many children from ages three to eight or so have these friends, usually in the form of another child or adult, but it can be an animal or some mixture of animal and person. The imaginary friend is always on the side of the child, although sometimes the child will describe it as being quite vicious to other people. Fictitious companions are a sign of a good imagination and the children who invent them tend to be creative and healthy. Sometimes it is hard for adults to tell if the child really believes in the companion. Of course, children understand that an imaginary friend is different from a real friend, but their belief in their imaginary friend may seem stronger in times of stress.

Self-Confidence

Schoolchildren become very involved in their activities. Often they approach even fun activities, such as learning to play baseball or swim, as though they were serious business. They associate work, in part, with fun, though some of it is also usually frustrating. The greater fun for the child, of course, is the satisfaction of mastering a game or task. Children's growth of identity during this stage centers on two types of feelings about themselves. Normally they strive to feel capable and industrious. On the other hand, they care about how they compare with other people and about whether or not they are inferior to other people. Most children experience both concerns at different times. The degree of support they receive from family and community at this stage may shape their identity. If other people make them feel capable, they will begin to acquire self-confidence.

Games and Mastery

Mastering tasks and controlling one's environment are important steps in emotional development during childhood. This development is observable in changes in the way a child plays. Whereas younger children tend to be spontaneous in their play or to act out themes, such as playing house or cowboys, elementary school children start to play traditional games, such as football, stickball, and checkers. They may spend more time arguing about the rules than playing the game. Even children who once played imaginatively with dolls, toy soldiers, and cars may start to spend much time arranging play equipment and deciding who should play with what. In the name of being "fair and square" with each other, two children may really battle over who gets how many pieces of play equipment or who really should go back to "start" on the game board. Some games, such as "the dozens" allow children to explore feelings in a con-trolled way. They have accepted "rules" about what is fair. Other games, like "buck-buck-how-many-fingers-up," allow one child to jump on and wallop another child in a way that their friends accept. These games help children express their feelings in a conventional manner. Games like these are possible during this developmental period because most children know how to bring their behavior under control during and at the end of the game. Knowing with whom you can play "the dozens" and when to stop requires intelli-gence, experience, sensitivity, and the ability for self-control.

During the middle years many children begin collecting things. This is another sign of increased interest in doing things in a regu-lated fashion.

Clubs

A club is a social unit that can have real meaning for a child for several reasons. It provides a way of organizing a variety of interests and needs. Many of the clubs that children start on their own have a relatively short life span. Sometimes, especially if an adult provides encouragement and support, a club can persist for a whole academic year or more. Like games, clubs have special rules, but many also involve secrets, intimacy, and a sense of being special. Children become quite aware of what it means to belong to a group during this period and what it means to be excluded from a group.

Children who are interested in acting like adults quickly pick up the moral and ethical values of their peers and community. Because children like to form clubs to which they can restrict membership, one unfortunate development in this stage may be behavior based on racial and economic discrimination if this is the model presented by adults.

General Development and School

Clearly, children are ready for school and formal education when they show natural curiosity, interest in learning rules, ability to control their impulses, pleasure in industry and activity, and increased capacity to think rationally. A school that is receptive to a child's needs and ambitions can become the most exciting and central concern in life.

For children to be successful and enjoy school, they must have a certain emotional, social, and intellectual maturity. Sometimes children need extra time and attention to develop the maturity they require for academic learning.

Sexual Development

Contemporary society is undergoing a reevaluation of traditional sex roles. Scientists and poets have known for a long time that men can have tender feelings and love flowers and that women can be strong-willed and love power. Nevertheless, social forces in the past have tended to stereotype people by sex just as they have tended to stereotype people by race, class, and ethnic background.

Elementary-school-age children have traditionally played in groups of the same sex and each sex has traditionally played its own kind of games, but their games seem to express many similar ideas about growing up, learning, understanding one's feelings, and the like. It is not clear how much the new freedom from established sex roles will change behavior patterns in children this age. Boys and girls may be slowly integrated into football or cooking groups. Already math clubs and baseball have been integrated, and we now realize that some boys may have a normal interest in cooking, whereas some girls may be interested in football. Old sex roles did not allow boys and girls this freedom to choose to participate in any activity.

During the middle-childhood years, boys and girls may love a person of the same or different sex who seems to respect and appreciate them and who is important in their eyes. It is common for schoolchildren to love their "beautiful" or "handsome" fourth-grade teacher, and a sensitive teacher knows how to handle children who have such feelings with respect and a sense of reality. Many a boy's first love outside of his home has come to grief when he realized that Miss Clary is Mrs. Clary.

Generally, boys and girls have nothing to do with children of the opposite sex when they are in the early grades in school. A boy may say "ugh" at the mention of a girl's name and be friendly only toward other boys. Usually, the boy will form a strong sense of himself as a man and develop an interest in girls a few years later.

There is nothing wrong with a child mooning over the teacher, avoiding children of the other sex, or becoming close to children of the same sex. It is also not abnormal for children in their early years of school to talk about their bodies or to compare themselves physically.

PROBLEMS DURING ELEMENTARY SCHOOL[9]

Teachers of elementary children should be able to detect major developmental problems that may show up in this age. Equipped with a knowledge of potential emotional, social, physical, and intellectual problems, they can help to solve children's difficulties by bringing them to their parents' attention.

Learning Problems

By far, the most common problems that bother children in this age group are school problems. The causes of learning problems are diverse. A child may be physically immature or emotionally not ready for school. Some children suffer from undetected physical problems, such as hearing and vision impairments. Anxiety about family life or one's own feelings, hunger, fatigue, and fright all may cause troubles in school, even for a child who is mature, intelligent, and capable of learning. Some children have specific problems with language. Others have general coordination problems, trouble telling their right hand from their left, and clumsiness, all of which can make reading and writing difficult. In certain situations bright children may act stupid, especially if they feel that what they do will not be appreciated, if they find the situation frightening, or if there is an emotional block to being active or creative.

School Fears

It is not unusual for a child to be frightened about going to school for the first time. Probably the majority of children are upset during the first weeks, and many children become upset once in a while during the whole first year of school and then at the start of each semester. Extreme school fears, sometimes called *school phobia,* are different from this normal worrying. Children with school phobia may be so terrified of going to school that they fight to stay home, collapse in tears in the school, and display panic when left in school. School phobia can take other forms. For example, a child with school phobia may act sick on school days, develop a headache, complain of a stomach ache, or vomit. Children who are school phobic may have accidents so that they can stay home, stay up all night so that they will be too tired to go to school the next day, or simply play hookey. Commonly, children with school phobia come from homes where they had little opportunity to act independently before the time came to start school.

Difficult experiences in school also may play a role in making a child frightened to attend. Faced with an overly strict or unsympathetic teacher, problems with other children in the school or class, racism, or any of a number of other factors, a child may feel out of place, worried, or frightened in school. To understand the fright some children experience when they go to school, teachers must evaluate and deal with these realistic worries.

Most frequently, school-phobic children and their parents need sympathetic and thoughtful help. Usually, both the parents and the child have difficulties separating from each other. Only by understanding these difficulties can the child return to school comfortably and develop well in other spheres. Staying away from school for a long time, however, can make a child frightened of returning and increase the general separation problem. Thus, most specialists feel that it is good for school-phobic children to come to school as soon as is sensible so that a pattern of staying away will not be set. A working parent may need help from an adult outside the family to get the child to school. The approach should not be angry or punishing. On the other hand, the adults should be firm. It is important for the parents and school to keep in mind that getting the child to school is not the end point. It may be only part of a process involving professional help for the child and parents.

Although children who are frightened to come to school because of difficulties with the teachers or other students may have a general emotional problem, this is not always the case. They may be in a realistically difficult situation in which any normal, healthy child would be frightened or worried and would want to escape. Children whose race or ethnic background sets them apart, sensitive children who are bullied by school toughs, and children whose teachers do not understand them, may have no problems with developmental problems or difficulties separating from their parents. On the contrary, these children are victims of social tensions that surround and disturb many children today. To be of help to the child who avoids school because of real problems there, teachers, parents, and the community must work together to bring about changes in the school and, at the same time, to provide alternatives for children who temporarily need special help.

Destructive Children

Many school-age children fight, break things, are bullies, tell lies, steal, cheat, or demand attention some other way. Sometimes called *externalizers* because they take out internal frustrations on the outside world, these children tend to be difficult to handle in school and elsewhere. Frequently, these same children reveal their problems in other ways, too. For example, they may suffer from speech problems, bedwetting, restlessness, and physical complaints. They may be inattentive in the same way as so-called hyperkinetic children and may need medical and educational help.

Children who are destructive and unsocial may have parents who are under too much stress to help them organize their behavior. They may themselves experience too much pressure from their own impulses. Or they may be children who, for a variety of complex reasons, are not "at home" in the school or program. The important point is that such children are not happy and could experience greater self-satisfaction with help and structure. Destructiveness and antisocial behavior may appear in children who have developed well when they experience stress. It is very important to make the distinction between children who have never had the opportunity to mature and normal children who have lost a degree of control due to stress. Some destructive and unsocial behavior is typical of the play in certain neighborhoods. In this case, the child needs the chance to learn from experience how to be "tough" and able in other ways.

What the immature child requires is firm structure and limits. Often specialized counseling will prevent immature children from developing long-term psychological problems. Children who have matured normally but who seem to be having temporary emotional problems may pull themselves back together with only warmth and comfort from others. Both kinds of children need help, but the help must suit the special problem.

Timid Children

Children who are sad, withdrawn, lonely, fearful, and submissive do not always elicit the adult attention that the overactive, destructive child does. Sometimes called *internalizers* because they keep their problems inside themselves, many of these children are underactive, pokey eaters, whiny, and friendless. In addition, they tend to show unusual concern for keeping everything too orderly. Parents of such a child may say that they wish he or she would "let go" once in a while and be messy. Teachers, however, are often too busy to notice timid children and may consider them "good students" even though they really are quite miserable.

Timid children may be afraid to do anything new. They may be afraid of their own, strong feelings or insecure in their relations with their parents. In addition, these children may have concentration problems. Sometimes, children who appear quiet and withdrawn simply cannot understand or pay attention to what is going on around them.

The best way of handling timid, quiet children depends on the nature of their problems. If they have never had the opportunity of expressing themselves because their house was too small and their parents overworked, they might need permission to move around a lot. Children who are insecure because of stresses in their lives may need emotional reassurance. Children with attention deficits may benefit from special educational and medical treatment. And those who show signs of emotional confusion may need psychotherapy.

The child who is "too good" may be as troubled as the child who is a "bad actor." Both kinds of children have real problems in working, making friendships, and feeling capable, and they are equally unable to develop the kind of personal identity that is appropriate for their age.

Sexual Problems

Sexual development sometimes concerns children during middle childhood. The boy who is a "sissy" or who takes unusual pleasure from dressing in girls' clothes may be troubled about his sexual identity and, therefore, might be headed for difficulty. If the boy shows no interest in assertive activities such as sports or participation in clubs, hobbies, or school activities with other boys, he may develop a lifelong sexual behavior problem.

Identifying sexual development problems in young girls is difficult, because the assertive "tomboy" may be developing just fine. We should show concern, however, about the girl who forcefully avoids friendships with girls, who seems deeply unhappy about being a woman, and who seems to have no close relationship with an adult woman. A girl who cannot love an adult woman, such as her mother, may come to feel that being a woman is not worthwhile.

For children who are having difficulty forming a sexual identity, special help is valuable. Some outdated, stereotyped sex roles are no longer applicable. On the other hand, happiness depends not just on the sorts of things that children do or like but also on the inner sense of personal worth.

For a more thorough discussion of this topic see Chapter 4.

THE SCHOOL'S RESPONSE TO DEVELOPMENTAL NEEDS[10]

As described above, the period called middle childhood, latency, or elementary school age is a period when children bring together the skills they acquired during preschool years and when they mature and learn new things. School can support this development and help children work through their difficulties.

Social Growth

School experiences must support each child's need for close relations with peers. During the five minutes between classes, the importance of interaction with other children is visible to any teacher. Children come to life in the corridors when they can talk with friends. Unfortunately, schools usually make little provision for this kind of peer group activity when no adult is present.

Teachers also have an important part to play in a young child's social growth. From them children learn about adults in a non-parental role.

Industry

Children need to work as much as infants need to suck. School can provide opportunities for different types of work. For some children, education is primarily work. But the school can encourage other types of work besides the usual schoolwork, including hobbies, crafts, sports, building, collecting, and inventing. The end product of this kind of activity is less important than the child's sense of mastery and industry, so it makes sense to tailor it to individual interests.

Developmental Problems

How should a school program relate to a child with problems? This is a tricky, sensitive question. Teachers must act thoughtfully when the need arises. Not all teachers can or should deal with some kinds of emotional or physical difficulties, but all teachers should have the ability to recognize when a child has a physical or emotional problem and should bring it to the attention of parents.

The child with hyperkinetic behavioral disturbance probably will need quiet, structured periods to do schoolwork and also may require medication, administered under a physician's guidance. The destructive, aggressive child and the timid, fearful child likewise may need special care from the teacher. The program may have to set limits to insure that the bully does not overstep bounds. On the other hand, the timid child may need time alone with the teacher to feel secure. For both the child who externalizes problems and the child who internalizes them, the teacher must cooperate with parents and specialists to devise a plan that supports the child's maturation.

The school program should allow a child to choose activities without forcing boys to do only "boy-like" things or girls to do only "girl-like" things. At the same time, sensitive professionals will accept the need to establish pride in one's sexual identity and will allow boys and girls to group themselves according to sex for some activities.

It is very hard for anyone to discuss a child's sexual development with a parent. Yet, teachers should be able to discuss their students' sex-related problems as freely with parents as they would be to talk about a child's squint or stealing.

Pubescence[11]

The word *puberty* refers to physical changes in a child's body. For a girl, puberty means the beginning of menstruation, breast development, and hair growth in her pelvic area. For boys, puberty involves an increase in the size of the penis, increased muscularity, and a deepening voice. Both boys and girls experience rapid physical growth, changes in hair quality and skin texture, new body odors, and new body shapes during puberty.

Adolescence is the time in a child's life when both emotional and physical changes occur. Puberty triggers this overall surge in development. Some children reach puberty at the very young age of six or seven. This experience is known as *precocious* or too early puberty. Children who experience precocious puberty may develop severe emotional problems, although, in terms of personal development, they are not yet adolescents.

Some children, especially those who are physically slow in maturing, begin to undergo adolescent changes before they are really in the full push of puberty. When puberty does not start until late in high school, the term *delayed* or late-onset puberty is applied. Everyone is familiar with the types of problems that face the short, beardless boy and the flat-chested girl in their junior year of high school. Nevertheless, some children experience adolescence relatively well when puberty is delayed.

What Is Puberty?[12]

Puberty is the sequence of events that transform the child into a young adult who is capable of reproducing sexually. During this period, the internal reproductive glands mature; boys begin to produce sperm cells and girls begin to release *ova,* or egg cells. The release of sex hormones begins, and the secondary sex characteristics develop: the testicles, penis, and breasts increase in size; pubic and facial hair appear; a boy's voice begins to "break"; and girls experience the first menstrual flow, or *menarche* (pronounced 'men-arkee) occurs.

In boys the first sign of puberty appears between 9.5 and 14 years of age. Approximately 95 percent of girls exhibit the first sign of puberty between 8.5 and 13 years of age. Menarche usually occurs at about 13 or 14 years, but there is considerable variation from child to child. Menarche occurs near the end, not the beginning, of puberty.

It is important to remember that the age at which puberty begins varies widely in healthy children. It is also important to realize that some normal children will complete the puberty phase in two years, whereas other normal children may take three or even four years.

The first sign of puberty in boys is usually an increase in the size of the testicles. Some scant growth of pubic hair may coincide with this, but it usually appears later, when the boy begins to grow rapidly taller. About 50 percent of boys also experience some enlargement of the breasts, with some accompanying tenderness, during puberty. This condition is called *gynecomastia.*

In girls the first sign of puberty is growth of the breasts. As in boys, pubic hair may also appear at this time, but pubic hair growth usually coincides with the adolescent spurt in height. Menarche invariably occurs after the peak rate of height growth, toward the end of puberty.

How Does Puberty Differ from Maturation?[13]

Puberty is simply one aspect of the body's overall growth and maturation process. *Maturation* is a catchall word for all of the developmental events by which a child becomes fully developed. So puberty could also be called *sexual maturation.* By the same token, we speak of *skeletal maturation,* which is the complete de velopment of the skeleton; maturation of the teeth, which is the complete development of the permanent teeth; and maturation of the nervous system.

Doctors find that the most reliable indicator of normal growth and development is not chronologic age but skeletal maturation. For this reason, they often use X-rays to determine a child's bone age. For example, X-rays may reveal that the ten-year-old who appears to be starting puberty too early may actually have a bone age of twelve and therefore is maturing normally. Particularly at the prepubertal and pubertal stages of growth, bone age and secondary sex characteristics are the best indicators of the total maturity status of a child. Each of the secondary sex characteristics is graded on a scale of one to five, on which stage 1 is prepubertal. Thus an individual child can have several maturity ratings, for example, "a twelve-year-old boy, bone age fourteen years, genitals stage 3, pubic hair stage 4."

How does Puberty Affect Growth?[14]

Puberty is the chief factor regulating growth in height and build during adolescence. In fact, the second most rapid period of growth that we experience occurs during time of puberty (the most rapid growth period occurs in infancy). The adolescent growth spurt is mainly due to the action of sex hormones. Approximately 95 percent of girls exhibit their peak rate of growth in height at twelve years of age. For most boys it occurs at age fourteen. For the average girl puberty occurs earlier than it does for the average boy in nearly all maturity indicators: the appearance of secondary sexual signs, skeletal maturity, and the onset of the adolescent growth spurt.

What Causes The Physical Changes of Puberty?[15]

Most pubertal changes result from the action of sex hormones released by the *gonads,* or sex glands (in boys the gonads are the testes; in girls, the ovaries). The male sex hormone is *testosterone.* In girls it is *estrogen.*

Two areas in the brain, the *pituitary gland* and the *hypothalamus,* control the release of sex hormones. The hypothalamus stimulates the pituitary to release two hormones that promote the function of the gonads. These hormones, or *gonadotrophins,* are *FSH* (follicle-stimulating hormone) and *LH* (luteinizing hormone). In turn, the gonadotrophins stimulate the gonads to release the sex hormones testosterone and estrogen.

DEVELOPMENT OF THE PREADOLESCENT CHILD (11–13 YEARS)[16]

During the last years of elementary school or the beginning of junior high school, children pass through a phase that is difficult to define. No longer the industrious, energetic, and sportsminded hobbyists who like an orderly and regular life, neither are they the croaking, gawky adolescent boys or the blushing, shapely adolescent girls. During this in-between period, children sometimes exhibit changes in personality that shock themselves, their parents, and other adults. Called *preadolescence,* this phase probably represents the very first changes of puberty. At this time the balance of hormones starts to change and children begin to have new body feelings and emotions. Only recently having become secure in their industriousness and capabilities, they now sense that a big change is coming. And they are right.

Upheaval

Preadolescents may seem to be moving backwards, although, in reality, they are moving ahead developmentally. At mealtime they may become greedy and almost grab food from the table or refrigerator. They may start to steal candies. Preadolescents' sloppy toilet habits are well known. They avoid baths and care little for clothing. They may be mean to younger children. At school and at home, they tend to lack consideration or empathy. Former good students may have no apparent interest in studies or any ability to concentrate on schoolwork. Some retain from middle childhood an interest in hobbies and the like and may become angry with peers who are no longer interested in collections.

In a way, preadolescence is a period when all of the good work of parents and educators seems to have been wasted. Preadolescents themselves do not know what is happening and may be frightened. This is also a challenging period for school planners. Helping children through this critical time is a special responsibility.

New Energy

The upheaval in a child's personality relates to the beginning of new types of energy. Although no special interest in the opposite sex may be evident, the level of interest in sex, in general, may increase. During this period, deviant behavior may develop, or a child may experience true anxiety.

At no other time is a child more in need of guidance than in preadolescence. Yet this is a phase when parents and teachers are perhaps least able to help. Younger children listen to and follow the suggestions of parents and teachers out of an emotional attachment to them. During preadolescence, old attachments loosen, and the children are less responsive to the criticism or praise of adults. They still care about their image with friends, but even their friendships may be less secure. Not yet ready to take on heroes and ideals, as they will later, preadolescent children often are rather self-centered, lonely, and unhappy.

Boy-Girl Relations

Preadolescent boys are usually uncomfortable with girls, but some boys already enjoy receiving attention and admiration from them. In a swimming pool, for example, a preadolescent boy may show off his diving skills in the hope that the girls will watch but walk past them later without lifting his eyes or saying "hello." He is more secure with other boys. At this time boys become curious about having babies and may yearn to be able to reproduce. A boy may experiment with this feeling by raising goldfish, mice, hamsters, or guppies and talk about the pet's pregnancy as though he himself were about to deliver.

Typical preadolescent girls tend to turn away from feminine interests and may become assertive and aggressive in new ways. For example, many girls around this time may become intensely interested in horseback riding and "tomboy" activities. On the other hand, some girls rush quickly forward into more traditional feminine activities, such as grooming or modeling classes.

Physical Exertion

Possessed of tremendous physical energy, preadolescents use sports and other physical activities to let off steam. If sports and other socially acceptable channels are not available to them, they find their own ways of reducing tension. To sustain their constant motion and to gain fuel for the oncoming spurt of physical growth they seem to eat all day.

At no other time in life is a period of upheaval so clearly a sign of developmental progress. The child who goes through this phase of "dirty" humor, messiness, boasting, unhappiness, sexual exploration, and greed—in so many ways a return to infancy—is preparing for the responsibilities and pleasures of adulthood.

Parents and Children

Parents are always the most important adults in a child's life. During certain developmental periods—for example, during middle childhood—a child and parent may get on quite well and experience general satisfaction and happiness with the relationship. Other times a certain amount of strain in the parent-child relationship is inevitable. These periods can be quite upsetting to the parent who has worked hard and successfully to be available and responsive to the child. The child may be equally upset. Normal development is not a smooth ride all the way. In the protection of the family characterized by special, close and secure relationships, a child can experiment with new feelings and try out new roles. Much of the child's personal growth affects relations with parents.

Parents naturally want to be helpful to the early adolescent who is suffering emotional difficulty. Why is it so hard for them to succeed? First, preadolescents eagerly want to separate themselves from their parents. A boy may want to be close to his mother, but because he also wants to grow up, he may feel uncomfortable when he is with her. Likewise a girl may want to snuggle with her father and sit on his lap, but sensing her own development into womanhood, she becomes aware of her father's maleness and thus cannot permit herself to continue this form of father-child contact.

Second, preadolescent children want to act grown-up. But they may try too hard. Not only do they want to be independent, they may try to make their parents behave as though they had no backbone by testing their patience. Sometimes it is hard to negotiate with a preadolescent who keeps pushing the limit. Perhaps they feel that in order for them to be big, they must make adults small. Preadolescent youths have some of the same feelings and go through some of the same problems as they did during the preschool years when they tried to act like their mothers and fathers. But parents and adults may find the imitation less cute in preadolescents experimenting with the same roles.

Third, parents and children may be embarrassed by sexual maturation. Probably most parents are uncomfortable when their children start to become sexually mature individuals. It may be hard for a parent to accept. In the one-parent family, there are some special problems. The mother who is raising a son may feel awkward when he begins to become a young man. She may not be able to discuss his bodily changes and new interests in the way she can with her daughter. The situation is the same for the father raising a daughter. Also, in a one-parent family a child whose parent is the opposite sex may feel uncomfortable being alone in the house with the parent or discussing personal issues with him or her.

Most children will keep puberty almost a secret from their parents.

More likely they will discuss physical and emotional changes with friends and explore these changes in privacy or with them. Children at this age become very curious about erotic books and magazines, medical books, sex education pamphlets, and each other's bodies. Although boys and girls love to talk about sexual activities they may utterly refuse to discuss them or effect stupid looks if a parent raises the subject.

For these reasons, preadolescent children may need guidance and help from adults other than their parents. But they are very hard to reach.

THE SCHOOL'S RESPONSE TO THE DEVELOPMENTAL NEEDS OF THE PREADOLESCENT

The preadolescent's needs are very different from those of a younger child. Teachers must be sensitive to each child's developmental needs, because some children enter this phase earlier than others. It is easy to recognize when a child begins to show increased appetite, unruliness, messiness, "dirty" humor, sexual curiosity, and social withdrawal, along with a fierce competitiveness on the ball field or in other activities.

Need for Communication

Preadolescents need adults who can help them understand what is happening to their bodies and emotions. At this time children turn away from parents and may turn to a teacher of the same sex for reassurance and information.

Parents will probably be happy to have a mature teacher available to their children for personal discussions. Of course these youths will not want to talk about most things, and when they do open up they may say their piece and then clam up.

Peer Relations

Peer group identification may cause real concern in a school program. Staff members will often feel uncomfortable about letting boys, especially groups of them, stay too long in a bathroom or locker room. Concern may also arise when a preadolescent boy becomes extremely friendly with a somewhat younger child and when some of the children appear to be indulging in sex play.

Teachers must distinguish maturely between the children's need for privacy and their need for adult structuring. Because preadolescents need time alone and crave opportunities to talk about what is on their minds with peers, teachers should not always be hovering about and supervising them. On the other hand, preadolescents should not be given to believe that they have no adult support or authority or, worse, that the adults want them to behave in a manner that would be very upsetting. Therefore teachers should take control of these children's activities only after careful consideration of the needs of the moment.

Activity

Preadolescents thrive on vigorous physical activities. In this area, the school program can most easily fulfill a developmental requirement. There can be nothing better than to allow the youngsters to exhaust themselves playing sports.

Often school fades into the background of a child's interests during these years. Perhaps in no other period of the educational process do children have so great a need for a break from studying. With so much to learn about themselves, preadolescents care little about learning what's in books. Some schools now appreciate this fact and let the children use much of their school time in self-directed or group activities. Unless schools are sensitive to preadolescent developmental needs, these children may temporarily or permanently lose interest in learning or going to school.

When a teacher notices that preadolescents have stopped doing their homework or that they do it in a hasty and sloppy way, it is important not to force them to sit and pretend to study, but instead to give them opportunities to learn about what interests them. Children turn away from school during this period. Many high school dropouts drop out of school mentally several years before they stop attending physically, although this is a problem that concerns junior high school more than it does elementary school.

OVERVIEW OF MIDDLE CHILDHOOD DEVELOPMENT

Every child is different, as every teacher and parent knows. But knowledge of the general stages of development is helpful in understanding and dealing with both everyday and occasional behavior. The following outlines, reprinted from *These Are Your Children,** present an overview of middle childhood development.

---

*From Gladys G. Jenkins, Helen S. Schactor, and William W. Bauer, *See How They Grow*, pamphlet reprinted from the 1966 edition of *These Are Your Children*. Copyright © 1966 by Scott, Foresman and Company. Reprinted by permission.

About Five

Physical Development

Period of slow growth. Body lengthens out and hands and feet grow larger. Girls usually about a year ahead of boys in physical development.

Good general motor control, though small muscles not so fully developed as large ones.

Sensory-motor equipment usually not ready for reading. Eye-hand coordination improving, but still poor. Apt to be far-sighted.

Activity level high.

Attention span still short, but increasing.

Little infantile articulation in speech.

Handedness established.

Characteristic Behavior

Stable—good balance between self-sufficiency and sociability.

Home-centered.

Beginning to be capable of self-criticism. Eager and able to carry some responsibility.

Noisy and vigorous, but activity has definite direction.

Purposeful and constructive—knows what he's going to draw before he draws it.

Uses language well, enjoys dramatic play.

Can wash, dress, eat, and go to the toilet by himself, but may need occasional help.

Individuality and lasting traits beginning to be apparent.

Interested in group activity.

Special Needs

Assurance that he is loved and valued.

Wise guidance.

Opportunity for plenty of activity, equipment for exercising large muscles.

Opportunity to do things for himself, freedom to use and develop his own powers.

Background training in group effort, in sharing, and in good work habits that he will need next year in first grade.

Opportunity to learn about his world by seeing and doing things.

Kindergarten experience if possible.

About Six

Physical Development

Growth proceeding more slowly, a lengthening out.

Large muscles better developed than small ones.

Eleven to twelve hours of sleep needed.

Eyes not yet mature, tendency toward far-sightedness.

Permanent teeth beginning to appear.
Heart in period of rapid growth.
High activity level—can stay still only for short periods.

Characteristic Behavior

Eager to learn, exuberant, restless, overactive, easily fatigued.
Self-assertive, aggressive, wants to be first, less cooperative than at five, keenly competitive, boastful.
Whole body involved in whatever he does.
Learns best through active participation.
Inconsistent in level of maturity evidenced—regresses when tired, often less mature at home than with outsiders.
Inept at activities using small muscles.
Relatively short periods of interest.
Has difficulty making decisions.
Group activities popular, boys' and girls' interests beginning to differ.
Much spontaneous dramatization.

Special Needs

Encouragement, ample praise, warmth, and great patience from adults.
Ample opportunity for activity of many kinds, especially for use of large muscles.
Wise supervision with minimum interference.
Friends—by end of period, a best friend.
Concrete learning situations and active, direct participation.
Some responsibilities, but without pressure and without being required to make complicated decisions or achieve rigidly set standards.
Help in developing acceptable manners and habits.

About Seven

Physical Development

Growth slow and steady.
Annual expected growth in height—two or three inches. In weight—three to six pounds.
Losing teeth. Most seven-year-olds have their six-year molars.
Better eye-hand coordination.
Better use of small muscles.
Eyes not yet ready for much close work.

Characteristic Behavior

Sensitive to feelings and attitudes of both other children and adults. Especially dependent on approval of adults.
Interests of boys and girls diverging. Less play together.
Full of energy but easily tired, restless and fidgety, often dreamy and absorbed.

Little abstract thinking. Learns best in concrete terms and when he can be active while learning.

Cautious and self-critical, anxious to do things well, likes to use hands.

Talkative, prone to exaggerate, may fight verbally instead of physically, competitive.

Enjoys songs, rhythms, fairy tales, myths, nature stories, comics, television, movies.

Able to assume some responsibility.

Concerned about right and wrong, but may take small things that are not his.

Rudimentary understanding of time and monetary values.

Special Needs

The right combination of independence and encouraging support.

Chances for active participation in learning situations with concrete objects.

Adult help in adjusting to the rougher ways of the playground without becoming too crude or rough.

Warm, encouraging, friendly relationships with adults.

Acceptance at own level of development.

About Eight

Physical Development

Growth still slow and steady—arms lengthening, hands growing.

Eyes ready for both near and far vision. Near-sightedness may develop this year.

Permanent teeth continuing to appear.

Large muscles still developing. Small muscles better developed, too. Manipulative skills are increasing.

Attention span getting longer.

Poor posture may develop.

Characteristic Behavior

Often careless, noisy, argumentative, but also alert, friendly, interested in people.

More dependent on his mother again, less so on his teacher. Sensitive to criticism.

New awareness of individual differences.

Eager, more enthusiastic than cautious. Higher accident rate.

Gangs beginning. Best friends of same sex.

Allegiance to other children instead of to an adult in case of conflict.

Greater capacity for self-evaluation.

Much spontaneous dramatization, ready for simple classroom dramatics.

Understanding of time and of use of money.

Responsive to group activities, both spontaneous and adult-supervised.

Fond of team games, comics, television, movies, adventure stories, collections.

Special Needs

Praise and encouragement from adults.

Reminders of his responsibilities.

Wise guidance and channeling of his interests and enthusiasms, rather than domination or unreasonable standards.

A best friend.

Experience of belonging to peer group—opportunity to identify with others of same age and sex.

Adult-supervised groups and planned after-school activities.

Exercise of both large and small muscles.

About Nine or Ten

Physical Development

Slow, steady growth continues—girls forge further ahead. Some children reach the plateau preceding the preadolescent growth spurt.

Lungs as well as digestive and circulatory systems almost mature. Heart especially subject to strain.

Teeth may need straightening. First and second bicuspids appearing.

Eye-hand coordination good. Ready for crafts and shop work.

Eyes almost adult size. Ready for close work with less strain.

Characteristic Behavior

Decisive, responsible, dependable, reasonable, strong sense of right and wrong.

Individual differences distinct, abilities now apparent.

Capable of prolonged interest. Often makes plans and goes ahead on his own.

Gangs strong, of short duration and changing membership. Limited to one sex.

Perfectionistic—wants to do well, but loses interest if discouraged or pressured.

Interested less in fairy tales and fantasy, more in his community and country and in other countries and peoples.

Loyal to his country and proud of it.

Spends a great deal of time in talk and discussion. Often outspoken and critical of adults, although still dependent on adult approval.

Frequently argues over fairness in games.

Wide discrepancies in reading ability.

Special Needs

Active rough and tumble play.

Friends and membership in a group.

Training in skills, but without pressure.

Books of many kinds, depending on individual reading level and interest.

Reasonable explanations without talking down.

Definite responsibility.

Frank answers to his questions about coming physiological changes.

The Preadolescent

Physical Development

A "resting period," followed by a period of rapid growth in height and then growth in weight. This usually starts sometime between 9 and 13. Boys may mature as much as two years later than girls.

Girls usually taller and heavier than boys.

Reproductive organs maturing. Secondary sex characteristics developing.

Rapid muscular growth.

Uneven growth of different parts of the body.

Enormous but often capricious appetite.

Characteristic Behavior

Wide range of individual differences in maturity level.

Gangs continue, though loyalty to the gang stronger in boys than in girls.

Interest in team games, pets, television, radio, movies, comics. Marked interest differences between boys and girls.

Teasing and seeming antagonism between boys' and girls' groups.

Awkwardness, restlessness, and laziness common as result of rapid and uneven growth.

Opinion of own group beginning to be valued more highly than that of adults.

Often becomes overcritical, changeable, rebellious, uncooperative.

Self-conscious about physical changes.

Interested in earning money.

Special Needs

Understanding of the physical and emotional changes about to come.

Skillfully planned school and recreation programs to meet needs of those who are approaching puberty as well as those who are not.

Opportunities for greater independence and for carrying more responsibility without pressure.

Warm affection and sense of humor in adults. No nagging, condemnation, or talking down.

Sense of belonging, acceptance by peer group.

NOTES

1. "Is Your Child Growing Up Normally," *Drug Therapy*, October 1976, pp. 55–58.
2. National Center for Health Statistics, "NCHS Growth Charts, 1976," *Monthly Vital Statistics Report*, 22 June 1976, pp. 11–16.

3. J.M. Tanner, "Earlier Maturation in Man," *Scientific American,* January 1968, pp. 21–27.

4. "New Growth Charts," *Medical World News,* May 1977, pp. 37–39.

5. Adapted from "Serving School Age Children—Child Development" (Washington, D.C.: U.S. Department of Health, Education, and Welfare 1973), p. 9.

6. Irving B. Weiner and David Elkind, *Child Development: A Core Approach* (New York: John Wiley and Sons, 1972), p. 346.

7. Mollie S. and Russell C. Smart, *Child Development and Relationships* (New York: Macmillan Co., 1972), p. 345.

8. Adapted from "Serving School Age Children—Child Development" (Washington, D.C.: U.S. Department of Health, Education, and Welfare 1973).

9. Ibid., pp. 10–14.

10. Ibid., pp. 15–16.

11. Ibid., pp. 16–17.

12. "Delayed Puberty," *Drug Therapy,* June 1977, pp. 34–35.

13. Ibid.

14. Ibid.

15. Ibid.

16. Adapted from "Serving School Age Children," p. 18.

CHAPTER 4
Development of Gender-related Role Behaviors

The apparently universal concern about the sexual behavior of children, particularly adolescents, suggests the desirability of giving the subject a separate chapter. Here the primary focus will be on the roots of sexuality, however. We will analyze the factors that seem to play a role in gender identification and the development of role-specific behaviors. In addition, we will examine the role of the school in a cooperative alliance with the home to impart to the child a healthy personal perspective in this dimension of life.

ROLE IDENTIFICATION

Considerable controversy exists about the relative importance of genetic and hormonal factors and social determinants in the sex role development. That hormones play a significant part is evident from studies in primates that reveal greater levels of aggression in males than in females.[1] Diamond believes that hormones provide both directional and activational effects on behavior, thereby imparting a distinct qualitative difference, both physiological and psychological, between maleness and femaleness.[2] On the other hand, Katz ascribes maleness to the effect of fetal androgens on brain centers that later promote pubescence. The androgens emanate from the fetal testes, which are a product of the genetic inheritance.[3] Not only do hormones influence physiological aspects of maleness and femaleness but apparently also color psychological qualities. Thus they give direction to styles of thought and behavior independent of, but usually harmonious with, psychosocial influences.[4]

From another point of view, social learning theorists state that, once the gender of a child has been established, society demands that the child learn gender-appropriate forms of behavior. The child thus becomes a "man" or a "woman" because social directives mold behaviors at progressive and succeeding stages of development.[5]

While the nature-nurture debate continues, educators, caught in the middle, do not know the degree to which their influence, both casual and educational, conflicts with biological determinants or simply contributes to the cultural thrust of a child's developing sexuality. Nevertheless, sensitive teachers can significantly reinforce children's yearning and striving in all dimensions of life if they understand the influences that affect who a child is and may become.

THE INFLUENCE OF THE HOME

Undoubtedly the home is the original source of a child's notions about maleness and femaleness and about where he or she fits into the picture. Sex-role learning takes place throughout the childhood years, but the period between age five and age six seems to be critical.[6] At this age, children are aware that mother and father are different in numerous dimensions. They may associate femaleness with higher voice, gentler touch, more frequent presence, food provision, and pain relief. Maleness, on the other hand, may be related to lower voice, rougher touch, and different clothes. In fact, characteristics such as clothing and mannerisms usually are such reliable clues to maleness and femaleness that a child can tell the gender of new acquaintances at a glance. But overlap, in behaviors at least, is so extensive among humans that children who couple gentleness with femaleness or roughness with maleness in the home may find that the association does not apply to all persons outside the home.

A critical consideration in the development of sexuality is identification. Specific factors help to determine which role a child will emulate. Present evidence seems to indicate that a child is more likely to identify with the parent who they think has greater power to give rewards, an ability that fathers more often display.[7] But the importance of other forces is evident from the observation that girls are more likely to imitate males than are boys to imitate females when parental roles are crossed. The reason may be that society still reinforces the masculine role.[8]

Adults also directly reinforce sex roles. Fathers tend to reinforce masculine roles in sons and feminine roles in daughters, in harmony with the parental roles as they exist in the home. They encourage boys to dress as they do and to do what they do, or would like to do. Likewise, parents encourage girls to imitate their mothers' way of dressing and to behave as their mothers do. The contrasts that parental behavior directly reinforces may not seem very great, but if you look at the traits listed for three children in Table 4-1, your impression would probably change. If you were asked to name children 1 and 2, you would be likely to call them Mary and Richard, respectively, rather than the other way around.

Most parents encourage the development of what they believe are gender-related qualities, characteristics, and behaviors, which they model and reinforce with considerable consistency. Even the boy raised in a fatherless home can receive sufficient masculine-behavior reinforcement from his mother to establish a male identity.[9]

Additional confirmation of the influence of the home comes from studies of hermaphroditic children. If a child is born hermaphroditic but assigned gender on the basis of external genitalia, it is apparent that some confusion could develop if examination of internal reproductive structures later revealed the child to be of the gender opposite to that assigned. In actual cases of this type gender reassignment was successful before age four, but in children older than four significant maladjustment followed the change.[10]

At least in the early years of life, then, children's sex identity seems to be a product of their ability to discriminate parental gender combined with gender assignment and reinforcement by the parents. As the child enters school we would expect the new exposure to modify and refine the home-established identity. Evidence suggests that this is the case, even for boys whose teachers are women who

TABLE 4-1. Parentally Reinforced Behavior Traits

Child 1	Child 2	Child 3
Neatly dressed	Sloppy dress	Long hair with permanent
Compliant or submissive	Aggressive	Slacks
Dependent	Autonomous	Make-up
Intellectual	Physical	Bracelets
Subdued	Boisterous	Necklace
Cries	Doesn't cry	Ruffles
Compassionate	Unyielding	Dirty
Sensitive	Stoic	Loud
Cleans the home	Cuts the grass	
Plays house	Builds forts	

reward them for feminine activities.[11] It may be that the home influence continues to predominate or that some principle of primacy is vindicated. It is also possible that peer expectations and pressures play a significant role in subsequent development.[12]

An observation that deserves study is the tendency, particularly in recent years. for cross-identification to occur, that is, for children to model behavioral elements more characteristic of the opposite sex. Interest centers not only on how it happens but also on the effects of crossover on personal and social functioning. The point made by Westlake is certainly pertinent:

> For in our culture, where masculine and feminine roles are not clearly defined, and are becoming even less so, a certain amount of cross-modeling seems to be desirable for boys. In the past, boys have been derided for having feminine traits, whereas girls have not been ridiculed for being "tomboys." For some traits commonly labeled feminine make society run more smoothly: sweetness, tact, the willingness to compromise, intuitiveness, sympathy, interest in people as well as things, and appreciation of the arts. These are traits as useful to the male as to the female.[13]

At this point, we can only guess about the impact of cross-identification on personal and social health. Carried to the point of confusion and conflict, it might encourage personal and social disorganization.

Although some psychologists, sociologists, and anthropologists, and even biologists maintain that sex-role assignment is simply a conservative convention, the majority of professionals still seem to feel that sex differences are as important today as in the past. Rosenberg states that, historically,

> Most cultures have preferred to maximize sex differences rather than reduce them. It could be, therefore, that though some of today's sex differences may disappear, others may arise, for men and women may well invent new techniques for polarization. Our present typology may not be simply a psychometric error or a cultural habit. It may be that a society without sex stereotypes is much less interesting and productive than societies with definition of sex role behavior.[14]

THE ROLE OF THE TEACHER

In school a child should find support for positive influences that are present in the home as well as additional encouragement to develop attributes that are necessary for responsible and charitable maturity. The teacher should be a role model who projects sensitivity and concern, as well as a source of praise to reinforce positive gender-specific behaviors generated by parental influences. For example, the boy who is dominant in kind and productive ways need not be remolded into a less assertive child simply because the teacher would prefer it that way. Parents and teachers alike must come to understand that children are affected by the composite of in-school and out-of-school learning experiences. Improved home-school relationships would optimize the impact of the total learning experience on the child's attitudes and behaviors.

For the teacher's part, it is important to understand differences in gender and sex-related knowledge and experience between boys and girls, among various socioeconomic levels and among diverse ethnic groups. Information, experiences, and even vocabulary are quite heterogenous in many classrooms, and if a teacher's background is different from that of the students, it is very probable that problems in expectations, understanding, and communication will develop. General knowledge of the information children receive from the home, peers, media, and other sources will help the teacher to identify and understand some of the students' attitudinal and behavioral problems and to adjust the classroom experience accordingly.

More difficult problems perhaps will revolve around the issue of what definitive information or activities the school should provide. Ethics, morality, and values all enter into the equation. And because no consensus exists in our pluralistic society about what is acceptable sexual behavior, it is difficult to plan an education program. It is wishful thinking to suppose that a community that cannot define pornography can effectively describe responsible sexual attitudes and behaviors in the face of many conflicting value systems.[15]

Children are too frequently the victims of a society that exploits sexual drives and devalues them as individuals. They are emotionally aroused by commercial enterprises that are insensitive to their needs and welfare or at least emotionally detached from their desire to be loved and respected as responsible and capable individuals. The impressionable youth is motivated to act but not educated to decide. Hence instruction should help young people learn to manage their feelings responsibly. They need guiding principles to govern not only sexual emotions but most other emotions as well.

There is scant evidence to suggest that educational programs directed specifically toward sexuality will provide the desired results, but perhaps we can learn a relevant lesson from Sweden's experiences in sex education and our own excursions into instruction about drugs. The effects of Sweden's long-term sex education program on sexual behavior and use of fertility control, for example, are not clear.[16] If the goal of direct instruction is to avert unwanted pregnancies or modify sexual behavior, the results are disappointing. In fact, Haag suggests that it does not work.[17] If the desired results are improved attitudes and responsible decision making and behavior, the whole instructional program must be effective in all dimensions.

Perhaps this observation is not surprising. American educators know that large-scale educational efforts to reduce tobacco and drug use have had little effect on the target age group. Current emphasis is on people rather than drugs, and the goal is to promote self-esteem, which enhances emotional control and helps to prevent and eliminate self-defeating behaviors. As a result, presumably the individual will avoid the disappointments associated with irresponsible activity in many facets of life including those more directly related to sexuality.

Attitude Development

The most important aspect of sex education consists of the attitudes that children develop about themselves and their sexuality. To a considerable extent, these attitudes will reflect those exhibited by the parents. Even in the absence of direct instruction, children perceive parental attitudes at an early age when they begin to ask questions about their bodies, especially if their questions make their parents uncomfortable. They may notice parental attitudes when they off-handedly relate their experiences with playmates. Parents should realize that first exposures create lasting impressions and should try to lay a firm foundation for the values and attitudes they want their children to have. If parents leave it to the schools to instill sex-related values, the results may not match parental expectations, in part because the diversity of value orientations in our society makes it almost impossible to formulate behavior standards that everyone would accept. Furthermore, attitudes are generally a byproduct of social interaction or personal experience, not the direct result of instruction. Kilander suggests that attitude formation occurs in several ways:

1. It may be the final result of a gradual accumulation of related experiences, including the acquisition of facts, over a period of time, giving us our likes and dislikes, interests, and prejudices toward food, people, exercise, and sexuality, as well as other things. Examples of attitudes acquired in this way are honesty, patriotism, affection, love, and fear. They develop in the daily atmosphere in which we live, work and play.
2. It may be the result of one sudden, dramatic, intense experience. Under such circumstances, the attitude can frequently become permanent. Seeing a person killed through the carelessness of a driver may make a person unusually careful (an attitude) about driving; a child may continue to fear (an attitude) the doctor because he used a needle that resulted in pain when the child was very young; and suddenly learning that one has VD may make a person despondent (an attitude).
3. It may have been taken over from other people in the form that was already held or developed. Examples include one's attitudes toward other races or creeds, toward certain sex practices, and toward love and mar-

riage. The pattern of acceptable behavior in a given social class is often called its subculture, such as of teenagers in a given age and place. Our cultural group or other groups determine our attitudes—what we think, what we expect.[18]

Attitudes motivate and direct behavior more than knowledge does. The way we feel about something is more likely to influence what we do than what we know about it. A child who knows the value of vitamin A in carrots is nevertheless more likely to eat them if he or she likes the way carrots taste. It is not easy to persuade a child to eat carrots if you dislike them yourself. If you believe that personal feelings should not prevent students from liking carrots, you may be able to influence the students to eat them. Unfortunately, separating desirable attitudes and personal feelings about sexual behavior is difficult and no one can say definitively what attitudes children should develop. The authors favor the following:

1. Gender is a quality of personality, not merely a physical attribute.
2. All gender-related behaviors should be regarded more as a means of giving than a means of acquiring.
3. Sexual behavior has interpersonal as well as personal consequences.
4. Social moral concern for behaviors related to the taking of life should extend to the creation of life.
5. Reverence and respect should replace the contemporary dehumanization of sexual behavior.

The goal of the instructional program should be to "contribute to family stability and to a healthy, positive attitude toward the sexual aspects of man's nature. When this is accomplished, hopefully the individual's sexual nature will contribute to his self-development and happiness and at the same time conserve and advance the welfare of society.[19]

What to Teach

The paradox of teaching isolated skills is evident in the accomplished student of mathematics who cannot balance a checkbook. Sex education should be integrated into a larger context of family life education. Sex education has been too closely associated with human reproduction to achieve the proper concept. Responsible behavior is not the product of lessons in anatomy and physiology. Rather, it is an amalgamation of attitudes, personal standards, and values applicable to interpersonal relationships. Therefore it is imperative, and really unavoidable, that the sex education program stress attitudes, standards, and values. The American School Health Association has stated:

> Many facts may be quickly forgotten, but the emotional responses and attitudes which accompany their learning tend to remain. It is hoped that these wholesome attitudes will have a favorable influence on and will result in desirable practices. Therefore, the way in which something is taught is even more important than what is taught.[20]

Furthermore, it is possible that elementary schoolchildren lack the experience and intellectual capacity to handle instruction on the complexities of heterosexual relationships, despite the insistence of zealots who feel that this information is essential to the fulfillment of the child's educational needs. Some educators believe that children are exposed to too much too soon with inappropriate attitudes. If we are not careful, the schools may contribute to the excesses rather than reduce them. Perhaps a point made by the father of Corrie ten Boom has not completely lost relevance:

> Oftentimes I would use the trip home to bring up things that were troubling me, since anything I asked at home was promptly answered by the aunts. Once—I must have been ten or eleven—I asked Father about a poem we had read at school the winter before. One line had described "a young man whose face was not shadowed by sexsin." I had been far too shy to ask the teacher what it meant, and Mama had blushed scarlet when I consulted her. In those days just after the turn of the century sex was never discussed, even at home.
>
> So the line had stuck in my head. "Sex," I was pretty sure, meant whether you were a boy or a girl, and "sin" made Tante Jans very angry, but what the two together meant I could not imagine. And so, seated next to Father in the train compartment, I suddenly asked, "Father, what is sexsin?"
>
> He turned to look at me, as he always did when answering a question, but to my surprise he said nothing. At last he stood up, lifted his traveling case from the rack over our heads, ands set it on the floor.
>
> "Will you carry it off the train, Corrie?" he said.
>
> I stood up and tugged at it. It was crammed with the watches and spare parts he had purchased that morning.
>
> "It's too heavy," I said.
>
> "Yes," he said. "And it would be a pretty poor father who would ask his little girl to carry such a load. It's the same way, Corrie, with knowledge. Some knowledge is too heavy for children. When you are older and stronger you can bear it. For now you must trust me to carry it for you."
>
> And I was satisfied. More than satisfied—wonderfully at peace. There were answers to this and all my hard questions—for now I was content to leave them in my father's keeping.[21]

PROBLEMS IN PSYCHOSEXUAL DEVELOPMENT

Elementary school teachers occasionally encounter students whose psychosexual development is proceeding in a way that may cause them significant problems as they continue to mature. Since many variables influence sexuality it is not surprising that some children have trouble maintaining consistent gender identities and sex roles and ultimately develop attitudes and feelings that will confuse adult mate selection and sexual behavior.

Gender Identity

Gender identity refers to our sense of our own sexuality, how we think of ourselves sexually as male or female. This self-concept of maleness or femaleness usually coresponds to our genetic, anatomic, and hormonal makeup and thus might be considered innate. Certain patterns of child rearing, however, can produce a gender identity that does not conform to biological sex. Gender identity has usually developed by the age of two or three years and is extremely difficult to change.

Sex Role

The concept of *sex role* includes everything we say or do that characterizes us as men or women—the way we walk, talk, act, dress, work, play, and relate to others. The rules governing these factors may vary considerably from place to place, within a culture, and over a period of time. As a result, social learning factors and interpersonal contexts sometimes outweigh biological factors in sex role development.

Mate Selection

Mate selection involves deciding what type of person we prefer and can accept as an object of sexual interest. Probably the most significant aspect of this choice is whether the chosen person is of the same or opposite sex. The importance of innate biological versus social and psychological factors in shaping mate selection continues to be a point of debate among behavioral scientists. Obviously the biological designation of male or female does not automatically determine the nature of an individual's sexual activity patterns.

Homosexuality

Ideally, from a health point of view, gender identity, sexual role, eventual mate selection, and sexual behavior are in perfect resonance. Unfortunately, this is not always the case. Among the alternatives to the typical heterosexual life-style, homosexuality is one of the most common choices.

Homosexuality is the condition of having a sexual attraction to members of one's own sex. The word "homosexual" derives from the Greek root *homo,* which means sameness. Homosexual behavior among females is often termed *lesbianism.*

No biological basis for homosexuality has been found. Studies have not established a link between hormonal aberrations and homosexuality, nor have researchers found any measurable physical characteristics that consistently differentiate homosexuals from heterosexuals.

Most authorities have concluded that homosexuality results from adverse life experiences and disturbed psychosexual development. Davenport states:

> The choice of sexual objects (heterosexual or homosexual) is not based upon instinct but is learned behavior derived from the culture and environment of each individual. According to most authorities, genetic, constitutional and glandular factors have little importance in the causation of homosexuality, whereas psychologic, social and cultural factors do play key roles.[22]

The chief causes of abnormal sexual adjustment, including homosexuality, are abnormal parental attitudes and behavior. The most common pattern of family life in case histories of homosexuality includes a father who is detached, disinterested, competitively hostile, and minimizing.

In regards to this, Bieber states:

> The profound disturbances in the father-son relationship play a determining role in a homosexual outcome and form the basis for the complex psychodynamics operant in the relationship of male homosexuals with other males.[23]

The father who is extremely harsh and suppressive when his son shows signs of masculinity can arouse fears which will prevent normal sexual adjustment.

The mothers of homosexual males are excessively intimate with the son, who is preferred by the mother to other offspring and to her husband. Such mothers tend to be domineering and overprotecting, such that the child fails to become assertive and independent.

Parents mold the homsexual pattern in the following ways:

1. They experience discomfort and nonacceptance of their own sexual identity and behavior thereby distorting the child's perception of the advantages of his or her own sexual identity.
2. They feel anxiety or guilt in response to their child's attention to his genitals as a source of interest and curiosity. They thus suppress the child's sexual curiosity, resulting in conflicts and

inhibitions which will influence reactions to sexual drives in later life.

3. They exhibit abnormal attitudes and behaviors which contribute to the child's behavior repertoire.

Both male and female homosexuality are thought to be a result of pathologic parent-child relationships. As in males, a daughter's attitude toward other females may derive from the personalities, character, and habits of her parents. Any heterosexual relationship that proves unacceptable to a female may cause a girl to reject men.[24]

The mothers and fathers of female homosexuals fall into two primary groups (as indicated in Table 4-2).[25] No one can pinpoint one cause of homsexuality, but the evidence is pointing more and more toward abnormal relationships between parents and their children. Not everyone accepts this theory, however. Perhaps the problem is too complex to be ascribed to one causative factor. Even though an individual's family may make him or her vulnerable to homosexuality, many other variables in the development of a homosexual life-style probably reinforce this kind of behavior.

Aside from abnormal family relationships, another point to consider is the effect of a first homosexual experience. If the experience is enjoyable and fulfilling, particularly interpersonally--a substitute for unmet needs in other dimensions of the person's life—the chances of engaging in further homosexual fantasy or behavior are great, even if the person was an active heterosexual prior to the experience.

TABLE 4-2.   Behavioral Groupings in Parents of Homosexual Females

	Mothers toward Daughter	*Fathers toward Daughter*
Group I	Rejecting Critical Competitive Defeminizing Emotionally cold Unaffectionate Discouarges feminine pursuits Jealous	Detached Rejecting Unaffectionate Submissive to wives Alienating
Group II	Possessive Dominating Controlling Discourages dating and romantic attachments	Possessive Seductive Intimate Binding Defeminizing Jealous of other males

A rewarding homosexual experience may even encourage an individual to enjoy sexual experiences with both sexes, that is, to be *bisexual.*

Several years ago *Time* magazine printed an article about homosexuality as a substitute for normal heterosexual behavior in which the following position was taken:

> As such it deserves fairness, compassion, understanding, and, when possible, treatment. But it deserves no encouragement, no glamorization, no sophistry about simple differences in taste—and, above all, no pretense that it is anything but a (sexual deviation).[26]

Dr. Harold M. Voth, psychiatrist and psychoanalyst at The Menninger Foundation, has said:

> In these times when some of the best human values are undergoing major changes, many of which reflect disintegration, it is imperative that there be complete clarity about what constitutes normal and abnormal sexual feeling and behavior. Young people are desperately in need of standards and guidelines, especially in the area of interpersonal relationships. Homosexuality is a form of pathologic sexuality; it is not a variant of normal sexuality.[27]

Dr. Lawrence J. Hatterer, a psychiatrist at Cornell University Medical School who has evaluated over 700 homosexual individuals, indicates that homosexuality results from inhibitions, disturbed patterns of gender identity, and other factors that are amenable to change and treatment.[28] Homosexuals who have a strong desire to become heterosexual are very treatable, particularly if they experience guilt, anxiety, or depression about their impulses or practices and have tried on their own to fight homosexual thinking and behavior. Their prognosis is favorable with competent help.[29]

Heterosexual Deviations

Deviant sexual behaviors tend to be symptomatic of significant and pervasive psychological disturbances and therefore represent a general developmental problem. Most have their roots in poor family relationships and inadequate instruction regarding appropriate sexual behavior in marital relationships.[30] Such circumstances block normal heterosexual development and may cause people to discharge sexual tensions in undesirable behavioral patterns.

HOME-SCHOOL RELATIONS

The foregoing suggests that the home influence is paramount in determining the child's gender identification and sex role behaviors. It would seem wise for the school to capitalize on that influence as much as possible. Parent-teacher conferences are excellent vehicles for airing children's problems and for soliciting cooperation in educational efforts.

Well-informed teachers must be familiar with both factual and value-laden dimensions of sexuality and family life education. Unfortunately, as we said earlier, sexual values, which have the greater impact on behavior, are almost as diverse as the people that hold them. Perhaps it would be more reasonable to expect responsible behavior if we could more explicitly define and teach it. A great leader, when asked how he governed his people so successfully, stated, "I teach them correct principles, and they govern themselves."[31] In family life education there seems to be some difficulty in determining what constitutes correct principles. In general, we might agree that attitudes and behaviors ought to exemplify selflessness and a commitment to be a blessing in the lives of others. From this perspective, any degree of exploitation is repugnant and disruptive of interpersonal relationships that would support and build feelings of self-esteem and self-worth in others.

NOTES

1. B.G. Rosenberg, Brian Sutton-Smith, *Sex and Identity* (New York: Holt Rinehart and Winston, 1972), p. 30.
2. M. Diamond, "A Critical Evaluation of the Ontogeny of Human Sexual Behaviors," *Quarterly Review of Biology* 40 (1965): 147–75.
3. J.L. Katz, "Biological and Psychological Roots of Psychosexual Identity," *Medical Aspects of Human Sexuality*, June 1972, p. 113.
4. Ibid., p. 116.
5. R.R. Sears, "Development of Gender and Role," in *Sex Behaviors*, ed. F.A. Beach (New York: John Wiley and Sons, 1965), pp. 133–63.
6. O.R. Matteson, *Adolescence Today* (Homewood, Ill.: Dorsey Press, 1975), p. 12.
7. Helen Gum Westlake, *Children, A Study in Individual Behavior* (Lexington, Mass.: Ginn and Co., 1973), p. 208. See also A. Bandura, D. Ross, S. Ross, "A Cooperative Test of the Status Envy/Social Power and the Secondary Reinforcement Theories of Identification Learning," in *Human Learning*, ed. Arthur Staats (New York: Holt Rinehart and Winston, 1964), p. 382.
8. "Sex-role Development in a Changing Culture, *Psychology Bulletin* 55 (1958): 232–42. See also K. Vroegh, "Masculinity and Femininity in the Elementary and Junior High School Years," *Developmental Psychology* 4: 254–62.
9. H.B. Biller, "Father Absence, Maternal Encouragement, and Sex Role Development in Kindergarten-age Boys," *Child Development* 40 (1969): 539–46.
10. J. Money, Joan G. Hampson, and J.L. Hampson, "Imprinting and the Establishment of Gender Role," *Archives of Neurology and Psychology* 77 (1957): 333–36.

11. B.J. Fagot and G.R. Patterson, "An In Viva Analysis of Reinforcing Contingencies for Sex Role Behaviors in the Preschool Child," *Developmental Psychology* 1 (1969): 563-68.
12. Ibid.
13. Westlake, p. 211.
14. Rosenberg and Sutton-Smith, p. 90.
15. For a brief discussion of contemporary value orientation, see Isadore Rubin, "Transition in Sex Values—Implications for the Education of Adolescents," *Journal of Marriage and the Family,* May 1965.
16. W.B. Haag et al. "Adolescent Fertility—Risks and Consequences," *Population Reports* J10 (July 1976): 157-75.
17. "Is School an Appropriate Place for Sex Education?" *Sexual Behaviors,* August 1971, pp. 64-73.
18. H. Frederick Kilander, *Sex Education in the Schools* (London: MacMillan Co., 1970), p. 25.
19. E.D. Schulz and S.R. Williams, *Family, Life and Sex Education: Curriculum and Instruction,* (New York: Harcourt, Brace, and World, 1968), p. 15.
20. "Growth Patterns and Sex Education—A Suggested Program Kindergarten Through Grade Twelve," *Journal of American School Health Association,* May 1967, p. 2.
21. *The Hiding Place,* by Corrie ten Boom and John and Elizabeth Sherrill. Published by Chosen Books Publishing Co., Ltd., Lincoln, Va. 22078. Used by permission.
22. Charles W. Davenport, "Homosexuality: Its Origins, Early Recognition, and Prevention," *Clinical Pediatrics,* January 1972, pp. 7-10.
23. Irving Bieber, "Homosexuality," *American Journal of Nursing,* December 1969, pp. 2637-41.
24. Harold K. Becker, "A Phenomenological Inquiry into the Etiology of Female Homosexuality," *Journal of Human Relations,* 1969, pp. 570-80.
25. Bieber.
26. "The Homosexual in America," *Time,* 21 January 1966, p. 40.
27. "Is Homosexuality Pathologic or a Normal Variant of Sexuality?" *Medical Aspects of Human Sexuality,* December 1973, p. 15.
28. Lawrence J. Hatterer, "Can Homosexuals Change?" *Sexual Behavior,* July 1971, p. 48.
29. Lawrence J. Hatterer, "Nine Myths About Homosexuality," *Medical Opinion,* January 1973, p. 46.
30. J.C. Coleman, *Abnormal Psychology and Modern Life* (Chicago: Scott, Foresman and Co., 1965), p. 415.
31. John A. Widtsoe, *Priesthood and Church Government* (Salt Lake City: Deseret Book, 1954), p. 100.

CHAPTER 5

Mental and Emotional Health

The major public health problem in the United States today is poor mental health, according to the National Institute of Mental Health. Even the children cannot escape the emotional implications of physical, social, and cultural problems; family strife; and language difficulties. As our society has become increasingly complex, the suicide rate among elementary schoolchildren has also increased.

It is estimated that anywhere from 10 to 25 percent of elementary children require psychiatric aid. Statistically, then, each elementary school classroom contains three to eight emotionally handicapped children.[1] Many more suffer emotional difficulties that cripple their learning skills. Elementary teachers who can recognize emotional problems and seek help for troubled children are extremely valuable. Equipped with a knowledge of mental and emotional health, both good and bad, elementary school teachers can positively influence the health of their students.

EMOTIONAL HEALTH—WHAT IS IT?

Personality development, which is the sum of our reactions to our environment, is an important part of mental health. Much of our personality development takes place early in life and parents play a key role in this process. As mature adults with harmonious personalities, parents provide the model for children to imitate. In the school setting, teachers play a similar role. Early developmental patterns involve three major periods of psychological growth: infancy, preschool, and middle childhood.

In infancy a warm, comfortable environment with physical closeness develops security, trust, and love. In the view of psychologists, love is one of the most crucial needs children have. Without it, they may physically or emotionally die.

Preschoolers develop new awareness of themselves and others as they venture to explore their environment. A three-year-old feels a surge of independence and desires some freedom but still has a great need to be loved and feel security or safety. The process of modeling is very important at this stage. It is a critical time for the right social and emotional training to occur. It is important to remember, however, that great variations in emotional development, as well as physical growth, are very normal. It is important to keep in mind the "different drum" concept while we discuss emotional health.

Now we approach the elementary school age. We base entry into school on chronological age, for example, entering the first grade at age six. Most children are ready for school at this age, but some are not emotionally and socially mature enough to handle the gap between home and school. Teachers who sense that a child is not ready for a particular grade level must patiently help the parents understand why. It is important for parents to understand that not being ready for the next step is not bad. Some parents will have to learn to socially wean their children and better prepare them for the school experience. Inadequate social skills can cause long-lasting problems that may hang over a child for life. Proper preparation makes going to school and learning basic skills, concepts, and value systems exciting for children.

GOOD MENTAL HEALTH

Even young children come to realize that life is a series of adjustments. Mentally healthy individuals are able to adjust to changes in their environment and to use coping devices in a positive way. Emotionally healthy students have positive self-concepts (they feel good about themselves) and feel good about others. They adapt well to change and are in control of their emotions. Most mentally healthy children greet the school day with eagerness and enthusiasm.

A definition of good mental health comes from the Committee on Mental Health in the Classroom:

> Mental health is that emotional adjustment in which a person can live with reasonable comfort, functioning acceptably in the community in which he

lives. The mentally healthy person is for the most part able to handle his emotions and cope acceptably with situations in his environment. The pupil who shows unacceptable behavior may be showing signs of emotional stress and may need specialized help.[2]

In addition, Rucker has abstracted (from several leading psychologists)* the following characteristics of people who have a "healthy, multivalued personality."

1. They acknowledge personal responsibility for their own actions (high rectitude status).
2. They are self-reliant (high status of self-respect). They are more independent in the solution of their problems than average or ill persons.
3. They deal with their environment in a creative manner (enlightenment and skill). They use their own skills and understanding to do those things necessary for their health and happiness.
4. Their concepts about other people are realistic and are not distorted by past experiences (Sullivan describes this trait as nonparataxic interpersonal relations). He says that such people are aware of these relationships and that their beliefs about themselves and other people are accurate (enlightenment and skill).
5. They have social feeling (love and respect). Adler says such persons are identified with mankind. He says that the unhealthy person spends all of his time competing for power in order to escape from his feelings of insecurity while the healthy person is free to love and to respect others.
6. They tend to realize their latent potentials in everyday activities (skills). They are not afraid to try out new ways of doing things for fear of failure (with consequent loss of respect).
7. They tend to see reality as it is and to be comfortable in their relationship with it. Such persons can more easily distinguish between the true and the false, the honest and the dishonest person. They do less "wishful" thinking than emotionally ill persons. They have less fear of the unknown and thus are relatively free to create new ways of doing things and to try them out with confidence (self-respect and skill).
8. They think and often act spontaneously. While inwardly despising the conventional, they will often accept it in order to avoid hurting people. Such persons can thus be said to have a social consciousness which forces them to think before they may act unconventionally (rectitude).
9. They are concerned with problems outside themselves rather than being concerned with self as are insecure people (rectitude, enlightenment, and skill). Such people, when they grow up, are concerned with the basic issues of life and work in the broadest frame of reference in thinking about values and their achievement.
10. They can be alone without discomfort (self-respect). Such people even have need of solitude or privacy more than the "average" or ill person who is usually uncomfortable when alone.

---

*Reprinted with permission from W. Ray Rucker, V. Clyde Arnspiger, and Arthur J. Brodbeck, *Human Values in Education,* © 1969 by Rucker, Arnspiger, and Bradbeck. Kendall/Hunt Publishing Co., Dubuque, Iowa.

11. They continue to get pleasure from the beauty of their environment throughout life. They respond aesthetically and with pleasure to a beautiful flower even though they have seen one almost exactly like it many times before (high status of aesthetic skill). This attitude of continuing appreciation is an index of good mental health.

12. They have democratic personalities. They demand that all values be shared. This is an index of high rectitude status. They will learn from the experiences of any person of good character regardless of political belief, class, religious persuasion, or nationality (respect and affection). They treat people courteously, have respect for people on the basis of merit rather than on the basis of family or other unearned status. They are ethical in their interpersonal relationships. They demand that others have the same access to values that they demand for themselves (rectitude).

13. They are able to distinguish between means and ends (enlightenment and skill). They always place the goals they seek above the means by which they seek to achieve them. This trait may often be displayed in the judicious management of personal finances.

14. They have an unhostile sense of humor (respect), do not laugh at misfortunes of others, and do not attempt to make people laugh by hurting others. Such people, however, are quick to see the humor in the errors of human beings in general, such as trying to feel important when this feeling is not justified. They can laugh at their own mistakes. Their humor is spontaneous rather than planned (well-being).

15. They offer intelligent and responsible resistance to many aspects of the cultural mold (rectitude). They conform with many of the observable symbols of conventionality but are really not conventional in the dependent sense. They accept conventional practices only to the degree to which they think they are good.

Another leading psychologist, Abraham Maslow, has developed an eclectic theory of human behavior that focuses on personality development.[3] His *hierarchy of needs theory* explains that human behavior is largely directed toward the fulfillment of basic needs and that personality evolves as these innate needs are satisfied. Believing that this evolution follows a fairly predictable sequence, Maslow has devised a ladderlike scheme for different degrees of personality development (see Table 5-1).

We are born with physiological needs, including hunger, thirst, the need for air, and so on. When we feel that our physiological needs are being satisfied, security or safety needs emerge. The physiological needs are most dominant, followed by the safety needs. Next come love, affection, and the need to belong. The gregariousness of human beings is evidence of this need. Satisfaction of all fundamental needs engenders a positive self-concept or sense of personal worth, which Maslow calls the esteem need. Meeting this need generates the need for self-actualization, or the need to achieve self-fulfillment or reach one's full potential. Maslow states that "What a man can be, he must be," yet he believes that only a very

TABLE 5-1.   Maslow's Hierarchy of Needs Theory

Self-actualization
   Reaching one's full potential
   A very small percentage of people reach this level

Esteem Needs
   Feelings of self-worth
   Having a positive self-concept

Love and Belonging Needs
   The need to be with people and to show and receive love
   Vitally needed from the moment of birth

Security or Safety Needs
   More easily abused in children
   Adults learn to mask it

Physiological Needs
   Need for air
   Satisfaction of hunger, thirst, sexual expression

Source: Abraham H. Maslow, *Toward a Psychology of Being,* 2nd ed. (Princeton. N.J.: D. Van Nostrand, 1968).

low percentage of people become fully self-actualized. Maslow does acknowledge exceptions to his general theory that people must satisfy lower-level needs before they can fulfill higher-level needs. For example, a mother may sacrifice her security need in order to save her child and a prisoner of war may sacrifice basic-level needs in order to attain higher-level needs.

Unsatisfied needs on any level (e.g., physiological needs) may be strong enough to push all other needs into the background. As lower-level needs are satisfied, higher-level needs emerge. A healthy, developing personality, therefore, will show need fulfillment emerging at the higher end of the hierarchy. This theory stresses the importance of basic need fulfillment, which is partially the responsibility of teachers.

Another psychological theorist who has had a great impact upon American education is William Glasser. His *reality therapy* stresses personal responsibility and a strong sense of responsibility toward others. Emotionally healthy students, according to Glasser, feel love, are able to give love, and have a sense of self-worth. Glasser suggests that we direct our behavior toward fulfilling needs and overcoming feelings of inadequacy.

Students who exemplify positive emotional health are enthusiastic and have a positive purpose for living. They feel good about themselves and others in their environment, and they adjust to the demands of life. Though occasional outbursts may occur, they remain in emotional control.[4]

POOR MENTAL HEALTH

To define poor mental health is a difficult and complex task, for we can express mental processes and emotions through overt behavior that is difficult to interpret. The ease with which we can mask many emotional problems makes it difficult to recognize them before they have become serious. A student's background and certain clusters of symptoms or behavioral signs may help teachers to spot a potentially serious problem early.

Poor emotional health has numerous causes. Physical problems, such as deafness, vision difficulties, physical abnormalities, and speech problems can all cause emotional problems and a real dislike for school. For example, a child may be too structured and over-worked because the parents demand excellence in too many extra-curricular or school activities. Consequently the child may be nervous and chronically fatigued (pale and constantly tired). Other causes may include parents whose expectations exceed the child's abilities, parents with emotional problems, a broken home, and lack of harmony in the home. When both parents work away from home, a child may develop an emotional problem because there is no one to turn to for support and comfort. For any of these reasons students may experience difficulty in learning, which can complicate and compound the original problem and result in antisocial behavior. Negative behavior, in turn, may cause tension and disruption in the classroom. Too often children with emotional problems are "pushed out." They become "delinquents" and later emotionally disturbed adults.

We tend to feel sorry for children who have physical handicaps, such as cerebral palsy. We fail to recognize that the child who lives with a divorced, single parent, suffers parental neglect, has a poor social environment or bad home life, or suffers emotional and physical abuse may have a slimmer chance of achieving a satisfying life than many physically handicapped children.

Society and science have assigned emotional disturbances and behavior problems many confusing labels. Behavior is quite complex, and judgments about the way people act are not always easy to make. To further complicate matters, the line between normal and abnormal behavior is very thin. The criterion for teachers to use in assessing behavior is whether it is destructive and harmful to the child or to others. Some behaviors are consequences of maturation, adjustment, emotional releases, and some stem from environmental upsets. Some behavioral problems may be outgrown, but many will lead to serious behavioral problems. To help distinguish between temporary, developmental problems and longer-term problems, we provide the following list of common characteristics of serious emotional problems from Kaplan:

1. Nervous behavior. Habitual twitching of muscles, scowling, grimacing, twisting the hair, continuous blinking, biting or wetting the lips, nail biting, stammering, blushing or turning pale, constant restlessness, frequent complaints of minor illnesses, head banging, nervous finger movements, frequent crying, body rocking, frequent urination.
2. Emotional overreactions and deviations. Undue anxiety over mistakes, marked distress over failures, absentmindedness, daydreaming, meticulous interest in details, refusal to take part in games, refusal to accept any recognition or regard, evasion of responsibility, withdrawal from anything that looks new or difficult, chronic attitude of apprehension, lack of concentration, unusual sensitivity to all annoyances (especially noises), inability to work if distracted, lack of objective interests, frequent affectations and posturing, inappropriate laughing, uncontrolled laughing or giggling, explosive and emotional tone in argument, tendency to feel hurt when others disagree, unwillingness to give in, shrieking when excited, frequent efforts to gain attention, sudden intensive attachments to people (often older), extravagant expressions of any emotion.
3. Emotional immaturity. Inability to work alone, tendency to cling to a single, intimate friend, inability to rely on own judgment, unreasonable degree of worry over grades, persistent inferiority feelings, unusual self-consciousness, inability to relax and forget self, excessive suspiciousness, overcritical of others, too docile and suggestible, persistent fears, indecision, compulsive behavior, hyperactivity.
4. Exhibitionistic behavior. Teasing, pushing or shoving other pupils, trying to act tough, trying to be funny, wanting to be overconspicuous, exaggerated courtesy, marked agreement with everything the teacher says, constant bragging, frequent attempts to dominate younger or smaller children, inability to accept criticism, constant efforts to justify self, frequent blaming of failures on accidents or on other individuals, refusal to admit any personal lack of knowledge or inability, frequent bluffing, attempting either far too little or far too much work.
5. Antisocial behavior. Cruelty to others, bullying, abusive or obscene language, undue interest in sex (especially efforts to establish bodily contact), telling offensive stories or showing obscene pictures, profound dislike of all schoolwork, fierce resentment of authority, bad reaction to discipline, general destructiveness, irresponsibility, sudden and complete lack of interest in school, truancy.
6. Psychosomatic disturbances. Reversals or complications in toilet habits, enuresis [bedwetting], constipation, diarrhea, excessive urination, feeding disturbances, overeating, nausea or vomiting when emotionally distressed, various aches and pains.[5]

These behaviors may well show up in normal children. At some ages they are more common that at others. The key is to look for combinations of these symptoms that are consistent and frequent and do not get better with time.

THE SCHOOL'S ROLE IN MENTAL HEALTH

How important is the school setting to the mental health of students? In the words of Dr. Robert H. Felix, former director of the National Institute for Mental Health, "Next to the family, the school is probably the most important unit of society as far as the protection of mental health is concerned."[6] Fulton and Fassbender enlarge upon this consideration:

> Between the ages of six and seventeen, most children spend more waking hours with their teachers than with their parents. Teachers, therefore, have a profound effect on both the social and emotional adjustment of children. . . .
> An emphasis on self-understanding, the development of a positive self-concept based on individually structured achievement and counseling to prevent emotional maladjustment, are all vitally important for the mental health of children.[7]

The teacher, then, has the opportunity to positively influence students' mental health. To establish students' trust the teacher has only to show real concern and caring love and to be patient in the face of the normal confusion of youth. A warm voice, inviting facial expression, friendly and communicative gestures and body postures are all elements of a positive emotional climate for good mental health. They project the message "I value you as a person" and enable the teacher to become more and more sensitive to the feelings of the students. The result is an ability to see through negative, defiant behavior to the underlying problems.

Many teachers are puzzled by the behavior of certain students and are not sure how to handle the ones who fail to adjust well to their classrooms. Many times the root of the problem lies in the way these children feel about themselves as people rather than a lack of ability to succeed or work with others. Therefore, teachers must understand the role they play in creating an atmosphere that promotes a positive self-image and good mental health. The school has a major responsibility to aid ego development in young children when problems with ego development seem to be having an adverse effect on learning.

Katherine D. Evelyn discusses five major "musts" in every child's life that directly affect mental health:[8]

1. All children must know and feel that they are integral members of the class. Young children need to feel at home in class, and older elementary children need to feel that they are important

members of their class. Children who feel wanted and believe they have the same rights and responsibilities as other class members are likely to develop a positive self-concept and to enjoy successful learning. Some children, however, have a difficult time in the average classroom. The disturbing bully, the sensitive, withdrawn child, and the psychotic child who lacks behavior control may all need specialized help outside of the regular classroom.

Elementary teachers are not diagnosticians. Rather than trying to label children whose behavior is unusual, they should seek the help of specialists.

2. Children must know what adults expect of them. Elementary schoolchildren need constructive adult guidance and control that is not restrictive or repressive. If children are unsure of teachers' expectations, they will push and test to find the boundaries of acceptable behavior. The resulting chaos will make learning difficult.

3. Children must interact with classmates. Students who participate successfully in the activities of the classroom know that their contributions have value and earn them respect. Each child's contributions are unique for each child is different and must have respect as an individual. Effective teachers respond to extroverted children without allowing them to monopolize classroom time and draw out the introverts without making them feel conspicuous.

A key to good mental health for a young child is a sense of mastery. Successful management of the life tasks that arise at different developmental stages is critical to mental health. Children who see peers ably mastering tasks that they cannot perform become ego-deflated. For example, a child who is having reading problems requires close observation and individual attention to special learning needs.

4. Children must learn self-discipline to be mentally healthy. The components of self-discipline are self-control, patience, an acceptable frustration-tolerance level, persistence at a given task, and the ability to control impulsive behavior. Encouragement at home is essential for the development of self-discipline. If the home fails in this task, the school has a tough, but possible job.

Teachers who attempt to instill self-discipline through punishment and harsh restrictions will find that they usually do not go hand in hand. Elementary schoolchildren respond to encouragement and understanding, behavioral limits, and lavish but sincere praise. The example and expectations of the teacher are also important. Another good technique for teaching self-discipline is to involve the child in satisfying activities and interesting experiences.

5. Children must achieve as much as their abilities permit. The real challenge for any teacher is to build a feeling of real accomplishment in each of the very different students in the classroom. That

is also a primary task, for a feeling of accomplishment is essential to good mental health. Constant failure cuts down motivation and generates a poor self-concept, both of which stunt learning. Parents and teachers must encourage and set the stage for children to realize their potential without pressuring or discouraging them with excessive demands. Failure, too, can be a good teacher if it involves the feeling and experience of being able to master a task after failing at it. In reality, we all need to learn how to cope with and overcome failure, and teachers can equip children to succeed after a failure.

6. Elementary children are very dependent on their teachers for security, learning, and the growth of a positive self-concept. The ideal guide is strong, controlled, and disciplined, on the one hand, and warm, sensitive, and supportive, on the other hand. Teachers are not pals but leaders who want children to grow and be successful. Not always approving, they are nevertheless understanding— not perfect, but emotionally controlled. Above all, successful teachers try to provide "good" school experiences.

Teachers may be the only stable adults a student knows. Therefore it is essential for them to show genuine affection and concern. A troubled child seeks protection and guidance from adults, no matter what they show on the surface. Bidwell states, "If his own parents or loved ones are not able to be with him, communications with them [teachers] as frequently as possible helps."[9] Furthermore, Bidwell maintains:

> A teacher can help eliminate external sources of tension by reducing pressures on the pupil. Perhaps she may tell the pupil who is concerned about poor spelling to enjoy writing compositions and just think about what he is trying to say and then when this comes more easily, it will be time to give attention to the spelling. It is important for a child to experience success in some area.[10]

Teachers can promote positive mental health also by helping parents understand that what they do at home has a real effect on their children's time in school. Charlotte Haupt gives this counsel:

> If a child is loaded with anxieties when he comes to school in the morning and you cannot alleviate them or at least let him know that you are in tune with him, he will learn nothing all day, no matter how hard you try to teach.[11]

Help parents appreciate the importance of sending happy children to school.

Experienced teachers can usually recognize children who are starved for love, security, and recognition. By noticing and treating the anxieties of these children, teachers can practice "preventive mental health." Through the use of value-clarification strategies and other "self-concept" programs, they can help students to sort out and understand themselves. Children need to experience success to know that they can succeed. "Success breeds success," as the adage goes, because it instills confidence and a positive self-concept, whereas failure lessens and beats down confidence, resulting in a negative self-concept. We can all take a lesson from Dale Carnegie, who suggests building confidence by giving lavish, sincere praise.

Seeing and teaching the whole child makes it possible to fit the curriculum to the individual. One way to understand the whole child is to observe how he or she functions, or acts and reacts, in a group setting. Sociograms, open-ended movies about life problems (e.g., Inside/out by A.I.T.), problem-solving discussions focused on behavior dynamics, unfinished stories, picture interpretation, role playing, and story reading all aid in removing teachers from the directive role and allowing them to be listeners.

The following list, adapted from Sorochan, summarizes what the teacher can do to effect good mental health in the classroom:*

1. Memorize your students' names as quickly as you can and call them by name.
2. Make sure you have everyone's attention before you begin to teach.
3. Give clear, explicit directions about what you want done.
4. Create a warm, friendly atmosphere in the classroom.
5. Be friendly and warm, but firm.
6. Be a good listener. This is a key point that Bidwell emphasizes:

   It is my hypothesis that if a program were organized to such a degree that the teacher would be able to see each child individually and listen effectively to what the child says, she would be able to promote positive mental health.[12]

7. Give each child recognition when appropriate and possible.
8. Use volunteer helpers and try to involve those who never volunteer.
9. Help your students understand the importance of good nutrition and a balance of work, play, exercise, and sleep.
10. Arrange frequent rest periods.
11. Allow for individual differences in academic assignments.
12. Help each child begin complex tasks and then gradually withdraw.
13. Provide for "reward from within" instead of extrinsic rewards and behavioral reinforcements.
14. Encourage hobbies, art, crafts, drama, music, and other interests.
15. Provide for more successes than failures. For example, a supportive administration will help you put less emphasis on grades (grade pressure can be too great) and more emphasis on personality-building experiences.
16. Involve parents actively in the school health program. If you successfully

---

*Sorochan/Bender, *Teaching Elementary Health Science*, © 1975, Addison-Wesley Publishing Company. Adaptation from pp. 103–104, Chapter 6. Reprinted with permission.

connect the home and school, children will not have to struggle with loyalties. One way to begin is to develop a questionnaire that will initiate an interviewing process between parents and children in the home.

Even the finest teachers occasionally have to deal with an emotionally disturbed child. The following points will provide guidance at these times:

1. Be an effective listener and observer, and discover what conditions caused the problem. (Refer to the earlier discussion of the causes of emotional disturbance.) Once you have learned what is behind the problem, develop a plan to help the child cope.
2. Find out whether group dynamics have contributed to the problem. For example, a child who is at the bottom rung of the social ladder may react by striking out in anger. This behavior upsets students on its receiving end and the cycle complicates itself. Program the child for success by developing activities that will bring success and admiration.
3. Ease classroom pressures that are pushing the child into a corner.
4. Consult mental health specialists, such as the school psychologist. Discuss the program with parents and the school nurse and refer the child to a community treatment center if necessary. Make sure parents understand that therapy need not disrupt the child's education.

Schools have a great potential for promoting and protecting emotional health as well as for damaging it. Teachers should strive to keep students healthy so they can learn and to help the emotionally stressed child. One of the surest ways to do that is to help the students develop self-control and disciplined ways of living.

DISCIPLINE AND SELF-CONTROL[13]

Children develop self-discipline if adults teach them well. Good school discipline means training that develops self-control in the child; it insures the healthy growth of the individual and the group.

The word "discipline" is not synonymous with punishment. Control that entails scolding and punishment is short-lived. Good discipline involves control and direction of behavior each minute of the day. It means listening, structuring, informing, and responding completely. The goal is self-control.

Harsh, scolding, angry teachers are not only unpleasant and unfair but also ineffective. Forcing children to solve puzzles without talking or to wait for long periods in line without pushing arouses children's resentment, which they will convert to rowdiness as soon as the teacher's back is turned.

On the other hand, a weak teacher is not very effective either. An anxious, unsure manner seems to encourage misbehavior. Indulgent teachers who allow children to leave unfinished work strewn about the classroom or to run in and out of the room as they please probably will have to put up with a lot of unruly behavior. Teachers who seem to be courting the children's affection with their indulgence probably will fail in the attempt. In fact, their classes may act as though they are desperate for steady rules.

A teacher's personality is the key to good discipline. Good teachers do not punish or push children around; neither do they give students free rein to do whatever they want to do. Affectionate and warm, effective teachers hold an unhappy child, pat a hard-working youngster on the back, and welcome a latecomer with a hug. Such communications have great meaning for teachers and children. Good teachers are firm without being harsh, gentle without being weak. They are friendly grown-ups, who nevertheless are clearly in charge. Adults who enjoy being with children, good teachers find them interesting conversationalists who are worth listening to. They confer with children and use their suggestions. They value children as people and take their ideas and feelings very seriously. They trust that each child will grow and mature. In exchange, each child trusts the teacher's patience, understanding, and firmness.

Because good teachers work with children rather than against them, the children reciprocate. They may dislike teacher demands—and say so. Likewise the teacher may disapprove of some of the children's behavior and let them know it. Good teachers and their pupils communicate well because they like and respect each other, because they are interested in each other, and because they believe in each other's worth.

The Importance of Mutual Respect and Interest

Teachers must show their respect for and interest in their students. For example, they build the morale and self-esteem of individual children by praising their work, by studying areas in which they are doing well—or at least are trying to do well—and verbally encouraging their efforts.

Empty praise demeans children. There is no point in calling an easel painting "pretty" without really examining it or in giving extravagant praise for a block building done halfheartedly or carelessly. Forced, sugary praise merely proves to children that the teacher's mind is elsewhere and that the words are insincere. But thoughtful encouragement and respect are another matter—they build cooperative attitudes. "That block building is really well-balanced. I like the way you used the column blocks on that side," a teacher might comment. Or when a child finishes a puzzle: "You

did it! It was a long, hard job; you must feel pretty good about that."
Experience shows that children who receive explicit, personal praise
behave much better than children who get attention only when they
misbehave.

Another way of showing respect and interest is to give children
some responsibility for running the room and the instructional
program. Children can do many tasks we often assign to adults.
Taking part in necessary work develops children's skills and self-
esteem, and thus it develops a desire to behave acceptably. Among
the jobs that children can do well are: washing tabletops and rear-
ranging settings for art activities or lunch, moving chairs, large
blocks, and outdoor equipment; preparing food; making placemats
or interesting centerpieces; washing dishes or paintbrushes and clay
equipment; helping each other with outdoor clothing; sanding
blocks; and sorting pegs or water-play supplies. Of course, all these
activities may seem like drudgery if teachers suggest them in a tired
voice or assign them as punishment or a moral duty. If the teacher
proposes such work enthusiastically, morale soars and children feel
more like cooperating than not.

Setting an example for good behavior is a third way for teachers to
show feelings of respect and interest. Children search hard for clues
to true feelings so adults have to be careful about how they speak
and what they say. Teachers need to be courteous as well as informative. Teaching children to say "please" and "thank you" has no value
if adults fail to practice what they preach. Good teachers speak
earnestly and warmly and in a polite way, no matter how others are
speaking. "Would you pass the basket over to Denise, please? May I
have it, then? Thank you." Children imitate; they bark and yell if
we do or speak with tact and decency if we do. Sometimes learning
by example takes a long time, but it finally works and sticks.

The same idea applies to the care of materials and rooms. If school
shelves are overflowing with scraps of paper, broken crayons, discarded pegs, and bits of chalk, children will not perceive or respect
the educational purposes of these materials. They will not care how
things are kept because their models—the teachers—obviously do not
care. If, on the other hand, teachers prepare table materials and
shelves in advance and faithfully involve all adults and children in the
upkeep and order of these materials, children will learn the habits of
helping to put things away and maintaining their room.

For instance, when it is time to put away the blocks some teachers
merely push a cardboard box over to the blocks and join the children
in tossing blocks helter-skelter into the box. Later they fuss at the
children for treating materials carelessly or putting supplies away in
messy condition. A much more sensible way to teach children to
pick up toys and equipment is to set the right example: the oblong
blocks go together here; arches go on the top shelf; small cars and

planes belong at the side, lined up carefully. If the teacher helps with this process and talks about it (not chiding or nagging), children catch the fun, aesthetic pleasure, and pride of the job.

Disciplinary Methods

Some trouble is inevitable despite the best planning, and the warmest and soundest relationship between teachers and children. To be sure, some days seem magical in their serenity and in the flowering of understanding and thought. But many days are full of frustration, stress, and incomprehension that leave teachers in despair about the children or about themselves and their profession. Between these two extremes are simply the many moments when plans go awry, schedules don't work, tempers flare, sarcasm erupts, and the supervisor is there witnessing it all. How should teachers deal with such disruptions?

Disciplinary requirements do not work without enforcement. Whether or not a requirement is too stiff, without enforcement it serves no purpose. That is why rules and regulations must be fair and just—and few. It is possible to make small children sit silently at desks for hours, but it is unfair and inappropriate, and the fact that this kind of force works does not justify it; it just demonstrates that big people can make smaller people do almost anything.

Let us take for granted that spanking and hitting, shaming and isolating, and all other humiliating techniques are taboo. Obviously what such measures teach is how to hit, shame and isolate—and those are not behaviors we want children to acquire. We cannot teach them to be decent unless we are decent. But we cannot help feeling frustrated or making strong demands sometimes. Children cannot help acting childish and unruly. What do we do? We stop forbidden behavior, all the while striving to accept children's feelings as being utterly real to them. For example: Richard hits Don over a coveted toy car. The teacher kneels down, Richard at one side, Don at the other. He takes Richard's hand, looks intently at him. "Richard, I know how you feel, but I can't let you hit Don like that. You must explain to him what's bothering you. Don, listen. Richard needs to tell you what's the matter." Open fights teachers must stop with physical force, sometimes stepping into the midst of it, sometimes removing one child bodily. Some people think that children should "fight it out". Sometimes this approach works and staying clear of the fight helps the fighters to clear the air by themselves and emerge with new understanding and mastery of their dispute. Usually, however, ample justification exists for stopping injury and aggression, stating the rules, and then teaching the children a better way to get what they want.

Words are better than blows in an argument. Words explicitly convey a person's resentment or rage. They let the other person know what the matter is in a way that blows do not. Of course, it takes children more time to formulate their emotions into words than it does to use force. Being primitive and quick, children naturally resort to blows. Indeed, many learn in their neighborhoods and at home to protect and even entertain themselves with aggression. School, on the other hand, is an environment established by society for symbolic learning, so within school walls, at least, children should find that words work better than force. The hope is, that by developing language skills, children will be able to control themselves—by talking and listening—even in the heat of anger and will progress from combativeness to insight and fair play.

Children are not born conciliators and teaching them to discuss their differences is a legitimate part of the curriculum: "Jane, you don't have to hit Brian and grab from him. You should tell him what you want. You just took it away from him, and he doesn't like that. Maybe Brian would be willing to give it to you if you ask him. Maybe not. But I won't let you just pull things away from people and hurt them. I won't let people do that to you, either." Because the teacher has not disgraced or punished Jane, she might accept the intervention without resentment. (Adults also find it difficult to comprehend a principle when they are seething with hurt feelings, or overwhelmed by guilt and disappointment in themselves.)

Sometimes it helps in these confrontations to skip the rules and admonitions for the moment and change the subject. If children are too tense to listen, the teacher can ease the situation by diverting the children's attention. After faces and bodies have relaxed, a discussion of the misbehavior will have more impact.

Sometimes teachers have to physically catch a child who is misbehaving. It is important to accomplish this action without scolding or seeming upset oneself. Having picked up the unruly child the teacher settles him or her in a comfortable spot. Once the child is quiet and calm, the teacher can explain the regulations. A light touch may help to restore the child's feelings of adequacy and faith in the teacher's affection. The following illustration suggests how effective this technique can be:

> Percy runs to the end of the playroom and tries to open the door to the kitchen. His teacher hurries over, grabs the doorknob, and says she cannot let him leave the playroom. He yells and tugs at the door. When she picks him up, he kicks and cries. Carrying him to the side of the room, the teacher sets him down. He angrily picks up a toy camera and brandishes it at her. In response, she asks him about the camera, makes a humorous remark about it, and smiles at him. Gradually Percy relaxes, puts the camera down, and walks with her to another activity.

Situations like this one do not always work out so nicely, however.

The incident actually happened that way, but it might have gone as follows:

> Percy tries to leave as described. The teacher removes him to the side of the room. Not only does he brandish the camera, but he also swings it at her. After taking the camera from him, she says she will not let him hit her no matter how upset he feels. She picks him up again, takes him firmly to a table or workbench activity, and works with him until he has forgotten his rage and become involved in his task. The teacher knows that coping successfully with a task will help set him straight. Percy knows that the teacher is still his friend in spite of the incident.

This kind of action is firm but not harsh. Rigid disciplinarians who never compromise, never forgive, never soften, never really care about understanding or humor or the childishness of children do not belong in the classroom. But harsh teachers may not recognize themselves as being too severe. Indeed, they often take pride in always being obeyed and never having to say things more than once. They never admit mistakes. These are the teachers who can make children stand in line without talking or shoving and who can get instant silence by calling for it or, for that matter, by looking at a child in a certain way. The memory of their "effectiveness" makes them smile, for they believe strict obedience has the utmost importance.

Proof of effective discipline, however, requires much more than the ability to make children stand in line or be silent. At least two questions beg for consideration: (1) Are these same children able to think for themselves and discipline themselves when their teachers are not there—on the playground, for example, or when the teacher is absent or in another part of the room and (2) do these children have a deep sense of self-respect and a growing ability to express their ideas verbally?

Harsh discipline ruins the preschool program. It harms young children. Confused, frightened, or humiliated by harsh teachers, they cannot learn. On the other hand, teachers who "lay down the law" as friends can reach an understanding with children. They can maintain order and control without being harsh.

Sympathy and understanding do not mean that "anything goes," however. Teachers should not be lax or overly permissive. Passivity and indecisiveness only lead to disorder and chaos. For example:

> Sixteen five-year-old children are having juice and crackers at the table with two teachers. One of the youngsters asks about a toy on a nearby table. One of the teachers, thinking he should respond to curiosity, gets up from the table, picks up the toy and holds it up in front of the children. All of them jump out of their seats knocking over chairs and chattering. As they crowd around the teacher, he tries to talk to them about the toy. While he holds it high in the air for all to see, the children clamor for it; after all, it is on display. Confusion follows. To quiet the group, the teacher tells them to finish their snack and then they will hear a story. One child asks to hear a favorite

record instead. Frazzled, the teacher agrees. A few children gather to listen. Others, confused, go to the usual story corner; no teacher is there. They mill around and a fight erupts.

This illustration of weak teaching by a truly earnest and hard-working person speaks of lack of conviction or experience. If it is time for a snack, then everyone snacks. The promise of a story requires fulfilling the promise. In other words, a failure to feel—and be—in charge means an unhappy teacher and unruly behavior, for which children themselves feel guilty or might be blamed. Meeting children's needs does not require that the teacher accedes instantly to each child's wish. Teachers respect feelings but need to squelch forbidden behavior. They are firm but friendly, not harsh or punishing nor lax and hesitant. Good teachers prepare for all children, not just the shy or volatile ones. They think not only about Tom or Sue or Helen or Charles, but about all the other children as well. Watching each face, noting each walk, listening to each voice, observing and pondering each nuance is how good discipline starts. It never ends.

In summary, elementary teachers can positively facilitate children's mental health through caring and loving them, firmly administering discipline, developing a proper emotional atmosphere in the classroom, and generally being consistent. Teachers who learn to design and teach a success-oriented curriculum and who praise the students for their success can effectively promote positive mental health.

NOTES

1. Walter D. Sorochan and Stephen J. Bender, *Teaching Elementary Health Science* (Reading, Mass.: Addison-Wesley Publishing Co., 1975), p. 93.
2. American School Health Association, "Report of the Committee on Mental Health in the Classroom," *Journal of School Health* 38 (May 1968): chap. 5a.
3. Abraham H. Maslow, *Toward a Psychology of Being,* 2d ed. (Princeton, N.J.: D. Van Nostrand, 1968), p. 97.
4. William Glasser, *Reality Therapy* (New York: Harper and Row, Publishers, 1965), p. 100.
5. Listing of behavior characteristics, pp. 283–284 (after pp. 16–17, *Resource Guide: Mental Health, Personality Growth, and Adjustment,* Minneapolis Public Schools, 1954) from *Mental Health and Human Relations in Education* by Louis Kaplan. Copyright © 1959 by Louis Kaplan. Reprinted by permission of Harper & Row, Publishers, Inc.
6. Robert H. Felix, cited in Jeanette Galambus, *Discipline and Self-control,* (Washington, D.C.: U.S. Department of Health, Education, and Welfare, n.d.), p. 81.

7. Gere B. Fulton and William V. Fassbender, *Health Education in the Elementary School* (Pacific Palisades, Calif.: Goodyear Publishing Co., 1972), p. 56.
8. Katherine E. Evelyn, *Developing Mentally Healthy Children* (Washington, D.C.: EKNE, 1970), p. 8.
9. Carrine Bidwell, "The Teacher as a Listener—an Approach to Mental Health," *Journal of School Health* 37 (October 1967): 373-83.
10. Ibid., p. 82.
11. Charlotte Haupt, cited in Fulton and Fassbender, p. 54.
12. Bidwell, p. 82.
13. Reprinted from Galumbus.

RESOURCES

Review all materials and preview all films.

Books

Arthur Alexander. *Hidden You*. New York: Prentice-Hall, 1962.
W.W. Bauer. *Moving into Manhood*. Garden City, N.Y.: Doubleday, 1963.
Jerrold Beim. *Laugh and Cry: Your Emotions and How They Work*. New York: William Morrow and Co.: 1955.
June Callwood. *Love, Hate, Fear, Other Emotions*. Garden City, N.Y.: Doubleday, 1964.
Rudolf Driekur. *Discipline Without Tears*. New York: Hawthorn Books, 1974.
Louis Dublin. *Suicide: A Sociological and Statistical Study*. New York: Ronald Press, 1963.
Ruth Fedder. *A Girl Grows Up*. New York: McGraw-Hill Book Co., 1957.
Ruth Fedder. *You, the Person You Want to Be*. New York: McGraw-Hill Book Co., 1957.
Sigmund Freud. *Psychopathology of Everyday Life*. New York: New American Library, 1951.
William Glasser. *Schools Without Failure*. New York: Harper and Row, Publishers, 1969.
Robert Goldenson. *All About the Human Mind: An Introduction to Psychology for Young People*. New York: Random House, 1963.
Mike Gorman. *Every Other Bed*. New York: Random House, 1963.
Vernon Grant. *This Is Mental Illness*. Boston: Beacon Press: 1963.
Arthur Gregor. *Time Out for Youth*. New York: Macmillan Co., 1965.
Eric Johnson. *How to Live Through Junior High School*. Philadelphia: J.B. Lippincott, 1975.
C.G. Jung. *The Undiscovered Self*. New York: New American Library, 1959.
Robert Loeb. *Manners for Minors*. New York: Associated Press, 1964.
Maxwell Maltz. *My Book of Secrets*. Texas: Goals Inc., 1975.
Karl Menninger. *Blueprint for Teenage Living*. New York: Sterling Books, 1958.
Karl Menninger. *Man Against Himself*. New York: Harcourt, Brace, 1938.
Diane E. Papalia and Sally Wendkos Olds. *A Child's World*. New York: McGraw-Hill Book Co., 1974.

John Powell. *Why Am I Afraid to Tell You Who I Am?* Chicago: Argus Communications, 1969.

Eleanor Roosevelt. *You Learn by Living.* New York: Harper and Row, Publishers, 1960.

Jerome H. Rothstein. *Mental Retardation.* New York: Holt Rinehart and Winston, 1961.

Noah Smaridge. *Looking at You.* Nashville, Tenn.: Abington, 1962.

Herbert Sorenson. *Psychology for Living.* New York: McGraw-Hill Book Co.,
1957.

Edward Strecker and Kenneth Appel. *Discovering Ourselves.* New York: Macmillan Co., 1957.

Readings for Children

Claire Bishop and Kurt Weise. *The Five Chinese Brothers.* New York: Coward-
McCann, 1938.

L. Dean Carper. *A Cry in the Wind.* (4-6)

Marguerite DeAngeli. *The Door in the Wall: Story of Medieval London.* New
York: Doubleday, n.d. (3-5)

Antoine de St. Exupery. *The Little Prince.* New York: Harcourt, Brace, and
World, 1971.

Don Dinkmeyer. *Manual: Developing and Understanding Self and Others.*
Circle Pines: American Guidance Service, 1970.

Paula Fox. Portrait of Ivan and the Stone. (5-6)

Laura French. "Getting It Together." In Fat Albert and the Cosby Kids, Racine,
Wis.: Western Publishing Co., 1975.

Irene Hunt. *Up a Road Slowly.* Chicago: Follett Publishing Co., 1966 (girls
6-10)

Lee Kingman. *The Year of the Racoon.* Boston: Houghton-Mifflin, 1966. (6-7).

Vladmir Koziakin. *Mazes for Fun Book 2.* New York: Grosset and Dunlap,
1973.

Ann E. Neimark. *Touch of Light: The Story of Louis Braille.* New York: Harcourt Brace and World, 1970. (3-6).

Margery Williams. *The Velveteen Rabbit.* New York: Avon Books, 1975.

Magazines

Public Health
Mental Health Association Quarterly

Pamphlets

Available from National Association of Mental Health, 1800 N. Kent St.,
Arlington, Va. 22209.
Growing Up Ain't That Easy
How to Deal with Your Tensions

Child Alone in Need of Help
Facts About Mental Health
Facts About Mental Illness
When Things Go Wrong
Mental Illness Can Be Prevented
Obsessive Children

Government Resource Materials

National Institute of Mental Health, *It's Good to Know About Mental Health.* For sale by: Superintendent of Documents, U.S. Government Printing Office, Washington, D.C. 20402, Stock #017-027-00337-9, Cat. #H.E. 20.3802: k 76. Price $.40.

About Mental Health, a 1976 scriptographic booklet by Channing L. Bete Co., Inc., Greenfield, Mass., #1109J-1-73.

Schizophrenia, Is There an Answer?, National Institute of Mental Health, OHEW Publication #(HSM) 73-9086, Revised 1974 (ADM) 74-24.

Alcohol, Drug Abuse and Mental Health Administration, 5600 Fishers Lane, Rockville, Md. 29852.

Stress—and Your Health. Available from: (1) Child Study Association of America—Wel-Met, Inc., 50 Madison Ave., New York, N.Y. 10003; (2) Family Service Association of America, 44 East 23rd Street, New York, N.Y. 10010; (3) Mental Health Materials Center, Inc., 419 Park Avenue South, New York, N.Y. 10016; (4) National Association for Mental Health, 1800 North Kent Street, Arlington, Va. 22209.

Health Education Texts

"Harlow Studies," Science Research Associates, Chicago, Ill.

Mental Health for Teachers and Pupils, U.S. Department of Health, Education and Welfare.

Justus J. Schifferes. *Healthier Living.* New York: John Wiley and Sons 1965.

National Association for Mental Health, Inc., Pamphlets.

C. Bauer and G.G. Jenkins, *The New Health and Safety,* Fairlawn, N.J.: Scott-Foresman, 1966.

Irwin, Cornacchia, Staton, *Health in Elementary Schools,* St. Louis: C.V. Mosby Co., 1974.

Films

Beginning Responsibilities, Coronet. (1) "Taking Care of Things" (2) "Other People's Things" (3) "Doing Things for Ourselves" (4) "Rules at School"
Your Study Methods, Coronet
Understanding Your Emotions, Coronet

Beginnings of Conscience, McGraw-Hill
High Wall, McGraw-Hill
Cipher in the Snow, Brigham Young University
Common Fallacies About Group Differences, McGraw-Hill
Everybody's Prejudices, McGraw-Hill
Stress, McGraw-Hill
Emotional Maturity, McGraw-Hill
Your Junior High Days, McGraw-Hill
Emotional Health, McGraw-Hill
Breakdown, McGraw-Hill
How to Succeed in School, McGraw-Hill
How to Take a Test, McGraw-Hill
Cheating, McGraw-Hill
Johnny Lingo, Brigham Young University
The Good Loser, McGraw-Hill
The Gossip, McGraw-Hill
The Hangman.
The Other Fellow's Feelings, McGraw-Hill
Outsider, McGraw-Hill
The Show Off, McGraw-Hill
Trouble Maker, McGraw-Hill
Understanding Other, McGraw-Hill
What About Prejudice, McGraw-Hill
Heredity and Family Environment, McGraw-Hill
Islam, McGraw-Hill
Age of Turmoil, McGraw-Hill
Home for Life, Drexel Home
Dialogue with the World Film Program, Films Incorporated
Mental Retardation Film List, Division of Mental Retardation, Social and
     Rehabilitation Service
Child Behind the Wall, Smith, Kline and French
Toymakers, Smith, Kline and French
Mirror, Mirror, Brigham Young University
Mr. Finlay's Feelings, Metropolitan Life Insurance Co.
The Time of Growing, Metropolitan Life Insurance Co.
The Last Leaf, Teaching Film Custodians
The Stratton Story, Teaching Film Custodians
Adolescence, National Film Board of Canada
Howard, National Film Board of Canada
Who Is Sylvia? National Film Board of Canada
Ages and Stages, National Film Board of Canada
He Acts His Age, National Film Board of Canada
From Sociable Six to Noisy Nine, National Film Board of Canada
From Ten to Twelve, National Film Board of Canada
The Teens, National Film Board of Canada
Growing Up—Preadolescence, Coronet
What About that Upset Feeling? (Primary) Coronet
Ways to Good Habits, (Primary) Coronet
The Key, National Association for Mental Health

Transparencies

School Health Education Study, 3M Company
The Use and Misuse of Drugs, FDA's Life Protection Series, DCA Educational
    Products

Sources of Free and Inexpensive Materials

Epilepsy Association
Public Affairs Committee, Inc.
Science Research Associates
National Education Association
Institute of Human Relations
National Association for Mental Health, Inc.
National Association for Retarded Children
U.S. Department of Human Resources
Metropolitan Life Insurance Co.
Mental Health Materials Center, Inc.

CHAPTER 6
Child Abuse*

Next to the family, the school is generally considered the most important influence on a child's life. The function of the school obviously goes beyond teaching children to read and add and memorize historical facts. In cases in which the family unit fails to protect a child or itself threatens the child's welfare, schools can play an invaluable role in saving or salvaging a life.

Before examining the role of the teacher and the school in relationship to child abuse and neglect we need to clearly understand the nature and incidence of the problem. The legal definition of child abuse and neglect is "the physical or mental injury, sexual abuse, negligent treatment, or maltreatment of a child under the age of eighteen by a person who is responsible for the child's welfare under circumstances which indicate that the child's health or welfare is harmed or threatened thereby."[1]

INCIDENCE

An estimated minimum of 700 children are killed by their parents or parent surrogates in the United States each year, approximately

---

*This chapter is adapted from *Child Abuse and Neglect—The Problem and Its Management*, vols. 1 and 2, available from the National Center on Child Abuse and Neglect, Publication No. (OHD) 75-30074.

10,000 children are severely battered, between 50,000 and 75,000 are sexually abused, and 200,000–500,000 are emotionally, physically, or morally neglected.[2] It has been suggested that for every case of child abuse that is reported, four go unreported. Of the more than 10,000 cases of battered child syndrome reported each year in this country, 50 percent involve children less than five years of age, 75 percent involve children less than ten years of age, 33 percent require hospital treatment, and up to 3 percent are dead on arrival at the hospital.

While the most severe cases of physical injury resulting from abuse or neglect tend to involve preschool children, particularly infants, the incidence of maltreatment among children aged five to eighteen is significant. Dr. C. George Murdock noted that, according to some surveys, children of school age are involved in only 20 to 30 percent of abuse cases.[3] Dr. David Gil, on the other hand, estimated that this age group accounts for about half of all incidents of physical abuse.[4] Based on estimates by school personnel, one survey concluded that 40 of every 100,000 school-age children are physically abused each year.[5] If this estimate is correct, more than 20,000 children between the ages of five and eighteen are abused annually.

The incidence of child abuse and neglect is difficult to ascertain, but there are indications of underreporting, particularly involving school-age children. Since preschool children are prone to more serious physical injury, they are more likely than older children to be taken to a doctor or hospital that will report the case. Physical signs of maltreatment may be covered by clothing. If bruises, welts, or other injuries are visible, the child may be kept from school until the "evidence" fades or the child may lie about the injury for fear of punishment.[6]

In the area of identification, teachers are laymen untrained to draw on medical or social work techniques to identify child maltreatment. Reading X-rays and diagnosing the pathology of the family are obviously beyond the teacher's professional scope. But because of their close daily contact with children in a setting that allows them to observe children, teachers are in a unique position to identify, report, and offer direct help to maltreated children and their families.

CHARACTERISTICS OF ABUSE AND NEGLECT

Recognizing a child's need for protection is obviously more important than determining the form of maltreatment involved. In confronting a possible case of child maltreatment, the operational problem is not how to classify it, but whether or not to report it. Unfortunately, many people who might report are not acquainted

child's family. Some 90 percent of the victims are girls, ranging in age from infancy through adolescence.

Since the sexually abused child lacks the telltale symptoms of battering, sexual abuse is difficult to identify and even harder to prove. Short of the child telling someone, the best indicators are a sudden change in behavior and signs of emotional disturbance. The child, for example, may unexplainably begin to cry easily and seem excessively nervous. Dr. Vincent De Francis reported that two-thirds of the children detected in a three-year study of sexual abuse in New York City displayed some degree of emotional disturbance.[7]

Behavioral indicators of possible sexual molestation include:[8]

1. Unwillingness to participate in physical activities: Young children who have had forced sexual intercourse may find it painful to sit during school or to play active games.
2. Indirect allusion: Sometimes sexually abused children will confide in teachers with whom they have a good rapport and who they feel may be helpful. The confidences may be veiled and vague but allude to a home situation, as does the statement "I'm going to find a foster home to live in" or "I'd like to live with you" or "I'm afraid to go home tonight."
3. Regression: Some sexually abused children, especially young children, will retreat into a fantasy world or revert to infantile behaviors.
4. Aggression and/or delinquency: The anger, hostility, and fear of the consequences of sexual abuse, especially in adolescents, may prompt delinquent, hostile, and/or aggressive behavior toward both people and property.
5. Status offenses: Children may run away from home to escape a situation over which they feel they have no control. The runaway child is asking for help and/or acting out hostile and aggressive behaviors, as previously noted.
6. Poor peer relationships: Isolation may follow feelings of guilt or serious emotional problems. Children seem unable to form stable and continuing relationships with others of their own age group.
7. Seductive behaviors: If children identify sexual contact as positive reinforcement for attention, they may adopt seductive behaviors with both peers and adults.
8. Drug use/abuse: Use of alcohol and/or drugs may represent a way of handling guilt and anxiety about having been sexually abused or perpetrating sexual abuse upon younger children.

Physical Neglect

Dr. Abraham Levine notes that, to some extent, neglect "defies exact definition, but it may be regarded as the failure to provide the essentials for normal life, such as food, clothing, shelter, care and supervision, and protection from assault."[9] Physically neglected children tend to exhibit at least several of the following characteristics:

1. They are often hungry. They may go without breakfast and have neither food nor money for lunch. Some take lunch money or food from other children and hoard whatever they obtain.
2. They show signs of malnutrition—paleness, low weight relative to height, lack of body tone, fatigue, inability to participate in physical activities, and lack of normal strength and endurance.
3. They are usually irritable.
4. They show evidence of inadequate home management. They are unclean and unkempt, their clothes are torn and dirty, and they are often unbathed. As mentioned earlier, they may lack proper clothing for weather conditions and their school attendance may be irregular. In addition, these children may frequently be ill and may exhibit a generally repressed personality, inattentiveness, and withdrawal.
5. They are in obvious need of medical attention for such correctable conditions as poor eyesight, dental care, and immunization.
6. They lack parental supervision at home. For example, they may frequently return from school to an empty house. While the need for adult supervision is relative, of course, to both the situation and the maturity of the child, generally a child younger than twelve should always have adult supervision or at least have immediate access to a concerned adult.
7. Their parents are either unable or unwilling to provide appropriate care. Some neglecting parents are mentally deficient; most lack knowledge of parenting skills and tend to be discouraged, depressed, and frustrated with their role as parents.

Emotional Abuse or Neglect

Emotional abuse or neglect is far more difficult to identify than its physical counterparts. Such maltreatment includes the "parent's lack of love and proper direction, inability to accept a child with his potentialities as well as his limitation . . . [and] failure to encourage the child's normal development by assurance of love and acceptance."[10] The parents of an emotionally abused or neglected child may be overly harsh and critical and demand excessive academic, athletic, or social performance. Conversely, they may withhold physical and verbal contact, care little about the child's successes and failures, and fail to provide necessary guidance and praise. Though emotional maltreatment may occur alone, it is almost always present in cases of physical abuse or neglect. Often the emotional damage to children who are physically abused or whose basic physical needs are unattended is more serious than the bodily damage.

The indicators of emotional maltreatment are often intangible, but sooner or later the consequences become evident. The child may be either "hyperaggressive, disrupting, and demanding . . . shouting his cry for help" or "withdrawn . . . whispering his cry for help."[11] In a class of psychologically healthy children, the emotionally abused child often stands out unmistakably. Emotional maltreatment has a decidedly adverse effect on a child's learning ability, achievement level, and general development. The strongest indicators are unaccountable learning difficulties and changes or unusual behavior patterns.

The parents of an abused or neglected child may exhibit any of the following traits:

1. They are isolated from family supports such as friends, relatives, neighbors, and community groups. They consistently fail to keep appointments, discourage social contact, and never participate in school activities or events.
2. They seem to trust no one.
3. They are reluctant to give information about the seriousness of their child's condition or injuries. When questioned, they are unable to explain, or they offer farfetched or contradictory explanations.
4. They respond inappropriately to the seriousness of the child's condition: either by overreacting, seeming hostile, or antagonistic when questioned even casually or by underreacting, showing little concern or awareness, and seeming more preoccupied with their own problems than those of the child.
5. They refuse to consent to diagnostic studies.
6. They fail to take the child for medical care (routine checkups, optometric or dental care, treatment of injury or illness) or they delay doing so. In taking an injured child for medical care, they may choose a different hospital or doctor each time.
7. They are overcritical of the child and seldom, if ever, discuss the child in positive terms.
8. They have unrealistic expectations of the child. They expect or demand behavior that is beyond the child's years or ability.
9. They believe that harsh punishment is necessary for children.
10. They seldom touch or look at the child, and they ignore the child's crying or react with impatience.
11. They confine the child—perhaps in a crib or playpen—for long periods of time.
12. They seem to lack understanding of children's physical, emotional, and psychological needs.
13. They appear to be misusing alcohol or drugs.

14. They cannot be located.
15. They appear to lack control or to fear losing control.
16. They are of borderline intelligence, psychotic, or psychopathic. While diagnosis is the responsibility of psychiatrists, psychologists, or psychiatric social workers, even the lay observer can detect whether a parent seems intellectually capable of child rearing, exhibits generally irrational behavior, or seems excessively cruel and sadistic.

THE ROLE OF THE TEACHER

Because of their daily contact with children, teachers sometimes cannot avoid wondering about their home lives. Perhaps one child continually has minor, untreated bruises, scrapes, and cuts or always seems hungry but never brings lunch or has the money to buy it. Disturbing as physical or emotional conditions that suggest poor parental care are, some teachers feel that these situations are outside their professional responsibilities. Others feel that calling attention to suspected problems is futile or will only create trouble for the child or themselves. But a teacher's responsibilities include concern for and involvement in any situation that gives reason to suspect child abuse or neglect. In fact, thirty-two states require teachers and other school personnel to report suspected cases of abuse and neglect. Nine other states, which do not specifically designate teachers and school personnel as mandated reporters, require "any person" to report. The laws of most other states either encourage or permit teachers, as private citizens, to report suspected child maltreatment.

In order to help children and families, teachers need the confidence of knowing that their observations are valid. They need a working definition of abuse and neglect, an understanding of the incidence and nature of the problem, and a knowledge of the characteristics and behavior that maltreated children and parents may display. They should also be familiar with their state's reporting law, particularly its definition of reportable conditions, the specified reporting procedure, and their obligations and legal protections in regard to reporting.

Most child abuse laws require a report when there is "reasonable cause to believe" or "to suspect" that a child is abused or neglected. Of course, there are degrees of suspicion. In cases of suspected violent physical abuse, when a child needs medical attention or possibly risks further abuse upon returning home, an immediate report is necessary. In such cases, teachers should not contact the parents about the child's condition. School officials sometimes assume that they can prevent further abuse by calling the parents and warning them that the school will report further mistreatment.

This measure not only fails to help the child or the parents, but also can place the child at greater risk for reabuse.

In marginal cases, a teacher's suspicions may build over weeks or months before there is reason to report. In these cases, a call to the home or a request to see the parents may help to reinforce or dispel the teacher's suspicions. There may be an entirely reasonable explanation for the child's appearance or behavior, such as a temporary family crisis that does not indicate a need to report or a need for services. In many familes, for example, a week-long hospitalization of the mother can result in a short-term breakdown of normal family functions. Moreover, it may be unfair to the family for the school to report questionable conditions, such as improper clothing or inadequate supervision, observed over a period of months or even years if the school has never expressed concern about the conditions to the parents.

A school psychologist or social worker can advise teachers if they suspect abuse or neglect. A teacher's proper professional stance, in terms of both the child and the family, is one of objectivity. For example, a teacher who questions a child about his or her condition should avoid probing or making the child uncomfortable. A psychologist or social worker is professionally within bounds to move closer to the situation and has the training to deal with hostile or defensive parents. But it is important to bear in mind that someone who is not in daily contact with the child may not have as much concern as the teacher about the child's condition. Therefore teachers should not feel that their responsibility ends when another staff member enters the case. They should make certain that appropriate action occurs, whether it be to report the case or to see that the family receives needed services.

Even if a report is not indicated or is subsequently invalidated, the teacher may be able to help the family gain access to services if needed. The school itself may have the resources to help parents with particular child-rearing problems. A teacher who is aware of the social and psychological services that are available may be able to help parents draw on the ones that would best foster understanding of the child's needs.

Professionals in the field of child protection offer the following guidelines to teachers:

1. You should be aware of the official policy and specific reporting procedures of your school system and know your legal obligations and the protections from civil and criminal liability specified in your state's reporting law. (All states provide immunity for mandated, good-faith reports.)
2. Although you should be familiar with your state's legal definition of abuse and neglect, you are not required to make legal distinc-

tions in order to report. Definitions should serve as a guide. If you suspect that a child is abused or neglected, you should report. The teacher's value lies in noticing conditions that indicate that a child's welfare may be in jeopardy.

3. Be concerned about children's rights (the right to life, food, shelter, clothing, and security), but also be aware of parents' rights, particularly their right to respectful treatment and to help and support.

4. Bear in mind that reporting does not stigmatize a parent as "evil." The report is the start of a rehabilitative process that seeks to protect the child and to help the family as a whole.

5. A report signifies only the *suspicion* of abuse or neglect. Teachers' reports are seldom unfounded. At the very least, they tend to indicate that a family needs help and support.

6. If you report a borderline case in good faith, do not feel guilty or upset if authorities dismiss it after investigation. Some marginal cases are found to be valid.

7. Do not put off making a report until the end of the school year. Teachers sometimes live with their suspicions while school is in session and suddenly fear for a child's safety during the summer months. A delayed report may mean delaying help for the child and the family. Moreover, reporting late in the school year will prevent you from giving continued support to both the child protective agency and the reported family.

8. If you remove yourself from a case of suspected abuse or neglect by passing it on to superiors, you deprive child protective services of one of their most competent sources of information. For example, a teacher who tells a CPS worker of a child who is especially upset on Mondays indicates that conditions in the home may be intolerable on weekends. Few persons other than teachers are able to provide this kind of information. Your guideline should be to resolve any question in favor of the child. When in doubt, report. Even if you, as a teacher, have no immunity from liability and prosecution under state law, the fact that your report is made in good faith will free you from liability and prosecution.

After filing a report, the teacher should continue to feel responsible for ensuring that the family gets help. If the child protective agency (or whatever agency investigates reports) does not provide feedback on the results of their investigation, the teacher should inquire whether the agency has investigated and whether the family is receiving help. Although many agencies refuse such requests on the grounds of confidentiality, the teacher should receive relevant information and advice, particularly if the child needs special care in the classroom.

In the absence of guidance from the protective agency, the teacher can rely on several general rules for dealing with the abused or neglected child:

1. Try to give the child additional attention.
2. Create an individualized program for the child. Lower your academic expectations and make fewer demands on the child's performance; he or she probably has enough pressures and crises to deal with at home.
3. Be warm and loving. If possible, let the child perceive you as a special friend in whom to confide. By abusing or neglecting the child, someone has said in a physical way, "I don't love you." You can reassure the child that someone cares.
4. Most important, remember that in identifying and reporting child maltreatment, you are not putting yourself in the position of autocrat over a family. The one purpose of your actions is to get help for a troubled child and family and to reverse a situation that jeopardizes a child's healthy growth and development.

In order to provide meaningful help to children and parents, teachers should be familiar with the types and quality of services in the community. They should know, for example, whether the protective service agency has sufficient staff to handle its caseload, whether appropriate diagnostic and treatment resources are available, and whether there are services for borderline as well as severe cases of abuse and neglect.

Although the individual teacher is not likely to be able to effect local changes, teachers working together often have considerable influence in the community. For example, to facilitate interagency coordination, the local teachers' organization could meet with social service representatives for the stated purpose of working together on mutual problems. They could develop a reporting procedure for the school that is suitable for both groups, discuss methods of providing feedback on reports, and establish general guidelines for teachers to use in dealing with the child in foster care, the child whose parents are in treatment, and children who have other special needs. In addition, the process of meeting can facilitate more personal working relationships. The protective service worker and the teacher who have participated in such a group are more likely to consult one another concerning the specific needs of individual children than are complete strangers.

There are various other ways teachers can help improve their community's system of managing cases of child abuse and neglect. But the classroom is where teachers play their most important role. Individual teachers should try to serve as examples for their students. The teacher-student relationship is only one model of adult-child relationships, but it can have lasting effects. Teachers who show honest respect for children by treating them with dignity, helping them with their problems, and showing appreciation of their successes present an example of adult behavior that they may duplicate with their own children.

THE ROLE OF THE SCHOOL

Perhaps the most basic responsibility of every school system is to have a policy and procedure for reporting child mistreatment. The school's policy should be more than a restatement of the state law. It should include clearly stated and detailed guidelines, including what, when, how and to whom to report. It should also include provisions for regular in-service training for all school personnel. School officials should make certain that the policies of the school are consistent with the policies of other community agencies in regard to the duties of each agency, the telephone number(s) for reporting, the type of information to report, and so on. If state law requires that reports be made in writing, reporting forms should be available in the school office. School administrators should also obtain legal consultation as to whether school personnel have immunity when they report.

Whatever the policies and procedures of the local school system, education of school personnel should be a top priority. The school should inform teachers and other staff members of the school's policy regarding child abuse and neglect and the provisions of the state's reporting law. Pupil personnel staff or social workers can conduct regular in-service courses to train the staffs of public, private, and parochial schools about the identification of abuse and neglect, the importance of reporting suspected cases, the local reporting procedure, the role of each community agency involved in case management, and the ways in which school personnel can help maltreated children and their families.

Thirty-two states currently mandate that schools and/or school personnel report suspected cases of child abuse and neglect. The balance of the statutes require either personnel serving in specified institutions or "any person" suspecting child abuse and neglect to report. Only Oklahoma makes no statutory guarantees of immunity from civil and criminal liability for those who report in good faith. However, in Maryland there is no immunity from civil suits for untrue statements made by one citizen against another.

In spite of the widespread existence of child-abuse and neglect reporting laws, few schools have established policies and procedures under which the employees of the school shall report.[12] Even though this number of schools is rapidly increasing, in only 17 percent of the states have state school boards established uniform reporting procedures.[13]

According to the Education Commission of the States,[14] 84 percent of the state departments of education, 56 percent of the largest school districts in each state, 71 percent of the smallest school districts in each state, and 90 percent of the largest private schools in each state have no policies regarding the reporting of child abuse and neglect.

On the surface, the data suggest that state and local boards of education and trustees of private schools have been relatively inactive or disinterested in the problem of child abuse and neglect. Nevertheless, it is true that no social reform has ever swept the country as rapidly as state and national legislative reform regarding child abuse and neglect, so it is unlikely that the data reported by the Education Commission of the States is still accurate. Since their report came out, in April 1976, two states (Nevada and Utah) have adopted statewide policies regarding the reporting of child abuse, and an increasing number of local and state school boards have adopted policies and procedures of their own volition.

Since a policy regarding child abuse and neglect is a commitment by the school (or other education group) to cooperate with other agencies, staffed by other professional personnel, in the identification, treatment, and prevention of this phenomenon, anything less than 100 percent is unacceptable. The guidelines that follow are practical suggestions to help education policy makers develop and implement policies suitable to their particular circumstances and state laws. They are the product of a task force of the Education Commission of the States' Child Abuse and Neglect Project. Some general suggestions regarding school policies and procedures for reporting child abuse and neglect are:

1. Since all states require or encourage school personnel to report suspected cases, every school system should adopt and issue to all school personnel and the constituents of the district a child abuse and neglect policy, particularly a policy on reporting.
2. The adopted policy should inform school personnel of their legal and professional obligations regarding child abuse and neglect.
3. The policy should inform all school personnel of immunities from civil and criminal liability provided in state laws when the report is made in good faith.
4. The policy should provide for periodic in-service education designed to assist school personnel in the identification of suspected cases of child abuse and neglect.[15]

Table 6-1 shows the critical elements of any school reporting policy and sample wording for each critical element.

The simple process of articulating a clear position on child abuse

TABLE 6–1. Critical Elements of School Policy on Reporting Child Abuse and Neglect

Elements to Be Cited	Sample Wording
1. A brief rationale for involving school personnel in reporting.	Because of their sustained contact with school-age children, school employees are in an excellent position to identify abused or neglected children and to refer them for treatment and protection.
2. The name and appropriate section numbers of the state reporting statute.	To comply with the Mandatory Reporting of Child Abuse Act (Section 350–1 through 350–5) Hawaii Revised Statutes (1968), as amended (Supp. 1975), . . .
3. Who specifically is mandated to report and (if applicable) who may report.	. . . it is the policy of the ____ School District that any teacher or other school employee. . .
4. Reportable conditions as defined by state law.	. . . who suspects that a child's physical or mental health or welfare may be adversely affected by abuse or neglect. . .
5. The person or agency to receive reports.	. . . shall report to the department of social services. . . OR . . . shall report to the principal, who shall then call the department of social services. . .
6. The information required of the reporter.	. . . and give the following information: name, address and age of student; name and address of parent or caretaker; nature and extent of injuries or description of neglect; any other information that might help establish the cause of the injuries or condition. School employees shall not contact the child's family or any other persons to determine the cause of the suspected abuse or neglect. It is not the responsibility of the school employee to prove that the child has been abused or neglected, or to determine whether the child is in need of protection.
7. Expected professional conduct by school employees.	Any personal interview or physical inspection of the child should be conducted in a professional manner. . .

(continued)

TABLE 6–1 (Continued)

Elements to Be Cited	Sample Wording
8. The exact language of the law to define "abuse" and "neglect"; if necessary, explain, clarify, or expand.	"Abuse" means the infliction by other than accidental means, of physical harm upon the body of a child. "Neglect" means the failure to provide necessary food, care, clothing, shelter, or medical attention for a child.
9. The method by which school personnel are to report (if appropriate, list telephone number for reporting) and the time in which to report.	An oral report must be made as soon as possible by telephone or otherwise and may be followed by a written report.
10. Whether or not there is immunity from civil liability and criminal penalty for those who report or participate in an investigation or judicial proceeding; and whether immunity is for "good faith" reporting.*	In Illinois, anyone making a report in accordance with state law or participating in a resulting judicial proceeding is presumed to be acting in good faith and, in doing so, is immune from any civil or criminal liability that might be imposed. OR In Maryland, there is no immunity from civil suits for untrue statements made by one citizen against another.
11. Penalty for failure to report, if established by state law.	Failure to report may result in a misdemeanor charge: punishment by a fine of up to $500, imprisonment up to one year or both.
12. Action taken by school board for failure to report.	Failure to report may result in disciplinary action against the employee.
13. Any provisions of the law regarding the confidentiality of records of suspected abuse or neglect.	All records concerning reports of suspected abuse or neglect are confidential. Anyone who permits, assists, or encourages the release of information from records to a person or agency not legally permitted to have access may be guilty of a misdemeanor.

*While every state provides immunity for those reporting child abuse, many do not provide immunity for reporters of child neglect. School systems in these states may be able to extend immunity to school personnel via the state public school laws. Many of these laws grant immunity to educators who act under a requirement of school law, rule or regulation. By enacting a regulation requiring school personnel to report suspected abuse and neglect, school systems can ensure full immunity to their employees who report.

Source: Reprinted from Education Commission of the States, Denver, Colo., *Child Abuse and Neglect Project—Educational Policies and Practices Regarding Child Abuse,* Report No. 85, 1976.

FIGURE 6-1. *Typical form to be completed by school personnel reporting suspected maltreatment. (Redrawn after Donald F. Kline,* Child Abuse and Neglect: A Primer for School Personnel *(Reston, Va.: Council for Exceptional Children, 1977), p. 33.)*

Child Abuse Neglect Reporting Form

Oral Report made to principal or designee: Date _____ Time _____

Child's name _____ / _____ / _____
                  Last name (legal)   First   Middle

Age _____ Birthdate _____ Sex _____

Child's address _____

Names and addresses of parents or other person(s) responsible for the child's care.

Father _____ Mother _____

Guardian or caretaker _____

Address_____ Telephone_____

Observations leading to the suspicion that the child is a victim of abuse or neglect. Supply time and date of observation(s).

Additional information. Interview with the child and name of other school employees involved.

Written report made to principal or designee: Date _____ Time _____

Signature _____ Signature _____
             Initiator of the report   Observer of the interview

---

To be filled out by the principal or designee:

Oral report made to: Written report made to:

Local City Police   ____   Local City Police   ____
County Sheriff   ____   County Sheriff   ____
Division of Family Service ____   Division of Family Services ____

Date _____ Time _____   Date _____ Time _____

Principal's signature _____

Distribute copies to: 1. Mail to agency receiving the oral report.
                         2. Mail to the district's pupil personnel office.
                         3. Place in principal's child abuse-neglect file.
                            (Not to be placed in the child's personal file.)

and neglect can go a long way toward establishing the educator's role in the multidisciplinary fight against the maltreatment of children. It can enhance the public's awareness and encourage primary prevention efforts. Certainly, a school policy regarding child abuse and neglect will encourage school employees, who have heretofore been reluctant to report suspected cases, to participate more willingly in the legal and professional obligations which they accept, not only as professionals but also as employees of an educational agency that has enunciated a clear policy on behalf of abused and neglected children.

Many educators have been concerned about violating privacy by reporting suspected cases of child abuse and neglect because of the Buckley Family Educational Rights and Privacy Act passed by Congress in 1974. This act requires schools to obtain parents' consent before sharing with a third party any information in the child's school record. The Buckley legislation excepts information that involves health or safety, however, and the Department of Health, Education, and Welfare has stated that child abuse is a matter of health and safety. Moreover, appropriate policies and procedures will exclude child abuse and neglect reports from the individual child's educational record (see Figure 6–1).

Even though most professionals are aware of the immunities provided by state statutes against civil or criminal liability, not all school personnel know that the majority of the states have enacted either civil or criminal penalties for failure to report suspected cases of child abuse and neglect. State-imposed criminal penalties range from $25 and ten days imprisonment to $1000 and one year imprisonment. Civil penalties extending the common law of negligence give any person the right to sue another person for damages resulting from negligence. If it can be established that any teacher or other professional school employee had knowledge of abuse and/or neglect and failed to report it, the child (or someone functioning in the child's behalf) could conceivably bring suit for damages.

NOTES

1. Reprinted from: Donald F. Kline, *Child Abuse and Neglect: A Primer for School Personnel* (Reston, Va.: Council for Exceptional Children, 1977), pp. 21, 26–30.
2. Frederick Green, "Child Abuse and Neglect," *Pediatric Clinics of North America,* May 1975, p. 330.
3. George C. Murdock, "The Abused Child and the School System," *American Journal of Public Health* 60 (January 1970): 105–9.
4. David G. Gil, "What Schools Can Do About Child Abuse," *American Education* 5 (April 1960): 2–4.
5. D.C. Drews, "The Child and His School," in *Helping the Battered Child and*

His Family, ed. Henry C. Kempe and Ray E. Helfer (Philadelphia: J.B. Lippincott Co., 1972), p. 117.

6. Ibid., p. 118.
7. Vincent De Francis, quoted in Herb Stoenner, *Plain Talk About Child Abuse* (Denver: American Humane Association, Childrens Division, 1972), p. 24.
8. Kline, p. 23.
9. Abraham Levine, "Child Neglect: Reaching the Parent," *The Social and Rehabilitation Record* 1 (July/August 1974): 26.
10. Henrietta Gordon, quoted in Robert M. Mulford, *Emotional Neglect of Children: A Challenge to Protective Services* (Denver: American Humane Association, Childrens Division, n.d.), p. 5.
11. Ibid.
12. Kline, p. 32.
13. Education Commission of the States, Denver, Colo., *Child Abuse and Neglect Project—Educational Policies and Practices Regarding Child Abuse,* Report No. 85, 1976.
14. Ibid.
15. Ibid.

RESOURCES

American Humane Association, Children's Division, P.O. Box 1266, Denver, Colo. 80201. (Extensive publications available.)

Child Abuse Listening Mediation (CALM), P.O. Box 718, Santa Barbara, Calif. 93102. (Volunteer program.)

Child Welfare League of America, 67 Irving Place, New York, N.Y. 10003.

Children's Bureau, Administration for Children, Youth and Families, P.O. Box 1182, Washington, D.C. 20013. (Federal agency.)

Day Care and Child Development Council of America, 1401 K Street, N.W., Washington, D.C. 20085.

National Center for the Prevention and Treatment of Child Abuse and Neglect, University of Colorado Medical Center, 1001 Jasmine Street, Denver, Colo. 80220.

National Committee for Prevention of Child Abuse, Suite 510, 111 East Wacker Drive, Chicago, Ill. 60601.

Parents Anonymous, 2801 Artesia Boulevard, Redondo Beach, Calif. 90278. (Parent self-help.)

National Center for Comprehensive Emergency Services to Children in Crisis, 320 Metro Howard Office Building, 25 Middleton Street, Nashville, Tenn. 37210.

CHAPTER 7
Drug Use and Abuse

Fifty years ago doctors could do little to help victims of the crippling disease known as polio. Serious cases usually ended in death. Slowly, progress was made in reducing both the death rate and the crippling effects of the disease although polio outbreaks increased at an alarming rate. Then, in 1955, a dramatic breakthrough took place. Scientists developed a vaccine that prevents the disease. As a result, polio is no longer a major health problem.

Similarly, other modern drugs can prevent or cure many illnesses that once caused disability or death. Drugs have radically changed medical practice over the years. Largely because of advances in drug technology, it has been said that the past twenty-five years have seen more medical progress than the previous twenty centuries. The life span of an average person has increased from about forty-seven years in 1900 to about seventy years today. Much of the credit for this amazing progress goes to modern drugs and improved medical care.

More than 90 percent of all prescriptions written today are for drugs that were not even on the market twenty-five years ago. In fact, many of the most important drugs that doctors prescribe today have been developed in the last twenty years. Used properly and only when medically necessary, modern drugs are one of the greatest blessings of our time. Elementary-age children need to develop an appreciation of and respect for the potential of drugs for good and harm.

DRUG PROBLEMS

The high incidence of drug abuse and misuse by young persons and adults has presented our school systems with one of their most puzzling problems. Clearly, no one preventive or rehabilitative program has been effective against all drug-related problems. Further, our attempt to solve the drug problem by disseminating drug information in our schools is not ultimately the answer to a serious problem. Homel has proposed a more realistic approach:

Communities across the country are concerned, confused, perplexed and anxious because of the behavior of young people and particularly their use of drugs. No longer can one presume that it is only the youngsters in another town who are toying with drugs while seeking thrills and kicks. Every community has its own number of people of almost all ages who, for a number of reasons, find the use of drugs appealing. This should not be surprising, for among any group of people young and old alike, there are those who are disturbed, immature, pressured, insecure or unprepared to benefit from past experiences and feel that they must try everything once to know what life is about. Some seeking identity feel that distortions of reality will generate insight into reality. Of course those seeking kicks and thrills are different from yesterday's thrill seekers only in the methods used to produce thrills desired.

It should not be surprising that young people use drugs because as a society we very definitely teach our young people to expect instant happiness, instant relief from tensions and anxieties, instant roots in life, instant relaxation and instant stimulation. The range of commercials presented via mass media, the content of the medicine locker and the behavior of society in general are all evidence of these facts.

Many are concerned over the drug problem. The concern seems to be misplaced. There is no problem with drugs; there is only a problem with people. People confronted with problems or needs, insufficiently prepared to understand themselves and seeking solutions through the self-administration of drugs. One often uses different expressions for these behaviors: drug misuse, drug abuse, etc. The fact remains that if one doesn't know what he is doing when administering drugs he is then abusing the drug and its recipient.

Before one can deal with drug abuse, one must be prepared to understand and deal with people and all of their dimensions. In spite of the fact that man is talked of in terms of his individuality, society relates to individuals primarily in terms of the physical dimension. While it is easy to demonstrate that people have physical, emotional, social, intellectual and spiritual dimensions, one would never guess as much from our disease-oriented, fear approach and biologically-centered programs for relating to man. The basic weakness in behavioral education and the study of related problems including drugs being abused is that people are not the frame of reference for prevention, rehabilitation or therapy; only their biologic dimensions are!

Changes in relating to young people are needed now before problems compound themselves geometrically. One of the major values of drug abuse has been the resultant look communities are taking at how children grow and mature, how young people develop attitudes and what factors pre-condition or precipitate behaviors in children, adolescents and adults. There is no questioning the need for a child, through adult multidisciplinary approach based upon the needs of the total person, to grow and mature.* There is no questioning that programs aimed at motivation, as well as behavior are needed now. There is no questioning that the problem isn't drugs; it's people![1]

This approach is applicable at the elementary school level.

The Five- to Eight-year-old[2]

At this stage of development children are very strongly influenced by the adult world. The drug experiences they are likely to encounter will occur around the house, since their social horizons are still narrow. They need to know about common medicines and their uses and about the chemical world they may find under the kitchen sink. They need to know the difference between candy and sugar-coated vitamins or aspirin. A seven-year-old living in an urban slum may already know about heroin, but most children who live in suburbia or in rural areas have little opportunity to know about, much less acquire, illegal drugs.

The primary developmental task during this period is learning to deal with others socially and cooperatively. This is the beginning of independence from the family, and the result is learning to function without direct supervision. Their concerns mainly include feelings about themselves, their skills, and their ability to get along with others. The building block for this period is the beginning acceptance of oneself as a person, someone who has unique talents and worthwhile skills. Both learner and teacher need to be able to say "I like me," followed closely by "I like you."

The Nine- to Eleven-year-old[3]

At this developmental level, children become aware of their growing responsibility for their own behavior and for decisions governing personal social drug use that they will be making in the near future. Many students may already be making such decisions, but the majority are probably still only in the awareness stage. Particularly toward the end of this period, children may be administering their own nonprescription medicines, such as aspirin or cough syrup. Some questions they may be considering include: Will I smoke when I grow up (enter high school)? What is alcohol like? Why can't I smoke and drink now? What does it mean when someone says that

---

*The Needs Approach to Health Education, copyright 1968 by Steven R. Homel, M.D., and Thomas W. Evaul, Pe.D.

Mr. Jones is an alcoholic? My big brother smokes pot, so what am I to do?

Some of the major developmental tasks for students in this age range are learning to be intimate, to share themselves with others and to understand sex-role identification. Consequently, they need such skills as the ability to determine what matters to others, social assessment, and the ability to cope with disapproval and rejection, particularly by peers. They must learn how to react to anger expressed toward them by friends and parents.

Other sources of information (peers, television, and older siblings) begin to rival the sole authority of parents, without necessarily encouraging consistent behavior. Media advertising encourages drug use. Mother discourages it, but mother uses drugs. Who is right and who is wrong, and how do I know? Taking sides may elicit disapproval from another side. If these children learn to live successfully with disapproval and rejection, they can begin to develop their own set of values because they can choose from alternatives what is important to them without fearing the reactions of others.

HUMAN NEEDS AND DRUG USE[4]

A person's most basic physiological drives are to meet physical needs: food, shelter, water, survival. The absence of any of these may so preoccupy a person that other needs recede into the background. For example, a hungry man might risk physical injury and arrest to steal food.

When basic physical needs are met, other needs assert themselves. We are not satisfied to know we have enough food and water for one day or shelter for a single night. We want some assurance of meeting basic needs on a regular basis. We need predictability. Thus, we have safety and security needs.

As the saying goes, "Man does not live by bread alone," not even daily bread. People need other people, who, in turn, need them. We need to belong, to be accepted. Everyone needs friends and close relationships. Even in a crowd, no one wants to be alone. Everyone has belonging needs.

In addition to basic physical needs, safety and security needs, and belonging needs, people have a need to do something worthwhile, to fulfill achievement or esteem needs. We all need a genuine sense of accomplishment whether in an occupation, child raising, artistic endeavors, or in some other aspect of life. Because we need to know that what we do is important, we need the respect of others for our deeds. From recognition, praise, and rewards for our achievements, we derive self-respect.

The most elusive of human needs is the need to be one's best self, or the need for self-actualization. As Sammy Davis, Jr., puts it in a popular song, "I've Gotta Be Me." Lacking a way to be all that they could be frustrates workers in unfulfilling jobs and rankles some housewives who feel chained to diapers and scrubbing. This need is at the heart of all genuine liberation movements. We all need to attain our potential, to have opportunities to develop talents and reach personal goals.

A number of principles underlie this theory of human needs. First, gratification of basic needs frees us to tackle higher levels of need gratification. A person who just satisfied the need for a job starts worrying about social needs with regard to fellow employees. Second, having met a need enables an individual to deal with still unmet needs. A person who has received frequent recognition of accomplishments has enough self-confidence to bear being overlooked on occasion. Third, we direct most of our activities toward frustrated or unmet needs rather than against already satisfied needs. For example, people who have worked their way out of poverty have more interest in further personal fulfillment than in reflection on past good fortune. They may find fulfillment in helping others free themselves of the bonds of poverty or strive to attain recognition in a field that holds special interest for them. Finally each individual is free to define personal needs at every level and to personally decide how to satisfy them. We must be careful, however, not to delude or lie to ourselves about what will really satisfy us.

Hierarchy of Human Needs

We encountered Maslow's theory of the hierarchy of human needs first in Chapter 5. You may recall that at the top of Maslow's hierarchy is self-actualization, or becoming everything one is able to become. This need for complete self-development lies deep in every person. Believing that we are progressing toward self-actualization is essential for human well-being.

Still, one person's security may be another person's achievement symbol. For example, a house to one of us may simply represent shelter, but to another it may represent achievement and accomplishment. We go about satisfying needs catagories in different ways, and what satisfies one may not satisfy another. Also, needs change throughout life. The levels of need are not all or nothing. Satisfying every belonging need, for example, is not necessary before we can attempt to satisfy achievement needs. The reverse is also true: we may be busy meeting our need for belonging when we must return to satisfying more basic needs.

The needs we have described are so essential that stress can develop when they are not reasonably met. The frustration of being unable to take care of these human needs can lead to conflict, stress, and anxiety. When a family cannot afford the basic requirements of human life, children may suffer and parents often experience mental anguish over their inability to provide the children's basic needs. The suffering of lonely people is no less acute because it is unseen.

People's Reactions to Stress

The way people respond to stressful situations varies from one person to the next. Some approaches are productive and useful. Others are destructive and ineffective. Generally, we can summarize people's reactions to stress as follows:

1. Ostrich approach: This approach to problems involves "hiding one's head in the sand" in order to avoid seeing the source of stress. The ostrich denies the existence of a conflict by avoiding the problem and pretending all is well.
2. Chicken approach: The chicken does not deny the problem. But knowing the problem is there recognizing the nature of the problem, it runs away from the problem. Since the problem won't leave, the chicken tries to escape it by running away.
3. Bulldog approach: The bulldog recognizes the problem. Instead of running away from it or attacking the problem itself the bulldog attacks and blames other people and causes for the predicament.
4. Ant approach: The ant is a realist. Unlike the ostrich, the ant understands that the mountain of sand will not disappear if it denies the existence of the mountain. Unlike the chicken, the ant confronts its problem and moves the mountain, one grain at a time. Unlike the bulldog, the ant assumes responsibility for its own problems. The ant doesn't just hope stress will go away. It doesn't blame others. It recognizes the problem and sets out alone, or with the help of others, to deal with the stress.

Continual recourse to drugs or alcohol to escape anxiety can lead to serious problems. It is not uncommon to hear people who have no apparent drinking problem say that they occasionally "drink to cope," and they seem to suffer no ill effects. But a person who continually uses alcoholic beverages in response to the frustration of human needs and hopes is in trouble. Repeated recourse to drugs as a way of dealing with stress is an ineffective and harmful way to try to cope with tension. Not only do drugs not resolve the stress, but they also can create new problems, as Table 7–1 shows. The practice of using drugs to reduce stress can be called *flight behavior*.

Most experts talk of escape as a totally negative response to frustration, stress, and anxiety. But there is another side to consider. In

TABLE 7-1. Problems that Arise from Drug Use Intended to Supplant Needs Fulfillment

Behavior	Need	New Problem
Drinking or drug taking because you can't be your best self	Self-actualization	Can cause you to be your worst self
Drinking or drug taking because you're not successful	Ego-status	Can cause you to be incapable of performing
Drinking or drug taking because you don't belong	Belonging	Can cause you to be more and more undesirable as companion
Drinking or drug taking because you hate your job	Safety and security	Can cause you to be unable to assume different responsibilities
Drinking or drug taking because of ill health	Basic	Can cause worse illness and can ruin health

some circumstances, getting away may be the only sensible thing to do. Many problems will disintegrate if people learn to cope, if they modify the way they respond to difficulties. Other problems are impervious to coping strategies and it would be folly to try to solve them by changing one's behavior. For example, you cannot teach a destitute person to cope with hunger, but you can teach ways of securing food. People who are well fed, safe, respected, and loved should be able to explore undeveloped capacities. Some problems require a change in people. Others require a change in the environment people inhabit.

Self-actualization

A great deal has been said about how forces outside of ourselves influence our thinking and sometimes get us into difficulties. We may forget the obvious fact that we have some control over the kind of people we are. Self-actualizing personalities are a good illustration of the way people make the most of this opportunity. Elementary-age children, although they have a way to reach the self-actualization stage, need help in developing the goals and concepts of the self-actualized person. And above all, their teachers should exemplify them.

1. Self-actualized people are realistic. They do not enjoy pipe dreams. They recognize their circumstances, but do not allow them to dictate their lives. Instead, they work to achieve their goals.

2. Self-actualized people take things in stride. They are down-to-earth and accept themselves, others, and the world as they are. They are aware of what is right, what is wrong, and what is possible.

3. Self-actualized people are spontaneous. They are not always tense. They are themselves, and they allow others to be themselves.

4. Self-actualized people do not indulge in ego trips. They do not begin every sentence with "I." Not self-centered, they are problem-centered.

5. Self-actualized people avoid being swallowed by life. They respect their own need for privacy and detachment. Knowing their own limitations, they pace themselves so that they will not burn out.

6. Self-actualized people are "awe-ful". They appreciate people and events in a fresh way. As beholders, they see a lot of beauty in the world.

7. Self-actualized people can run deep. They do not focus constantly on the superficial. They can see below the surface of things.

8. Self-actualized people have a few profound relationships. They are known and loved deeply by a few special people.

9. Self-actualized people are democratic. They elicit respect and take into account the feelings, desires, and aspirations of others, even when it is not necessary.

10. Self-actualized people laugh at life situations not people. Their sense of humor is philosophical rather than hostile.

11. Self-actualized people are open to new experiences. They are creative and like creative people and their creations. They are not easily threatened.

12. Self-actualized people do not follow the Joneses. They do not conform but have their own standards to which they adhere.

13. Self-actualized people rise above problems. They are not submissive, nor are they satisfied simply to cope with problems. They endeavor to solve them.

HIGH-LEVEL HUMAN NEEDS AND DRUG USE[5]

Most Americans—about 80 percent of those who live in families in which one or both parents have jobs—do not have to worry about meeting their lower-level needs. Consequently the behavior of many Americans is subject to the influence of some of the higher-level needs in Maslow's hierarchy, such as the need for love and companionship and the need for personal self-esteem. Nevertheless, it is characteristic of American society, especially on a technological level, that we continue to concentrate most of our time, energy, and skill on meeting lower-level material needs long after they have been adequately met. At the same time, emotional neglect of one another has become widespread. Husbands and wives ignore each other's emotional needs, and parent-child relationships often collapse. The result is that middle-class Americans are able to meet their physical needs with superabundance and yet many of these same people suffer emotional starvation.

Sometimes world conditions aggravate the situation. News reports of political unrest, social upheaval, and economic instability complicate our emotional distress with feelings of disorder, confusion, and uncertainty. Thus we are surrounded by an environment that seems fundamentally out of step with meeting our needs. Surely we can explain at least some drug-using behavior as a response to some of our neglected upper-level needs, needs that families ought to be helping members meet in wholesome ways.

Because our concern here lies with elementary-age children, habitual drug use is outside our purview. We should take a look, however, at the emotional needs that pull people toward drug dependence. Children in whom these needs suffer neglect are the ones who require help learning to respond to their own needs in other ways. The list that follows is not exhaustive or conclusive, but perhaps the act of identifying and describing them will suggest ways for families to fulfill some of them without using drugs and thus help to prevent chemical dependence.

Need for Adventure

Human beings resist boredom. Everyone wants variety, excitement, change, and challenge in life. Incredibly some people are bored in today's exciting world in which new opportunities develop almost daily. But the fact is that many people are.

One attempt to explain the paradox of multitudes of bored people in a world full of exciting opportunities suggests that we are actually so flooded with exciting stimuli—sensory, emotional, and intellectual—that we simply deny attention to some of them to protect ourselves from being overwhelmed. In addition, we also lower the intensity of our responses to those stimuli that do penetrate our awareness. Thus, by numbing ourselves psychologically, we suppress enthusiasm, initiative, creativity, and our capacity for excitement. We become bored. But we do not lose our basic need for adventure. Some people choose chemicals as an artificial way to restore the capacity for excitement, even though the range of alternative possibilities is almost infinite.

Need for Relief from Anxiety

Our modern world has a variety of ways of making people uncomfortable. At times all of us experience feelings from which we desire relief. Some of these feelings are easy to identify. Others are vague but nevertheless real. Many of them we might describe as feelings of anxiety. When they become intense enough to disturb normal living, we usually refer to them as emotional problems.

There can be no question of the ability of some drugs to provide temporary relief from uncomfortable feelings before they turn into problems. For years doctors have been prescribing them to otherwise healthy people for just that reason. Although drugs merely relieve or change feelings rather than solving problems, some people undoubtedly use chemicals to gain temporary freedom from psychological discomfort.

Need for Meaning

Beginning in adolescence everyone seeks satisfactory answers to such basic questions as "Who am I?" "Why am I here?" "What is the meaning of life?" These are difficult questions and finding answers to them is complicated by the many impersonal ways in which our way of life tends to ignore people or to turn them into numbers, animals, or machines.

In an impersonal world, some people find mind-altering drugs useful in their search for meaning. Drugs easily and promptly turn a person inward where "I" is a significant person and where the present moment is all that matters.

Need for Growth

The ability to grow and adapt to change is vital throughout life. Adults require growth as much as children do.

The teenage years are especially tumultuous in terms of change and the need to experiment with adaptive mechanisms. Teenage behavior often disturbs adults because they interpret youthful experimentation as rebellion. Alarming as the word "rebellion" sounds, rebellious teenagers may be entirely normal.

Unfortunately, use of drugs, often illegally, seems to be a part of so-called teenage rebellion. Young people try to justify their behavior by accusing the over-30 generation of being materialistic, enslaved by technology, hollow, phony, narrow, hypocritical, unaware of their own dependencies and insensitive to nature, beauty, silence, wonder, and people.

Some adults understand that young people are not rejecting all of the adult world but are striving to satisfy their need for authentic new adult growth. In their need to grow in ways different from their parents, some young people turn to drugs as a convenient way of experimenting with inner experiences completely removed from the materialism of the adult world. They see drug use as an exciting and immensely satisfying kind of growth experience, at least momentarily. And many of them do not care to look any further ahead than right now. In one moment drugs allow them to edge closer to self-fulfillment. Never mind that the stay is temporary.

In younger children the need to grow shows up in the anticipation of growing up, as they begin to covet the rights and privileges of older brothers and sisters and adults. To children who look forward to their initiation into the adult world, it must become obvious long before adolescence that the use of drugs, especially alcohol and tobacco, is an intimate part of adult social life. Add to this awareness the seldom considered fact that our drug laws subtly define society's initiation rites into the mysteries of adulthood by setting the age at which individuals can legally smoke and drink alcohol and it should not be surprising that children think that using drugs makes people grown up.

Need for Acceptance

One of the subtle ways in which people respond to the deeply rooted need for acceptance or belonging is to submit to the so-called "pressure to conform." Though this pressure may seem real, it may actually be more self-induced than it is imposed upon us by others in our society. If we are honest, we will not deny that conformity is a personal response to the need to feel accepted by significant persons or groups that have special meaning for us.

Sometimes we are certain that society exerts pressure on everyone to conform or "keep up with the Joneses." Sometimes the pressure seems to come from a segment of society and burdens only a few people or a particular person. Peer pressure, for example, encourages young people to wear similar clothes, speak a similar vocabulary, adopt the latest fad, or experiment with drugs to avoid losing the approval of other young people. Very often, among young people and adults, acceptance seems to hinge on the adoption of a life-style that includes the use of drugs.

The fact that people submit to this pressure is evidence that the need for acceptance is universal. Conformity is the price people pay to fulfill this need. Once a person has submitted to the pressure to conform, the pressure to continue paying the price may increase rather than decrease.

Need for Pleasure

The human need for pleasure is a higher-level need that we should not ignore. Every person has a need and a capacity for having fun.

An obvious fact about the use of chemical substances, yet one that people who are preoccupied with the "drug problem" often overlook, is that drug taking can be and often is pleasurable. At least momentarily and temporarily the experience is fun. What virtually all drug users have experienced and tell their friends is that the prompt, predictable, effect of certain chemical substances is a sensation of pleasure that no other experience can duplicate. Even though they know about all the possible long-term bad effects, they consider them remote and easily worth the risk to gain the benefit of immediate pleasure.

The traditional preoccupation of our society with the long-range destructive effects of habitual drug use usually ignores or denies the short-range rewards that users experience. Surely pleasure is a strong motivation for using chemical substances. Remarkably, by taking a drug into the body, we can overwhelmingly replace many kinds of personal distress with pleasure.

Other Needs

Doubtless there are many other needs to which people can respond by taking drugs. A summary of the experiences people claim to be seeking when they use drugs reflects some of them: to be happy, to be sociable, to calm down, to relax, to feel worthwhile, to be creative, to experience a sense of personal identity, to feel intimately accepted as a person among friends, and to experience a sense of freedom.

ALTERNATIVES TO DRUGS

Individuals can learn to respond in healthy ways to each other's needs so that it is unnecessary to turn to chemicals. If families and schools meet the needs that might motivate children to use drugs, there is less likelihood that they will become drug dependent.

The first step in establishing alternatives to drug use is to identify the needs that need to be met. To accomplish this purpose the family or class should meet to discuss individual and group needs. If the effort is sincere and everyone strives to be keenly sensitive to each other recognition of many needs should emerge from the discussion. Ideally, needs identification skills will develop and group members will continue applying them after the meeting has ended.

The second step is to communicate needs. Even after people have identified certain needs they experience them in different forms from time to time. Thus, if we want others to know what our needs are when we are experiencing them, we must communicate them.

Freedom to communicate depends upon the practice within the family or school of talking openly, honestly, and often about important matters. People who can level with each other learn about each other's needs promptly and hence are able to respond quickly. Hiding a need seldom fulfills it. Sharing it usually helps.

The third step in the process of needs fulfillment is to respond to others' needs in an appropriate, meaningful manner. When someone in a caring environment communicates a need, it is vitally important for people to help that person come up with a creative response to that need. That caring persons communicate understanding, support, and emotional nourishment is as important as clear communication of a need, for it helps the individual resolve the problem.

Thus, if a child feels a need for acceptance by a peer group, it would not be creative for the family to interpret the child's behavior as a rejection threat and to respond by rejecting the child. Much more creative would be the family's continued acceptance and understanding, which would encourage the child to believe that there need be no conflict between family acceptace and peer-group acceptance.

To a person who needs meaning and identity, the family and school should communicate that every person counts. This kind of response will help the person to experience meaning. If the need is for excitement or for fun, the family and school can communicate that these experiences are indeed important enough to search for together. In response to the need for relief from uncomfortable feelings, the family and school can communicate that in these environments powerful feelings of aggression can be safely expressed and relieved, and crippling feelings of depression will be met with loving support. In response to the need for companionship and love, the family and school can communicate that they will always share warm, good feelings. If the need is for growth—even the kind that seems rebellious—the family and school can communicate that it is all right to struggle to become your own person. Thus, the challenge to families and schools is to demonstrate through daily exercise of the process that there are better ways to experience need fulfillment (meaning, identity, acceptance, variety, adventure, pleasure, and so on) than by using drugs.

A BRIEF PHARMACOLOGY OF SELECTED DRUGS[6]

For our purposes, pharmacology is the science of how chemical substances interact with the human body. As a science, it is objective, highly technical, and extremely complex. Although it may be of interest to some, a knowledge of pharmacology is not absolutely essential to understand the role of drugs in society, nor is it particularly important to the purpose of education. Nevertheless, a brief pharmacology is a useful reference. A few definitions precede our brief pharmacology.

Glossary

Habituation   is a condition resulting from the repeated consumption of a drug. The word implies (1) a desire (but not a compulsion) to continue using the drug to achieve a sense of improved well-being, (2) little or no tendency to increase the dosage, (3) some degree of psychic dependence but little or no physical dependence, and (4) detrimental effects, if any, primarily only to the user.

Addiction   is an ambiguous term that changes meaning in different situations. One definition describes addiction as a state of periodic or chronic intoxication produced by the repeated consumption of a drug. Usually, however, the word implies (1) a strong, almost overpowering psychological dependence on a drug and hence a compulsion to continue its use and to obtain it by any means, (2) a physical dependence that produces withdrawal symptoms with abstinence, (3) a tendency to increase the dosage, and (4) detrimental effects on both the user and society. Because of the often sensational connotations and ambiguous meaning of the term "addiction," it seems to be increasingly appropriate to substitute the term "dependence."

Dependence   is a condition of psychological and/or physical dependence on a drug following periodic or continued use of that drug. Specific characteristics of dependence vary from one substance to another. For clarity, descriptions of dependence should refer to the specific drug under consideration.

Physical dependence   is a physiological condition of adaptation to the continuous use of a drug. Characterized by the development of tolerance and consequently, the need for increasing dosages to produce the same effect, genuine physical dependence produces withdrawal symptoms when the use of the drug ceases.

Psychological dependence (sometimes also called *psychic dependence*) is a condition of dependence on a drug to produce a feeling of satisfaction or well-being, to create pleasure, or to escape discomfort. It varies in intensity from a mild preference to a strong craving or compulsion to use the drug. In severe cases, what may be thought of as withdrawal symptoms—in the form of unpleasant psychological disturbances—may develop if use of the drug ceases.

Tolerance is a condition in which the response to a specific drug decreases with repeated use so that increasing amounts are necessary to create the same effect.

Withdrawal symptoms (also called *withdrawal syndrome*) are a characteristic set of unpleasant physiological and psychological symptoms that occur after the development of dependence if the regular administration of a drug ceases (or its effect is counteracted by an antagonist). The characteristics of withdrawal vary with different drugs and with the individual patterns of use associated with the dependent person. Severe instances of withdrawal symptoms may be fatal, especially in the case of alcohol and barbiturate abuse.

Classification of Drugs

There are many ways to classify drugs. The bases for several classification schemes are: the system or portion of the human body on which a drug acts, physical structure or chemical properties, the chemical mechanism by which a drug acts, the ultimate effect, or use against particular diseases or symptoms. Of primary concern here is the mind-altering or consciousness-changing properties of drugs that people use with the intent of bringing about pleasure, even though this is not always the effect. We will divide these drugs into four broad categories, according to the type of action and reaction they produce on the body—namely, stimulants, depressants, miscellaneous drugs that both stimulate and depress or have neither effect, and tobacco. In describing representative drugs from each category we will consider general characteristics, method of use, short-term effects, duration of action and effect, physical risks, and psychological risks.

Stimulants

Stimulants are mind-altering drugs that stimulate the brain and the central nervous system and consequently accelerate or increase functional activity. The most commonly used stimulant, caffeine, is the active chemical in coffee, cocoa, cola soft drinks and over-the-counter sleep preventatives. The average cup of coffee or tea, depending on the method in which it was brewed, contains 150 milligrams of caffeine, which usually increases the flow of thought, relieves drowsiness and fatigue, and permits more sustained intellectual and motor activity. When the respiratory center has been depressed by drugs such as morphine, caffeine by injection is of therapeutic value in increasing the rate and depth of respiration.

Caffeine also has strong effects on the circulatory system. Because it stimulates the heart and dilates the coronary and other arteries, and therefore increases the flow of blood to the brain, caffeine is therapeutically effective against some headaches.

Caffeine also lessens the susceptibility of skeletal muscles to fatigue, thereby increasing the body's capacity for muscular work. In addition, it increases urine production and the basal metabolic rate, as well as the secretion of hydrochloric acid in the stomach (which helps to develop and maintain peptic ulcers). In humans, the fatal oral dose of caffeine is estimated to be about 10 grams (10,000 milligrams), but no deaths from the drug are known. Tolerance develops with regular daily use and so does habituation (psychological dependence). Doses of 1 gram or more (about six cups of coffee) often produce toxic symptoms, including insomnia, restlessness, and excitement. In time, perceptual distortions, tremors, and accelerated breathing and heart rate may occur. Many people develop symptoms of a withdrawal nature, most notably headaches, if they stop using it.

Cocaine, a white crystalline powder that doctors once used as a local anesthetic, is the most potent stimulant. Recreational users snort it or inject it to experience effects similar to those of strong amphetamines. As tolerance develops, the user might shift to intravenous injections. Injected in combination with heroin, it becomes a *speedball.* Though it is uncertain whether cocaine produces physical dependence, the craving for its extreme high does constitute psychological dependence.

Amphetamines are synthetic stimulants that have been used medically to inhibit appetite and relieve mild depression. They are useful in treatment of hyperkinetic (hyperactive) children and in management of narcolepsy. The most commonly used amphetamines are dextro-amphetamine sulphate (Dexedrine or bi-phetamine), methedrine or Desoxyn, and Benzedrine. Amphetamines are popularly known as *pep pills. Methamphetamine,* especially in injectable form, is often referred to as *speed, crystal,* or *meth.* Usually sold in tablet or capsule form, amphetamines are also available in white powder form or in solution (in ampules for injection).

Shortly after taking moderate oral doses, users become more alert and energetic and can carry on activities for longer than normal periods before becoming tired. The larger the dose, the greater the effects. A large intravenous injection produces a *rush*—a sudden, overwhelming euphoria.

Many users report that these drugs increase concentration. Other psychological effects may include a sense of power or superiority, nervousness, irritability, anxiety, memory lapses, or hallucinations. Sometimes amphetamines heighten sexual desire and sometimes they eliminate it. Unusually large doses may cause rapid-fire speech, blurred vision, dizziness, tremors, headache, diarrhea, palpitations, and cardiac arrhythmias.

Ordinary dosages usually affect people for 3 to 4 hours. Abusers, however, may begin with a massive intravenous dose and take more every few hours to maintain a *run.* Some stay awake and high for as long as 72 hours before *crashing,* that is, sinking into a long sleep, usually followed by depression. Chronic, high-dose oral users may stay high for several weeks, during which time they sleep only occasionally.

The physical risks of frequent and heavy amphetamine use include weakness, skin trouble, nutritional problems, ulcers, pneumonia, and convulsions. Serum hepatitis, sometimes a result of using un-sterilized needles, can cause permanent liver damage, that, in turn, may produce chronic illness and premature death. Particularly large doses of amphetamines occasionally cause fatal cerebral hemorrhage or cardiovascular collapse. Use of amphetamines to increase stamina may impose strain on systems of the body by artificially prolonging stress.

When taken as usually prescribed, people slowly develop tolerance to amphetamines. With larger doses, it develops more rapidly. Soon it takes more amphetamine to produce the same effect. Some people take increased doses to heighten the experience. Those who inject amphetamines are especially likely to become dependent. Some users develop a *needle habit*—dependence on the act of injecting.

Depressants

The second general classification of mind-altering substances comprises the *depressants,* which depress or decrease bodily activity. *Alcohol* is the most commonly used depressant. Although alcohol may seem to stimulate some people, it is a primary depressant of the central nervous system, as are general anesthetics, narcotics, and barbiturates and other sedatives to which it is biologically equivalent.

When injected locally, alcohol blocks nerve conduction and hence is sometimes used to treat severe nerve pain. The drug has little effect on the heart or blood vessels. Specifically it does not dilate coronary arteries as commonly believed. Ingestion of alcohol brings about heat loss by the body and a fall in temperature, which contradicts the myth that consuming alcohol in cold weather has a warming effect on the body; it will actually make a person colder. Alcohol strongly stimulates salivary and gastric secretions, and higher concentrations of the drug in distilled beverages irritate the lining of the stomach, produce inflammation. Continued consumption can cause gastritis or ulcers. Alcohol causes fat to accumulate in the liver, where it eventually impairs liver function and possibly accelerates the development of hepatic cirrhosis seen in alcoholics. In addition, alcohol increases urine production. Even in moderate amounts, alcohol raises the levels of two chemicals—epinephrine and norepinephrine—circulating through the body. This effect, in turn, may be responsible for the observed increase in blood sugar, dilation of the eye pupils, and the modest increase in blood pressure observed with ordinary consumption of the drug.

The most pronounced effects of alcohol occur in the central nervous system, particularly in the area that coordinates the complex activities of the different regions of the brain and nervous system, but it also seems to depress the frontal cortex of the brain. This dual action results in disorganization and disruption of ordinary thought and motor activity. It also has an effect on judgment, memory, reasoning, self-control, speech, and mood. As measured by a variety of tests, mental and physical efficiency decreases when a person is under the influence of alcohol, unless he or she has inhibitions that impede optimum performance, inhibitions that alcohol diminishes.

Alcohol can be a source of caloric energy for the body, but it contains no proteins, vitamins, or other essential elements. Therefore people for whom alcohol is the primary source of nutrition or who combine alcohol with inadequate diets are susceptible to malnutrition, vitamin-deficiency diseases, and cirrhosis. Psychological dependency commonly develops with regular use of the drug and both tolerance and physical dependency occur with daily heavy use.

Approximately 90 million Americans use alcohol, including threefourths of all adults of all socioeconomic and occupational groups. An estimated 90 percent of college students are users of alcohol.

The *barbiturate* family includes many different drugs. The most common barbiturate preparations are phenobarbital (Luminal), Ambital, Nembutal, Seconal, and combinations of these drugs, such as Tuinal.

In medical practice, barbiturates are used to treat insomnia, anxiety, nervous tension, and epilepsy. Barbiturates are also used and abused by people who want to experience effects similar to those produced by large doses of alcohol, such as euphoria and relief from daily worries or concerns. A person who is high on barbiturates will exhibit many of the same symptoms that characterize alcohol intoxication. Usually taken by mouth, barbiturates also may be taken rectally or injected.

Generally speaking, a small dose of barbiturates will produce calmness, relieve anxiety and tension, and relax muscles. The effects of slightly larger doses resemble those of alcohol intoxication: if kept awake in a social setting, the user will exhibit slurred speech, staggering gait, sluggish reactions, exaggerated emotional states, and sometimes irritability and hostility. Some users experience a high degree of euphoria. In a quiet setting, a small dose induces sleep.

Much larger doses produce anesthesia. Very large doses cause respiratory failure and death.

Prescribed doses of long-acting barbiturates affect most people for about eight to twelve hours. Effects of prescribed doses of short-acting barbiturates last about four to six hours.

Barbiturates can induce both psychological and physical dependence. In a physically dependent barbiturate abuser, abrupt withdrawal is extremely dangerous. In the first eight to twelve hours of withdrawal the user may seem to improve, but very severe symptoms may portend delirium, hallucinations, and extreme depression followed by exhaustion. Sudden withdrawal from heavy use of barbiturates can cause death.

Narcotics, most Americans believe, are the most dangerous group of depressants. Narcotics consist of opiates and opioids—meaning opium—its derivatives and synthetic equivalents. Used in medicine mainly as analgesics (pain relievers), these drugs have several other important medical purposes.

Although opium has been used for thousands of years for both medical and psychological effects, it was not until the mid-nineteenth century that it came into widespread medicinal use around the world. Its neurophysiological, biochemical, pharmacological, behavioral, and sociological effects have been more studied than any other drug, mind-altering or otherwise. Opiates are absorbed from the gastrointestinal tract but in a manner so variable that they are almost always injected subcutaneously (under the skin).

The opium derivative *morphine* has been the subject of much study since it was first isolated from opium in 1800. In addition to what is known about the complexities of its mind-altering ability— its ability to affect the underlying personality and mood—the fact that it is a pain modifier is an additional determinant in its use. Average painkilling doses of morphine (about ten milligrams) also produce euphoria. Given to an individual who is not in pain, the same dose may act as a mood depressant and anxiety reducer. Morphine reduces most kinds of pain without interfering with other sensory modalities, such as sight and hearing, but some clouding of consciousness accompanies its use along with drowsiness, loss of energy, nausea, and sometimes loss of appetite. With larger doses, sleep occurs and respiratory depression becomes pronounced. This effect on respiration is the most serious potential toxic effect of excessive doses of morphine and its chemical relatives (e.g., heroin). Unlike barbiturates or general anesthetics, narcotics do not have anticonvulsant effects and do not impair coordination as alcohol and barbiturates can. Other effects of the drug include a decrease in urine production, a mild decrease in body temperature, constriction of the pupils, suppression of cough, and dilation of the blood vessels of the skin accompanied by sweating and itching.

Heroin is a narcotic drug that has long had a fearsome reputation. Users buy the fine tan powder in cellophane bags called *glacines*. Some individuals begin using it by snorting the grains into their noses through straws or glass tubes. It is more common to melt the powder by holding it over a match or candle in a cooker—a spoon or bottle cap. Injecting, or mainlining this form directly into the vein with a hypodermic needle produces a rush of excitement that some describe as the equivalent of sexual orgasm. Within a few minutes, the effects of the regular heroin high set in: feelings of physical warmth, peace, and increased self-confidence. Large doses can sufficiently slow bodily functions to cause death.

A regular user of heroin—or any of the opiate drugs—develops the familiar symptoms of physical dependence: tolerance and withdrawal. Although doctors report rare cases of occasional users who do not develop a heroin habit, a large majority of all people who try it on any regular basis become physically dependent.

Miscellaneous Drugs

The third general drug classification of interest to us includes drugs that have mixed effects. We will look at hallucinogens, volatile substances, and marijuana. One noteworthy fact about the so-called hallucinogenic drugs (LSD, mescaline, psilocybin, etc.) is that scientists know little about their chemical effects inside the human body.

D-Lysergic acid diethylamide, commonly known as LSD, is an extremely powerful synthetic hallucinogen. In fact, LSD is 4000 times more powerful than any other hallucinogen. Seventy-five micrograms (0.000075 gram), an amount that is almost invisible to the naked eye, will produce a mild experience in most people. To appreciate how potent LSD really is, consider that an amount of LSD equivalent to two aspirin tablets would provide normal 100-microgram doses for 6500 individuals.

Tolerance to LSD develops rapidly if used daily (a highly unusual pattern of use). Cross-tolerance to mescaline and psilocybin also occurs, but it disappears soon after use of the drug is discontinued. Physical dependence is unknown and psychological dependence, as it is understood with the other mind-altering drugs, is much less common with LSD.

There is no evidence of deaths or damage to body organs as direct results of LSD use even with large doses or chronic use. What makes it a significant drug is the intensity and pervasiveness of its perceptual and psychological effects on the central nervous system.

Before discussing the effects of an LSD high, it is appropriate to point out again that they are not consistent in all individuals. The effects are highly dependent on the dose, the physiological and psychological state of the individual, the setting in which it is taken, the tasks set for and by the individuals, the reasons for taking the drug, user expectations, and the expectations of the person who administered the drug.

An LSD trip is a highly personal experience, but it does have several common potential effects. Perceptual changes may be dramatic. Of all the senses, vision seems to be most affected. Objects and patterns may seem to come alive, shift and become wavy. Colors may seem very vivid, intense, and beautiful. The perceived intensity of white light may increase and it may seem to be surrounded by numerous colors. Colors may take on emotional meaning. Depth and figure-ground relationships change, causing texture to become important and fascinating. Taste, smell, hearing, and touch may seem more acute, and music may be richer than ever. True hallucinations are relatively rare on LSD, but *pseudohallucinations* are common. The individual experiencing a pseudohallucination has a visual experience without appropriate sensory cues but is usually well aware that the vision is subjective and a product of the drug. The more structured of these experiences often consist of dreamlike sequences or fantasies related to previous life experiences. They may be pleasant or horrible. Intensification of experience may be facilitated by the occurrence of *synesthesia,* the translation of one type of sensory experience into another. As a result, the LSD user may hear or feel light or color, see sounds, or feel music. Color may merge with emotion or mood.

Rapid shifts of emotion and extreme mood swings are common effects of an LSD experience. Within the eight to fourteen hours of the trip profound depression, anxiety, terror, euphoria, serenity, and ecstasy may all occur. Suspiciousness or hostility may also develop.

Many individuals can think and function adequately when pressed to do so, but they prefer not to do so. After taking LSD, an individual may sense thoughts moving much more rapidly than usual, and it may become very easy to deviate from normal logic and normal causal relationships. Past, present, and future may become confused. Depersonalization and distortion of the body image reminiscent of Alice in Wonderland are not uncommon. Such distortion may be amusing or bizarre and frightening. Most experiences assume increased meaning and increased importance to a person having an LSD experience.

Proponents of LSD stress the powerful emotional and philosophical-religious impact of the experience triggered by the drug. As they see it, the trip is beneficial to the individual and, in the long run, to society. Opponents stress the "bad effects," which proponents call "side effects." Unquestionably some reactions most people would consider bad. That these effects are truly bad has been questioned. Some would argue that only people who have basic personality problems have had bad trips and that bad experiences may be the bases of meaningful rebuilding or therapy.

Mescaline, which is chemically similar to amphetamines, is a derivative of the peyote cactus, a cucumberlike plant native to the Southwest. Mescaline profoundly stimulates vision, which becomes more acute, so that colors seem extremely bright and profuse. Overstimulation of the visual cortex by mescaline results in wavering outlines and other distortions similar to those that LSD generates.

The big difference between mescaline and LSD is that mescaline does not seem to provoke the rapid emotional changes often experienced with LSD. A feeling of peace and openness is a common experience among mescaline users. Due to this controlled trip and concern about possible chromosomal damage from LSD mescaline has become very popular, more in demand than LSD. Most of what is sold as mescaline, however, in fact is LSD, PCP (phencyclidine, a veterinary anesthetic, or one of the other hallucinogens. The true mescaline trip lasts four to twelve hours, depending on the amount taken.

Phencyclidine (PCP) was originally developed as an animal tranquilizer and is still utilized extensively for that purpose. Based on its effects on the human body, it is hard to classify PCP as a stimulant, depressant, or hallucinogen, although it acts pharmacologically as both a hallucinogen and a central nervous system stimulant. Originally used as a human anesthetic agent, PCP produced so many ill effects that in 1967 its use was restricted to animals.

The first appearance of PCP on the streets of San Francisco in 1967 met with displeasure among users, so it disappeared rapidly. Now purveyors often mislabel it or use it to extend other drugs such as LSD, cocaine, and tetrahydrocannabinol (THC), the active component of marijuana. It is generally taken orally although, as "angel dust," it may be inhaled with marijuana or other smokeable drugs.

Reported effects of PCP are mainly unpleasant and nondescript. Subanesthetic doses induce these stages of sensation: (1) changes in body image and depersonalization, (2) perceptual distortions, and (3) feelings of apathy or estrangement, feelings of drowsiness, "nothingness," or "emptiness." Secondary effects include flushing, profuse sweating, mild relaxation of the arteries, analgesia, involuntary eye movements, muscular incoordination, double vision, dizziness, nausea, and vomiting.

Psychomotor agitation, incoherent speech, unpredictable destructiveness, and impairment of mental functioning may also follow PCP use.

Psilocybin may be synthetically produced or naturally derived from mushrooms that grow in Mexico. Taken orally, psilocybin can produce four- to fourteen-hour hallucinogenic trips that are similar to mescaline highs, but more visual.

Most *volatile substances* are not commonly classified as drugs at all. They include modeling glue, paint, paint thinners, gasoline, aerosol propellants, and many others. They are generally easy to obtain at prices even lower than those of marijuana, and consequently, inhalation of volatile substances often appeals to junior high students and younger children. The physical effects of these substances vary considerably and are not well documented.

Marijuana is the last, but certainly not the least, in our catalog of miscellaneous drugs. The active component of marijuana is tetrahydrocannabinol (THC). Its effects are so diverse that it is easier to say what marijuana is not than to describe what it is. Not a narcotic or a hallucinogen or a tranquilizer, it nevertheless has tranquilizing, sedating, psychedelic, intoxicating, and many other effects in different people. In terms of present knowledge, marijuana is best described as a mixed sedative-stimulant drug. Many drug laws, however, still classify marijuana as a narcotic, which is what authorities believed it to be thirty years ago.

The once fearsome reputation of marijuana, based on outdated alarmist attitudes has come under reexamination. Though we can hardly dismiss marijuana as harmless, it comes as a surprise to some adults that many authorities no longer consider it to be as significant a problem as other drugs, some of which we have chosen to virtually ignore in spite of the mammoth proportions of their abuse.

Marijuana itself is not a plant but a preparation of black and brown flakes—the dried and powdered flowers, stems, and leaves from the female hemp plant, called Cannabis sativa. The active ingredients are present in the resins that collect in the leaves and flowering tips of the plant. Its strength varies widely with the climate and soil in which the plant grows.

Currently, most American users of marijuana inhale it in the form of homemade cigarettes. On any given occasion, an individual user usually smokes between one-half and one cigarette to achieve the optimal desired effects and then stops. Heavier doses frequently diminish the pleasurable sensations sought. The effects become noticeable within a few minutes after smoking and thirty to sixty minutes after oral ingestion, and they last somewhere between two and four hours.

Primarily marijuana affects the brain, but it also causes a mild increase in pulse rate and blood pressure, dryness of the mouth and throat (perhaps because of the generally irritating effect of smoke), reddened eyes, and increased appetite. No evidence has been found of damage to body organs from short-term use but from chronic use, and no deaths have occurred even from large doses. In ordinary doses, marijuana acts on the brain and interacts with the mind of the average person to induce mild euphoria, relaxation, increased flow of ideas, sometimes increased volubility and hilarity, and specific changes in the perception of time that makes minutes sometimes seem to be hours. Like other drugs, in large doses marijuana can cause temporary illusions, hallucinations, and personality disorganization. Psychological dependence can occur with regular use, but no physical dependence and probably no tolerance arise from use of the drug.

Marijuana users report lightness in the head, feelings of total relaxation, peacefulness and serenity, some loss of bodily coordination, intensified sensory perceptions, and a distortion of time. Inexperienced users and chronic abusers who smoke too much have reported that marijuana produces swings of mood—between great joy and extreme anxiety—and hallucinations in which objects change shapes and colors or unreal visions occur. Most authorities agree that marijuana has no inherent aphrodisiac properties, but in some users it does lower inhibitions and increase sensory pleasure. In others, it seems to numb the body and decrease sexual stimulation. At one time people believed that drug use was the cause of sexual promiscuity, but most authorities now believe that is is more often a result of broader social mores and changing social attitudes. Likewise, marijuana itself does not stimulate crime and violence, although some violence-prone individuals use it. Instead authorities feel that persons under the influence of marijuana tend to be passive, more so than persons under the influence of alcohol.

A review of the anthropological and medical literature from around the world, combined with the preprohibition experience in this country, indicates that cannabin (marijuana) preparations has potential as a treatment for depression, anxiety and tension, poor appetite, headache and other forms of pain, possibly some symptoms of the withdrawal illness from alcohol or narcotics addiction; cough; impaired respiration, and hypertension. It may also be valuable as an investigative tool for understanding brain function, an adjunct to psychotherapy, and an antibiotic (the non-THC components of the plant).

The most serious effects of marijuana, aside from the possibility of psychological dependence, are indirect. Recent studies show that marijuana can affect an automobile driver's judgment much as alcohol does. Thus, many researchers recommend that if you smoke pot, don't drive. Another indirect effect may also be considered serious: in most states, you can be arrested for using it.

Tobacco

Smoking behavior usually begins during youth, frequently during middle childhood. When a person starts smoking depends on the availability of cigarettes, on the degree of curiosity about what smoking is like, and the extent to which it is a mode of expressing either conformity to the behavior of others (parents, older siblings, or peers) or rebellion against the imposition of what seem to be proscriptions against smoking.

Smoking is much more common in children of parents who are themselves regular smokers. This fact is partly due to the ready availability of cigarettes to children because there is already a smoker in the household. In addition, older members of the family who smoke cigarettes communicate by their example that it is acceptable behavior and stimulate curiosity about what makes the cigarette so enjoyable. Thus, when smoking first begins to be popular in a culture, it tends to be taken up with increasing frequency by successive waves of young people.

In certain respects, tobacco smoking parallels the use and abuse of other drugs. Attempts to limit its use or to change the behavior of those who use it provide insights into the problems inherent in attacking the general problem of drug abuse. Without a doubt, chronic cigarette smoking is a form of drug dependence. Some researchers believe that the nicotine in tobacco is the key to dependence. The fact that only nicotine-containing tobacco has been acceptable to smokers supports the hypothesis that it is nicotine that provides the tranquilizing effects sought by smokers. But as with other types of drug abuse, habit formation and social factors play major roles in perpetuating the behavior. Certainly a large percentage of those who smoke more than just a few cigarettes a day tend to develop patterns of chronic heavy use, and most of them find it very difficult to stop smoking permanently once they have developed this pattern.

It is evident that tobacco use over long periods of time produces great tissue damage. Smoke from cigarettes is believed to be the chief cause of lung cancer as well as a major factor in heart disease, chronic bronchitis, and emphysema. In other words, cigarette smoking mainly affects the respiratory and circulatory systems. Eighty percent of the deaths linked with this habit are caused by these diseases.

Among people aged 35 and older the death rate is higher for both men and women cigarette smokers than for nonsmokers. And the differences are striking. Among men between the ages of 45 and 54, the death rate for smokers is almost three times that of nonsmokers.

As might be expected, cigarette smokers have more disability and illness than nonsmokers. They suffer more frequently from chronic conditions and spend more time sick in bed than nonsmokers. One estimate is that 77 million workdays are lost each year in this country because of the higher rate of illness among smokers.

The more one smokes, the greater the risk of serious consequences. Compared to the nonsmoker, the two-pack-a-day smoker is more than twice as likely to die of heart disease and twenty times more likely to die of lung cancer. The effects of smoking do not strike only the heaviest smokers, however. The average smoker (one pack a day) and the fairly light smoker (one-half pack a day) also can suffer significant consequences.

Laboratory studies have isolated from tobacco smoke a number of *carcinogens,* chemical compounds that can cause cancer. In addition, smoke also contains *cocarcinogens,* substances that interact with other compounds to promote cancer.

NOTES

1. Steven R. Homel, M.D., "The Problem Isn't Drugs, It is People." (unpublished manuscript), copyright 1973 by Steven R. Homel, M.D.
2. National Institute on Drug Abuse, *Doing Drug Education—The Role of the School Teacher* (Washington, D.C.: U.S. Department of Health, Education, and Welfare, 1976).
3. Ibid.
4. Adapted from: National Institute on Alcohol and Alcoholism, "How You Think Is How You Drink," *An Ounce of Prevention.* (Washington, D.C.: Department of Health, Education, and Welfare, 1977).
5. Adapted from: National Institute on Drug Abuse, *A Family Response to the Drug Problem* (Washington, D.C.: U.S. Department of Health, Education, and Welfare, 1976), pp. 33-38.
6. Ibid.

RESOURCES

Do It Now, Box 5115, Phoenix, Ariz. 85010. (Materials on drug abuse mostly aimed at "street" people or youth.)

Drug Abuse Council, 1828 L Street, N. W., Washington, D.C. 20036. (A private foundation doing research, policy evaluation, and program guidance in drug use and misuse.)

Drug Enforcement Administration (formerly Bureau of Narcotics and Dangerous Drugs), 1405 I Street, N.W., Washington, D.C. 20537. (Materials are available at the Preventive Programs Division, 2nd floor, telephone (202)382-4315, and in an extensive library in Room 601 [telephone (202)382-5706].)

Educational Resources Information Center, U.S. Office of Education, 400 Maryland Avenue, S.W., Washington, D.C. 20202. (Materials and information on all aspects of education.)

National Clearinghouse for Drug Abuse Information, 11400 Rockville Pike, Rockville, Md. 20852, telephone (301)443-6500. (NCDAI distributes materials produced by the Federal Government. Single copies are free. Write or call for information on any aspect of drug abuse.)

National Coordinating Council on Drug Education, 1211 Connecticut Avenue, N.W., Suite 212, Washington, D.C. 20036. (NCCDE is a private, nonprofit drug education consortium. It publishes *National Drug Reporter, Drug Abuse Films, An Evaluation,* and other drug abuse materials.)

National Institute of Alcohol Abuse and Alcoholism, 5600 Fishers Lane, Rockville, Md. telephone (301)443-1273. (Alcohol Clearinghouse, telephone (301)948-4450.)

National Library of Medicine, 8600 Rockville Pike, Bethesda, Md. 20014. (Medical aspects of drugs and drug abuse.)

Non-medical Use of Drugs Directorate, 365 Laurier West, Ottawa, Ont. KIA 1B6 Canada, telephone (613)996-7680. (Canada's national resource and information body on drug abuse.)

Special Action Office for Drug Abuse Prevention, New Executive Office Building, 17th and Pennsylvania Avenue, N.W., Room 3227, Washington, D.C. 20506.

STASH, 118 South Bedford Street, Madison Wis. 53703, telephone (608)251-4200. (Publishes *Capsules* (a newsletter), *Grassroots,* and other drug-related materials.)

CHAPTER 8
Disorders of
Learning and Speech

CHARACTERISTICS OF
LEARNING DISORDERS

Observant elementary teachers may discover among their pupils a variety of specific learning disabilities or perceptual problems that make learning a very difficult process. Probably 9 to 20 percent of the school population experience learning disabilities.[1] The National Advisory Committee on Handicapped Children defines learning disabilities as follows:

> Children with special learning disabilities exhibit a disorder in one or more of the basic psychological processes involved in understanding or in using spoken or written languages. These may be manifested in disorders of listening, thinking, talking, reading, writing, spelling, or arithmetic. They include conditions which have been referred to as perceptual handicaps, brain injury, minimal brain dysfunction, dyslexia, developmental aphasia, etc. They do *not* include learning problems which are due primarily to vision, hearing or motor handicaps, to mental retardation, emotional disturbance, or to environmental disadvantage.[2]

The concept of learning disabilities is fairly new. Current ideas date from the 1930s and 1940s, but many learning disorders still lack clear definitions. They tend to occur in children of near-average or above-average intelligence who also show evidence of behavior or learning abnormalities. Associated with subtle malfunctions of the central nervous system, they range in seriousness from mild to severe. Children suffering from learning difficulties characteristically experience problems in thinking, listening, talking, reading, writing, spelling, and arithmetic. Other symptoms are poor attention, memory control, and motor function. In essence, the problem lies in the child's functioning capabilities and does *not* come from organic eye and hearing problems, motor handicaps, mental retardation, or environmental retardation.

Freeman identifies more specific signs and symptoms of learning disabilities.[3] For instance, learning-disabled children have trouble with associations and cannot categorize, conceptualize, or draw conclusions. A low level of awareness prevents them from keeping up with their peers. They frequently experience confusion and need constant attention. In addition, they have trouble focusing their attention and usually experience hyperkinesis along with easy distractibility. They also may seem to lack motor coordination.

Visual perception in learning-disabled children usually is faulty. Unable to comprehend sequencing exercises, they tend to confuse letter sequences in words (e.g., spilt for split). They also mistake one letter for another when writing and reading (e.g., b instead of d or p rather than g). Their handwriting is generally poor and they have trouble discriminating between shapes and colors.

Certain hearing characteristics are associated with learning disabilities. Hearing association is abnormal. Poor auditory memory prevents learning-disabled children from repeating even at one-second intervals. Auditory sequencing is poor, and these children have a hard time hearing consonant sounds. They have a hard time expressing themselves and become easily confused when trying to follow directions. Poor sound discrimination causes them to confuse words and to miss rhymes.

Murphy summarizes the characteristics of learning disabilities as follows:

1. Poor visual discrimination: Difficulty distinguishing between
   *squares and rectangles
   *circles and ovals
   *m and n
   *h, n, and r
   *p, b, d, g, and q
   *6 and 9, 12 and 21
2. Poor visual memory
   *forgetting what he has seen
   *not remembering what he has read

3. Poor auditory discrimination: Inability to distinguish between different, but similar, sounds and words.
4. Poor kinesthesia: Difficulty distinguishing between familiar objects by feeling, such as
   *a penny and a nickel
   *a dime and a quarter
   *cardboard cutouts of letters of the alphabet
5. Poor eye-hand coordination: Difficulty making his hand do what his eye sees, such as
   *copying
   *tracing
   *hitting a ball with a bat
6. Poor spatial orientation: Difficulty remembering the differences between
   *right and left
   *up and down
   *over and under
   *outside and inside
   *horizontal and vertical
   *on top of and underneath
7. Poor figure-ground: Difficulty selecting one thing from a group, such as
   *a particular letter in a word
   *his cubby hole from other children's cubby holes
   *a triangular block from a square block
8. Perseverance: Difficulty shifting from one activity to another. (Once he has learned the answer to a question, he may give the same answer even when the question changes.)
   *What color is the grass? Green
   *What color is the sky? Green
   *What color is the snow? Green
9. Hyperactivity: Inability to concentrate on a structured activity, because almost any lesson bewilders a child with a learning disability. This might result in
   *talking at any time
   *touching everything
   *inattention
   *distracting other children
10. Disinhibition: Tendency to be lethargic or hyperactive, with an "I don't care about anything" attitude.
11. Poor self-image: As a result of the reaction of parents, teachers, and classmates to one or more of the above symptoms, a child may see himself as anything but "normal."[4]

Obviously, most of us at one time or another display some of these symptoms (you may become hyperactive or lethargic during a dull speech). But children with learning disabilities exhibit many of these symptoms most of the time, and they interfere with everyday life and performance.

FIGURE 8–1. *Complex vicious cycle originated by minimal brain dysfunction. (Redrawn after L. E. Arnold, "Is This Label Necessary?"* Journal of School Health *43 (October 1973): 53.)*

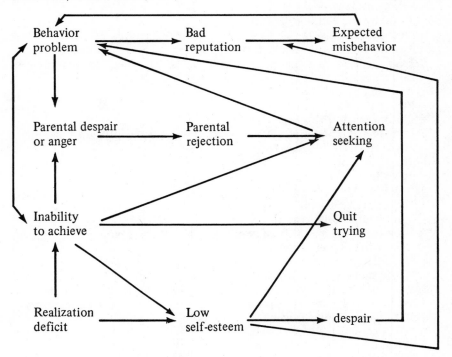

CAUSES OF LEARNING DISABILITIES

The cause of a learning disability is sometimes difficult to establish, but probable attributions include congenital developmental problems, trauma during birth, and infections and injuries early in life. Typical behavior patterns of children who have suffered such difficulties include:

1. Emotional instability, such as emotional overreaction to environmental stresses, continual temper tantrums and crying, almost uncontrollable emotional states, extremely gullible, and not usually accepted by their peers.
2. Hyperactive, with a short concentration or attention span. Always on the go, constantly talking and moving about.
3. Very impulsive, is easily distracted and blurts out in class.
4. Continuous, abnormal repetition of an action or response which has previously met with success.
5. Unpredictable in actions, with an explosive temper and mood swings.[5]

Figure 8-1 shows the characteristic cycle of problems and responses experienced by a child with minimal brain damage. The left-hand side of the diagram names three major problems of minimally brain-damaged children, which Arnold identifies as behavior problems, inability to achieve, and realization deficit. Because these problems disturb others in the child's environment they increase the number of problems the child faces. Parental despair or anger may cause rejection, which causes the child to resort to attention-seeking

FIGURE 8-2. *Williams's natural history of learning disabilities. (Redrawn from J. Floyd Williams, "Learning Disabilities: A Multifaceted Health Threat,"* Journal of School Health *96 (November 1976): 9.)*

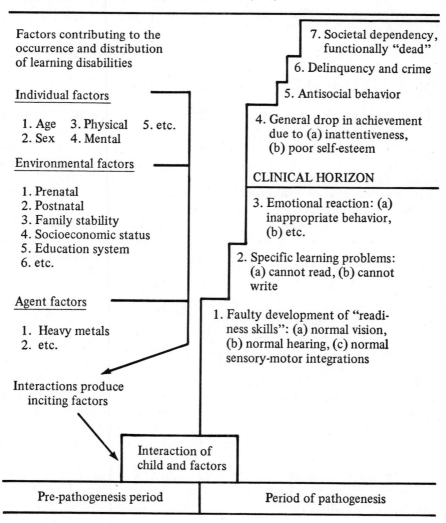

Factors contributing to the occurrence and distribution of learning disabilities

<u>Individual factors</u>

1. Age   3. Physical   5. etc.
2. Sex   4. Mental

<u>Environmental factors</u>

1. Prenatal
2. Postnatal
3. Family stability
4. Socioeconomic status
5. Education system
6. etc.

<u>Agent factors</u>

1. Heavy metals
2. etc.

Interactions produce inciting factors

Interaction of child and factors

7. Societal dependency, functionally "dead"

6. Delinquency and crime

5. Antisocial behavior

4. General drop in achievement due to (a) inattentiveness, (b) poor self-esteem

CLINICAL HORIZON

3. Emotional reaction: (a) inappropriate behavior, (b) etc.

2. Specific learning problems: (a) cannot read, (b) cannot write

1. Faulty development of "readiness skills": (a) normal vision, (b) normal hearing, (c) normal sensory-motor integrations

Pre-pathogenesis period   Period of pathogenesis

devices. The attention-seeking behavior, in turn, may lower the child's self-esteem and compound the behavior problem. As a result, the child acquires a bad reputation, and a vicious failure cycle develops.

According to Williams, the "natural history of learning disabilities" has two phases (see Figure 8–2). The pre-pathogenesis period is that time between the conception of a child and the event that causes the disability. Various individual environmental and agent factors may interact to produce one or more learning disabilities. During the subsequent period of pathogenesis the learning disabilities manifest themselves. As the interaction of the child and the causal factors continues, additional problems arise, Williams says. At the "clinical horizon" outside professional help can be of tremendous value. Without it the learning-disabled child may develop the serious problems numbered 4 through 7 on the chart.

HELP FOR CHILDREN WITH LEARNING DISABILITIES

Teachers who observe some of the foregoing characteristics in their students should notify the school nurse or physician, who will probably call upon a medical specialist or team of specialists to diagnose the problem. This team will closely examine the medical history of the child and conduct a thorough physical, neural, and psychological examination before offering a diagnosis. Usually they will order an electroencephalogram for the child, too.

If the child does have a learning disability, a special treatment program should commence. Chemotherapy is a common treatment in cases in which drugs (stimulants, antidepressants, tranquilizers, antihistamines, and anticonvulsants) will give the patient more control and greater ability to communicate. For example, Harbin reports that certain symptoms of hyperkinesis (e.g., learning, social behavior, and physical control) may improve with amphetamines.[6]

Some specialists disapprove of chemotherapy. The possibility of negative side-effects is one argument against drugs. In addition, children vary a great deal in their response to medication. Criticism of the regular use of drugs, especially amphetamines, has been strong in regard to treatment of hyperkinesia, in particular because no one knows precisely how they affect the brain. Still another objection to drug therapy is that teachers may be using drugs to stifle spirited, creative children, or that the children may turn into speed freaks or become drug dependent.

To evaluate criticism of drug therapy for children The Department of Health, Education and Welfare conducted a study and drew some important conclusions:[7]

1. Stimulant drugs, carefully prescribed and supervised, do produce major improvements in many children with hyperactivity and certain other learning and behavior disabilities.
2. No evidence was found that the "proper use of amphetamines to treat children could lead to drug addiction in the teen or adult years."[8]
3. The use of stimulants does not suppress, slow down, or overstimulate the energy capacity of the child.
4. HEW suggested that the "paradoxical effect" of stimulants in children is appropriate. Stimulants appear to "mobilize and to increase the child's abilities to focus on meaningful stimuli and to organize his bodily movements more purposefully." The panel went on to enumerate positive secondary effects, which include a joy in increasing competency, better relationships with other children, and an improved self-image.

From one-half to two-thirds of children who experience hyperkinesia benefit from stimulant drugs, according to HEW, although further research is necessary to establish the type of drug and dosage that best meet the needs of these children. An important point of the HEW study is that hyperactive children seem to outgrow the need for medication by eleven or twelve years of age. If loving parents and positive environmental experiences can help the troubled child to maintain a positive self-concept during adolescence, adulthood may be normal.

Special education programs can help learning-disabled children to overcome problems with perception, written and oral language, and conceptualization. Learning disabilities need not handicap children if teachers will approach the process in ways they will understand. It is also important to structure the program so that children in the program will not have to contend with labels like "dumbbell," the effects of which could be negative and long-lived.

Teach Through Activity

Children—all children, but especially those with learning disabilities—learn best through activity, through doing something rather than sitting back passively and being told or shown. It may be partly because doing, touching, handling makes things less abstract; it may be because of the element of discovery that doing brings; it may be because impulses from the muscles to the brain facilitate the learning process.[9]

Teach Through Many Senses

Teaching through as many senses as possible seems to work best with learning-disabled children. Even when the teaching material seems to involve only one sense it is possible to bring in other senses. Tracing a letter and feeling a letter made out of sandpaper, as well as looking at it, sometimes help to fix it in a child's mind. For children who have trouble following spoken language to visualize a story or a series of verbal directions, augment the presentation with pictures or charts.

Teach at the Appropriate Level

Three teaching levels are especially important to consider in programs for learning-disabled children:

1. A tolerance level at which it is easy for the child to work, (using skills which the child has already attained)
2. A level at which it is a challenge for the child to apply himself
3. A level at which it is frustrating for the child to try[10]

Everybody, adults included, learns best at the first two levels. Children enjoy activities that they can do as well as those that challenge them. More difficult tasks overwhelm and frustrate them and are no fun at all. The following illustration demonstrates how real the difference is for a child:

> One mother decided to teach Lennie how to tie his shoes. She knew where he was—he knew his right shoe from his left and how to put them on—but he wasn't yet able to tighten up the laces or actually tie the knot and bow. She elected to spend some time on the lace-tightening stage before she went on to the knotting and bowing steps. This tightening stage might seem insignificant (why spend time on something so easy?), but it was a challenge for Lennie, who had very poor hand coordination. He had trouble concentrating on pulling both laces with both hands at the same time. To try teaching Lennie how to tie the bow without first teaching him the preceding steps would have been a very frustrating experience for him.

Use Repetition[11]

> Children with learning disorders often have very short attention spans, which means they don't learn well in activities which require a lot of concentration and time. They learn best when they have short doses of activities, repeated many different times. Repetition doesn't have to be boring; these children need the security of doing something over and over again. They also have difficulty generalizing from one situation to another. Once they seem to have mastered a particular skill, they can try doing it with different materials. A boy might learn how to tie his brown shoes but be lost when asked to tie his sneakers. Practicing with different kinds of shoes is the kind of repetition he'll need.

Avoid Drastic Changes of Gears

Children with learning difficulties may find it hard to change from one kind of activity to another—from drawing to water play, from quiet to noisy play, and so on. These changes in activity can't and shouldn't be avoided in a regular day care program—they provide a varied, exciting curriculum. But drastic changes of pace for a special child can be avoided. For instance, if the child is playing a quiet game by himself, he shouldn't immediately be asked to plunge into a noisy, active game with a large group of kids. Include him first in an activity with a small group, then later move him into the larger group.

Give Directions in Small Steps

Many times children with learning disabilities cannot follow multistep directions. They are usually capable of performing each step involved, but the directions are told to them in a way that throws them off. If a whole series of steps are involved, ask them one at a time, not simultaneously. For example, instead of asking John, "Could you close the door and then come into the kitchen and get out the cookies?", ask him in three consecutive steps: 1. "John, could you close the door?" (John closes the door.) 2. "John, please come into the kitchen." (John goes into the kitchen.) 3. "Please get the cookies out." (John gets the cookies out.) This is easier for John to understand and follow than asking all three steps at once.

Give Directions Without Clutter

Children with poor auditory memory often have difficulty screening out the unimportant words that are not necessary in sentences. You can help by giving directions using only necessary words. Here is an example of a cluttered direction: John, **could you** close the door **so it won't be cold in here** and then help Susie and me **in the kitchen to** get the cookies and milk ready **for snack time?** (Bold phrases point out clutter.)

Reduce Distractions

Many learning disabled children may be easily distracted by outside stimuli. They may not be able to put into perspective every sound and sight that they hear and see around them. They can't filter out all the details and therefore find it hard to concentrate or focus on the important stimuli. For example, when you show Keith the picture of a little boy on a book cover, he might not "see" the little boy but rather will become distracted by the shiny cover. Reduce all possible distractions.

Success-assured Activities

Failure breeds failure. If a child has too many bad learning experiences he'll be afraid to try new things. Plan a number of success-assured activities—ones the child can't help but do well—to give him the confidence he'll need for new and more challenging ventures. Things with no "right" and "wrong" about them are reassuring to the child with learning problems. They can be as simple as asking, "What do you think of when you hear that music?" or "Which book would you like me to read today?"

Praising the efforts of any child is important in teaching—only more so for children with learning difficulties. They need frequent positive encouragement. They're often timid about entering new activities for fear they won't be good at them, so your job is reassurance that they're doing a fine job with the tinker toys and that it's wonderful that they can climb the jungle gym.

If a child is learning a particular skill step by step, such as tying his shoes, he must be praised at every step. When he learns to tighten up the laces, make him feel he's accomplished a very important task—he has. Waiting to praise him until he's learned the whole sequence will be too defeating. If you want him to move on to the others, he must be praised for what he's already mastered. However, don't praise children for no reason. Unwarranted praise can be smothering and may even encourage a child to stop trying altogether. Again, there's a middle ground.

TYPES OF LEARNING DISABILITIES

Hyperkinesis

Hyperkinesis is one of three specific learning disabilities; dyslexia and autism are the other two. It is a condition that causes children to be hyperactive or to overreact. Symptoms of hyperkinesis are excessive restlessness or overactivity, impulsiveness, irritability, a short attention span, inability to work in a group, and usually poor coordination. Not all children whose behavior includes these characteristics have hyperkinesis.

It is not uncommon to find schoolchildren who have no minimal brain dysfunction classified as hyperkinetic or hyperactive simply because they are extremely active or disruptive. Anxiety, boredom, temperament, training, a chaotic or disorganized family, and a lack of practice in mental activities are other possible causes of overactivity in children. It is a grave mistake to label all overactive or normally active children hyperkinetic.

Hyperkinetic children have learning problems because they cannot sit still or pay attention long enough to learn. It is important to diagnose this problem early, for untreated hyperkinetic children tend to exhibit severe psychiatric symptoms even after they have matured.

Although hyperkinesis is not usually a direct cause of psychological problems, it is not always easy for hyperkinetic children to cope with their own unexplainable behavior and the reactions it produces in other people, so it is not surprising that emotional problems sometimes develop.

An estimated 500,000 to 1.5 million hyperkinetic children attend elementary schools in the United States. Thus, in any classroom 4 to 10 percent of the students might be hyperkinetic.[12] The diagnosis itself can be tricky because the disorder is not attributable to one cause, nor is there a fixed set of symptoms. We do know, however, that an early diagnosis, followed by treatment, can help these children lead well-adjusted and productive lives. The earlier the diagnosis, the more favorable the results.

The treatment for hyperkinesis involves parental counseling, school assistance, and possibly chemotherapy. First, the parents need to understand that their child has a developmental lag, but that potential for full development is very good. Some tips for parents of hyperkinetic children are:

1. Know what behavior requires control and control it *early* before the child veers off the track.
2. Keep the child out of large groups of people (department stores, big parties, etc.).
3. Build the child's self-concept with lavish but sincere praise.
4. Control your own anger in a mature way.
5. Practice being a good listener.
6. Work with a nutritionist and physical educator for body fitness, development, and coordination. Directed physical activity provides an excellent emotional outlet.

Second, the schools can help by providing special classes and teachers to give hyperkinetic children success experiences. An environment conducive to growth is essential. For example, behavior modification programs have proven beneficial for some hyperactive children.

Specialists prescribe chemotherapy for about one-half to two-thirds of the children diagnosed as hyperkinetic. Because stimulants have proven to be effective and to have the least side effects of the drugs used to treat hyperkinesis, they are usually the first choice. Other drugs used commonly with smaller groups are antidepressants and tranquilizers. The purpose of chemotherapy is not just to mask the symptoms but also to help hyperkinetic children successfully interact with their environment. If these children can learn to cope with this early stage of life without developing any major psychological problems, they will probably calm down around the age of puberty and emerge as normal, productive adults.

Dyslexia

The term *dyslexia* characterizes a delay or dysfunction in the mental processing of language symbols. Dyslexic children experience difficulty in processing language because of poor symbol interpretation when they read. They may be victims of "congenital word-blindness," minimal brain dysfunction, or psychomotor (coordination) problems. Specifically, dyslexia makes it unusually difficult to copy figures and words accurately, to write and draw, to order letters and numbers in the desired sequence, and to speak in a controlled, regular manner. Dyslexia sometimes has physiological correlates, such as hearing and vision problems, glandular dysfunctions, and poor nutrition, the correction of which should eliminate the dyslexia.

Not surprisingly, dyslexia poses special learning difficulties that need specific attention. Dyslexic children need the same kind of support as the hyperactive child. The main goals are early diagnosis, correction of any physiological problems, and a specific plan to overcome the difficulty.

Autism

Autism is not a well-defined disorder but is a syndrome characterized by personality disorganization. Jones et al. define autism in the following way:

> The patient is overly absorbed with himself, or silly, or he has bizarre delusions and incoherent speech and apparent indifference to social mores or standards. He is inert or mute, has hallucinations, or displays occasional sudden, impulsive outbursts of speech or actions.[13]

Autistic children engage in ritualistic stimulation by self-punishment (slapping themselves or banging their heads against the wall), pacing, or rocking back and forth. They do not attempt to explore their environment or make contact with people and therefore are very unsociable. Unloving, they seem to have no desire to receive love. Apathy is commonplace, and autistic children seldom make eye contact with other people, even with those who are trying to communicate with them. Autistic babies may go rigid when they are being cuddled and throw tantrums at the slightest frustration. Many autistic children are totally mute, but some will parrot what they hear. Most are evidently not mentally retarded but they may not recognize their names or learn to dress themselves. Interestingly enough, many have excellent memories and spatial skills.

Traditional treatment methods have not been very effective. The success rate for the usual self-concept–building strategies and psychotherapy has been very small. Behavior modification programs designed to punish bad behavior and reward good behavior were somewhat more successful at teaching some autistic children how to behave civilly, to show and accept affection, and even to speak. In the late 1960s and early 1970s scientists began to use sign language as an alternate communication tool. Some autistic children who have learned to communicate through sign language have been able to move into classes for learning-disabled children in public schools. As a result, the picture for autistic children and their families is somewhat brighter.

PRESCRIPTION FOR MINIMIZING LEARNING DISABILITIES

A learning disability is a lot like a disease in that it robs a child of being able to take full advantage of life's opportunities. Learning-disabled children become academic cripples and they suffer mental and social handicaps, as well. They may become juvenile delinquents and thus a burden to society and their families.

In order to minimize learning disabilities we need to catch them as soon as the child enters school, if not earlier. So many children have faulty readiness skills when they begin school and are not able to follow basic educational instruction. Some of the problems center on vision and hearing—the ability to match what they see with what they hear. Academic failure causes many children to react emotionally. They may become excessively active, lose interest in school, and eventually drop out.

Learning disabilities comprise one of the most prevalent childhood afflictions. Failing prevention or detection coupled with unsuccessful treatment, the outcome for the child and for society could be disastrous. Generally we cannot pinpoint one specific cause of a child's learning problems, except in the case of disadvantaged children who received inadequate verbal and perceptual stimulation from infancy through childhood. Hereditary influence appears to be substantial, however.

Perhaps only 10 percent of learning-disabled children show signs of actual brain damage. In many cases, a delay in the development or maturation of parts of the brain that control skills necessary for learning to read well seem to contribute to the child's problem. These developmental delays may be genetic, organic, or environmental in nature. Language function seems to be the most vulnerable skill.

Strong evidence suggests that the lack of essential prereading skills is readily detectable in kindergarten-age children and probably in much younger children. Training programs to coordinate eye, hand, and brain may prove to be an effective way to prevent learning disabilities in children who seem likely to suffer from them.

As mentioned, most learning disabilities come to light only after some deviant behavior has occurred. Usually behavior problems appear after the patterns have become set. At this stage it is much more difficult to rectify the situation and help the child. Thus it is very important that parents and teachers observe their children carefully and seek solutions for learning problems at the preschool level, if possible.

CHARACTERISTICS AND CAUSES OF SPEECH DISORDERS

Speech and language skills develop in distinctive and fairly orderly stages. Tables 8–1 and 8–2 detail these stages.[14]

Sometimes abnormal conditions interfere with the orderly development of communication skills. The extent of the problem depends on the severity of the abnormality, the stability factor in the total development of the child, and the environment in which the child develops. Also, the earlier in life the abnormal condition occurs, the more severe and long-lasting the disruption of language development and speech is likely to be.

There are several common types and causes of speech and language disorders. They are:

1. Premature birth and low birth weight: Premature birth or low birth weight is a very common causal factor in children with communication disorders. Preverbal communication activities are usually delayed because the baby has problems adjusting to early life and perhaps began life in a confined environment. Premature and low-birth-weight babies are more vulnerable to infections and other illnesses as well as to neurologic damage. Attainment of normal speech and language development by two to three years, greatly lessens the chance of serious communicative disruption.
2. Mental retardation: Mental retardation is the most common cause of speech and language development problems. The speech and language of a retarded child develop late and usually do not follow a normal pattern to normal modes of communication because of reduced brain function and an abnormal environment. Specific problems include faulty articulation, symbolic concepts, and deficient vocabulary.
3. Delayed maturation: Some children experience an overall delay in development for reasons ranging from prolonged illness and hospitalization or malnutrition and physical abuse to psychological, social, and cultural deprivation. Preverbal development (babbling, cooing, etc.) usually encounters interference, which can lead to serious speech and language development disruption. Articulation problems combined with reading and writing problems are signs of this particular problem.

TABLE 8-1. Pattern of Normal Language Development in Articulation and General Intelligibility

Age in Years	Articulation	General Intelligibility
1–2	Uses all vowels and consonants *m, b, p, k, g, w, h, n, t, d.* Omits most final consonants, some initial. Substitutes consonants above for more difficult ones. Much unintelligible jargon around 18 mo. Good inflection rate.	Words used may be no more than 25 percent intelligible to unfamiliar listener. Jargon near 18 mo. almost 100 percent unintelligible. Improvement noticeable between 21 and 24 mo.
2–3	Continues all sounds above with vowels but use is inconsistent. Tries many new sounds, but poor mastery. Much substitution. Omission of final consonants. Articulation lags behind vocabulary.	Words about 65 percent intelligible by 2 yr.; 70 to 80 percent intelligible in context by 3. Many individual sounds faulty, but total context generally understood. Some incomprehensibility because of faulty sentence structure.
3–4	Masters *b, t, d, k, g,* and tries many others including *f, v, th, s, z,* and consonant combinations *tr, bl, pr, gr, dr. R* and *i* may be faulty, so substitutes *w* or omits. Speech almost intelligible. Uses *th* inconsistently.	Speech usually 90 to 100 percent intelligible in context. Individual sounds still faulty; some trouble with sentence structure.
4–5	Masters *f* and *v* and many consonant combinations. Should be little omission of initial and final consonants. Fewer substitutes, but may be some. May distort *r, l, s, z, sh, ch, j, th.* No trouble with multisyllabic words.	Speech is intelligible in context even though some sounds are still faulty.
5–6	Masters *r, l, th,* and such blends as *tl, gr, bl, br, pr,* etc. May still have some trouble with blends such as *thr, sk, st, shr.* May still distort *s, z, sh, ch, j.* May not master these sounds until age 7.5.	

Herold S. Lillywhite, Norton B. Young, and Richard W. Almsted, *Pediatricians Handbook of Communications Disorders* (Philadelphia: Lea and Febiger, 1970), pp. 76–78. Reprinted from Herold S. Lillywhite, "Doctor's Manual of Speech Disorders," *Journal of the American Medical Association* 167 (1958): 850. Copyright © 1958 American Medical Association.

TABLE 8-2. Pattern of Normal Language Development in Expressive Speech and Comprehension of Speech

Age in Years	Expressive Speech	Comprehension of Speech
1-2	Uses 1 to 3 words at 12 mo., 10–15 at 15 mo., 15–20 at 18 mo., about 100–200 by 2 yr. Knows names of most objects he uses. Names few people, uses verbs but not correctly with subjects. Jargon and echolalia. Names 1 to 3 pictures.	Begins to relate symbol and object meaning. Adjusts to comments. Inhibits on command. Responds correctively to "give me that," "sit down," and "stand up" with gestures. Puts watch to ear on command. Understands simple questions. Recognizes 120–275 words.
2-3	Vocabulary increases to 300–500 words. Says "where kitty," "ball all gone," "want cookie," "go bye-bye car." Jargon mostly gone. Vocalizing increases. Has fluency trouble. Speech not adequate for communication needs.	Rapid increase in comprehension vocabulary to 400 at 2.5 yr., 800 at 3. Responds to commands using "on," "under," "down," "over there," "bye," "run," "walk," "jump up," "throw," "run fast," "be quiet," and commands containing two related actions.
3-4	Uses 600–1000 words, becomes conscious of speech. 3–4 words per speech response. Personal pronouns, some adjectives, adverbs, and prepositions appear. Mostly simple sentences, but some complex. Speech more useful.	Understands up to 1500 words by age 4. Recognizes plurals, sex difference, pronouns, adjectives. Comprehends complex and compound sentences. Answers simple questions.
4-5	Increase in vocabulary to 1100–1600 words. More 3–4 syllable words. More adjectives, adverbs, prepositions, and conjunctions. Articles appear. 4-, 5-, 6-word sentences, syntax quite good. Uses plurals. Fluency improves. Proper nouns decrease, pronouns increase.	Comprehends 1500–2000 words. Carries out more complex commands requiring 2–3 actions. Understands dependent clause, "if," "because," "why," "when."
5-6	Increase in vocabulary to 1500–2100 words. Complete 5–6 word sentences, compound, complex, with some dependent clauses. Syntax near normal. Quite fluent. More multisyllabic words.	Understands vocabulary of 2500–2800 words. Responds correctly to more complicated sentences, but is still confused at times by involved sentences.

Herold S. Lillywhite, Norton B. Young, and Richard W. Almsted, *Pediatricians Handbook of Communications Disorders* (Philadelphia: Lea and Febiger, 1970), pp. 76–78. Reprinted from Herold S. Lillywhite "Doctor's Manual of Speech Disorders," *Journal of the American Medical Assocation* 167 (1958): 850. Copyright ©1958 American Medical Associaton.

4. Illness, injury, and congenital anomalies: Congenital problems that affect speech include cleft palate and other orofacial anomalies and moderate to severe cerebral palsy. Besides marked delays in speech and language development, a child may also have an inadequate voice, articulation problems, and hypernasality.

5. Neurologic dysfunction: The child with neurologic dysfunction, or damage to the brain centers of language and speech, may show any of the speech and language disorders previously discussed. The key symptom, however, is the inability to organize the symbols of communication in relation to their proper meanings and sequences.

   Unable to communicate with language, these children may develop deviant and bizarre behavior. Time, space, and form disorganization may occur. Hyperactivity, inability to concentrate, and obliviousness to reward and punishment are other characteristics.

6. Hearing impairment: Deafness always causes communication disorders to some extent. Because of their predictability, these problems generally receive corrective attention. Communication disorders caused by mild to moderate hearing loss present a greater problem among school-age children. Communication problems coupled with school failure are a reliable indication of hearing loss and always suggest the need for a hearing-screening test.

7. Anomalies of the tongue: The tongue is rarely a speech problem. In those rare cases, the problem may be a structural defect or some actual tongue paralysis. The tongue can be restricted by the lingual prenulum, which is easily taken care of by surgery.

   Some children develop a "tongue thrust" problem. They strongly force the tip of the tongue between the teeth or against the upper incisors while swallowing or speaking. Usually this behavior ceases by age seven or eight. If it does not, buck teeth and articulation problems may result. Evidence of this problem is poorly articulated *s, sh,* and *z* sounds.

8. Enlarged tonsils and adenoids: Enlarged tonsils and adenoids may give the voice a denasal quality, but they do not impair speech development. The big threat is an infection spreading to the middle ear and consequent hearing loss. Middle-ear infection, termed *otitis media,* is very common among elementary-age children.

9. Social, psychological, and environmental conditions: Stress can cause communication disorders. Examples of stressful situations that may impair speech development are wartime bombing, violent social upheaval, and residence in a riot-torn community. They can cause language delay, stuttering, and language deficiencies.

   An oppressive or rigidly restrictive environment may also disrupt the orderly development of speech and language skills. A bilingual family environment can cause problems if there is language inconsistency in the home and the community, for example, if parents punish a child for using the community language at home.

Stuttering

Perhaps the most puzzling of all communication disorders is stuttering. A variety of circumstances and conditions seem to be responsible for stuttering behavior. Environmental stresses, emotional reaction to delayed speech, and immaturity of certain organ systems all may play a part.

Whatever the cause, most stuttering begins between the ages of two and five. As stuttering becomes more complex, the child becomes increasingly aware of it and the problem grows worse. Verbal avoidance of the troublesome consonants or syllables may even affect physical posture and cause a child to effect facial grimaces.

Teachers and parents must learn to ignore this speech problem and treat stuttering children as though their speech were normal by not hurrying or demanding repetition and by giving them full attention while they are speaking. Ninety-nine percent of children pass out of this developmental stage and develop normal speech.

Help for Children with Speech Problems

The normal tendency of parents and teachers who want to eliminate children's speech problems is to interrupt and correct them when they make mistakes. Some may even use scolding and punishment to try to bring a child's speech and language to their standards. Far more effective and less stressful methods include the following:

1. Understand expected normal development by becoming familiar with average norms of speech and language development.
2. Many parents whose children have speech and language problems hear misinformed reassurances that nothing is really wrong and that they will outgrow the problem. Basically, children learn language and speech through hearing, so problems may stem from an organic difficulty or poor sound discrimination. Sound discrimination develops at different rates. For example, young children may say "goggy" for "doggy" because they hear g instead of d. This practice is perfectly normal for a certain age, but if the problem persists, the child is still hearing the sound incorrectly. Therefore, use the correct sound repeatedly to make sure the child hears it ("This is a doggy. Would you like to pet the doggy. Good doggy"). This way the child will not become oversensitive to making errors. Oversensitivity makes the problem worse. Go slow and stick with one or two sounds at a time.
3. Speech problems will worsen if children are excited or anxious or if they think you aren't listening to them. Therefore, give speech-disordered children your full attention during conversation. Adopt a warm, "slow-down" attitude, which will be extremely helpful.

4. Help these children occasionally when they get "stuck" on a word.
5. Do *not* use exaggerated facial expressions when mouthing words for children who have hearing problems.
6. Do not hesitate to refer a child for professional help if you feel the speech problem is not improving. Any of the following conditions warrant a professional evaluation (symptoms a–g, of course, would occur prior to a teacher's involvement):
   a. If the child is not talking at all by age two.
   b. If speech is largely unintelligible after age three.
   c. If there are many omissions of initial consonants after age three.
   d. If there are no sentences by age three.
   e. If sounds are more than a year late in appearing according to development sequence.
   f. If there is an excessive amount of indiscriminate, irrelevant verbalizing after eighteen months.
   g. If there is consistent and frequent omission of initial consonants.
   h. If there are many substitutions of easy sounds for difficult ones after age five.
   i. If the amount of vocalizing decreases rather than steadily increases at any period up to age seven.
   j. If the child uses mostly vowel sounds in his speech at any age after one year.
   k. If the word endings are consistently dropped after age five.
   l. If sentence structure is consistently faulty after age five.
   m. If the child is embarrassed and disturbed by his speech at any age.
   n. If the child is noticeably nonfluent (stuttering) after age five.
   o. If the child is distorting, omitting, or substituting any sounds after age seven.
   p. If the voice is a monotone, extremely loud, largely inaudible, or of poor quality.
   q. If the pitch is not appropriate to the child's age and sex.
   r. If there is noticeable hypernasality or lack of nasal resonance.
   s. If there are unusual confusions, reversals, or telescoping in connected speech.
   t. If there is abnormal rhythm, rate, and inflection after age five.[15]

A speech problem may lead to reading difficulties and a poor school experience, both of which would greatly hamper a student throughout life. In addition to the causes discussed in this chapter, other sources of speech and language disturbances include cultural background, inadequate patterns and methods of teaching, and psychological and environmental stresses. Whatever the cause, early discovery, early diagnosis, and early help are critical to normal development and learning.

NOTES

1. Floyd J. Williams, "Learning Disabilities: A Multifaceted Health Threat," *Journal of School Health* 96 (November 1976): 515.
2. "Definitions of Learning Disabilities Used in the United States," *Journal of Learning Disabilities* 9 (June/July 1976): 378.
3. Stephen W. Freeman, "Learning Disabilities and the School Health Worker," *Journal of School Health,* 42 (October 1973): p. 68.
4. John F. Murphy, *Listening, Language and Learning Disabilities: A Guide for Parents and Teacher* (Cambridge, Mass.: Educators Publishing Service, 1970), p. 1.
5. Herold S. Lillywhite, Norton B. Young, and Richard W. Almsted, *Pediatricians Handbook of Communication Disorders* (Philadelphia: Lea and Febiger, 1970). pp. 85–87.
6. V.K. Harbin, "The Hyperkinetic Child," *School Health Review* 4 (March/April 1973): p. 4.
7. "Serving Children with Special Needs," U.S. Department of Health, Education, and Welfare, p. 54.
8. "Definitions of Learning Disabilities," p. 379.
9. Margaret Golick, *A Parent's Guide to Learning Problems* (Montreal: Quebec Association for Children with Learning Disabilities, 1970), p. 12.
10. Marylou Ebersole, Newell Kephart, James Ebersole, *Steps to Achievement for the Slow Learner* (Columbus, O.: Charles Merrill Publishing Co., 1968), p. 4.
11. This and the following five methods are reprinted from: Day Care Office of Child Development, U. S. Department of Health, Education, and Welfare, *Serving Children with Special Needs* (Washington, D.C.: U.S. Government Printing Office, 1972), pp. 53–54.
12. Brent Q. Hafen, *The Hyperkinetic Child Syndrome: A Behavioral Disorder,* (Provo, Utah: Brigham Young University Press, 1974), p. 3.
13. Kenneth L. Jones, Louis W. Shaunberg, and Curtis O. Byer, *Health Science,* (New York: Harper and Row, Publishers, 1974), p. 22.
14. Lillywhite et al., pp. 76–78.
15. Ibid., p. 96.

RESOURCES

Virginia Apgar and Jean Beck. *Is My Baby All Right?* New York: Trident Press, 1973.

"Definitions of Learning Disabilities Used in the United States." *Journal of Learning Disabilities* 9 (June/July 1976): 378.

Marylou Ebersole, Newell Kephart, and James Ebersole. *Steps to Achievement for the Slow Learner.* Columbus, O.: Charles Merrill Publishing Co., 1968.

Stephen W. Freeman. "Learning Disabilities and the School Health Worker." *Journal of School Health* 42 (October 1973): 521-22.

Margaret Golick. *A Parent's Guide to Learning Problems.* Montreal: Quebec Association for Children with Learning Disabilities, 1970.

Robert H.A. Haslam. and Peter J. Valletutti. *Medical Problems in the Classroom.* Baltimore, Md.: University Park Press, 1975.

Brent Q. Hafen. *The Hyperkinetic Child Syndrome: A Behavioral Disorder."* Provo, Utah: Brigham Young University Press, 1974.

V.K. Harbin. "The Hyperkinetic Child." *School Health Review* 4 (March/April 1973).

Herold S. Lillywhite, Norton B. Young, and Richard W. Almsted. *Pediatricians Handbook of Communication Disorders.* Philadelphia: Lea and Febiger, 1958.

John F. Murphy. *Listening, Language and Learning Disabilities: A Guide for Parents and Teacher.* Cambridge, Mass.: Educators Publishing Service, 1970.

Day Care Office of Child Development, U.S. Department of Health, Education, and Welfare. *Serving Children with Special Needs.* Washington, D.C.: U.S. Government Printing Office, 1972.

Floyd J. Williams. "Learning Disabilities: A Multifaceted Health Threat." *The Journal of School Health* 96 (November 1976) p. 515.

CHAPTER 9

Postural Development

The growth of the bony framework, or skeleton, of a child has life-long importance. Soft tissues of the body are responsive to regulation and change through diet and exercise, but irregular skeletal growth may produce permanent deformities. Elementary school teachers are in an excellent position to teach good posture and observe irregularities in skeletal structure. For this purpose, an understanding of bone growth, good posture, and postural problems is essential.

DEVELOPMENT OF THE SKELETON

Our genes determine the general size and proportions of our skeletal framework, but responsibility for the implementation of our genetic "blueprint" rests with the endocrine system, which secretes the hormones that regulate bone growth. A baby's skeleton is largely cartilaginous and soft. Only the middle sections of the bone shafts are hard, or *ossified*. During the course of development, *epiphyses*, or ossification centers, appear in the cartilage near the ends of the bones, where they create colonies of spongy bone. As ossification continues, these spongy bone colonies gradually merge and proceed along the shaft of bone toward the center section. Growth in length occurs in the cartilaginous ends of the bones. When ossification, or *calcification,* of the bones is complete, growth ceases. After a bone has completely ossified, its shape changes only as a result of disease or injury. It is for this reason that proper skeletal development in the growing years is vital. It is also essential to realize that a skeletal deformity is more easily correctable in youth, when the bones are still somewhat cartilaginous.

POSTURE

Posture is the alignment of body parts to achieve balance in walking, running, sitting, standing, or any other physical activity. The skeletal system and muscular system govern balance. Poor postural habits established in the early years carry over into adult life and bring corresponding difficulties of vertical alignment and body movement. In addition, posture studies have found a significant association between poor posture and physical, mental, and emotional problems. An estimated 70 to 80 percent of all people have some degree of postural malalignment.

The normal spinal column, viewed from the back, forms a straight line. When viewed from the side, however, it shows mild natural curves in the neck (cervical), chest (thoracic), low back (lumbar), and pelvic (sacral) regions (see Figure 9–1). An exaggeration of one or more of these curves can result from poor posture (see Figure 9–2). An abnormal forward angulation of the thoracic vertebrae is called a *kyphosis* (hunchback, humpback). *Lordosis* (swayback) describes an increased, inward curve, usually in the low back. A lateral deviation (side-to-side curve) of the spinal column is called *scoliosis.* These conditions may occur when the skeletal muscles and skeletal system are not in balance. Months or years of poor posture can cause this kind of imbalance to occur.

It is important to understand that children do not assume the same stance as adults and should not be expected to. Whereas the center of gravity in an adult is in the umbilical and pelvic region, in young children the head is larger in relation to the body so the center of gravity is in the upper part of the trunk. Children have a tendency to throw the trunk back upon the pelvis, thereby showing some lordosis. During adolescence, developing strength and coordination of the spinal cord and muscles produces a proper erectness.

Teachers can examine posture by imagining a straight line (plumb line) running through the following body points, shown in Figure 9–3:

1. Ear lobe
2. Center of the shoulder

FIGURE 9-1. *The spinal column viewed from the side.*

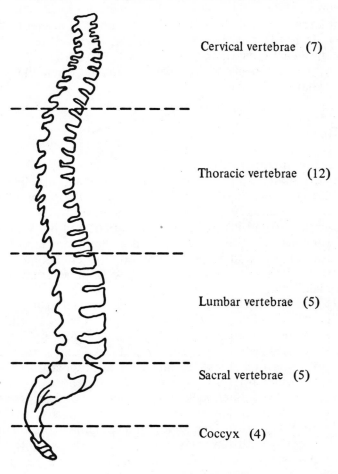

Cervical vertebrae (7)

Thoracic vertebrae (12)

Lumbar vertebrae (5)

Sacral vertebrae (5)

Coccyx (4)

3. Hip joint
4. Just behind the knee cap
5. Through the lateral (outside) ankle

Inspected from the front and rear as well as the side, children should show alignment of the head, neck, and balance in the height of the shoulders and hips. A child whose one shoulder or hip is lower than the other has postural, and possibly structural, problems. Progressive structural deformity could cripple a person.

Postural defects usually develop in combination with defects in other areas of the body. For example, lordosis (an exaggerated curve in the lumbar region) is usually accompanied by compensatory deviations, such as a forward head, round shoulders, flat chest, and

FIGURE 9-2. *Common spinal aberrations.*

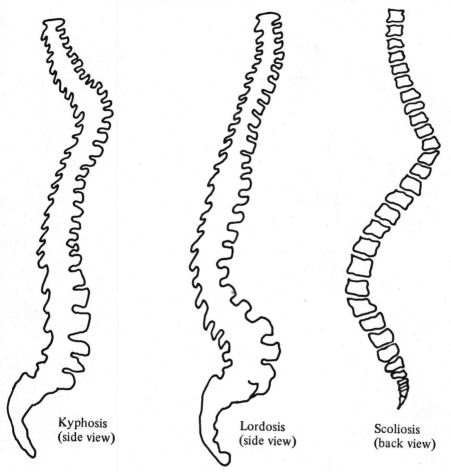

Kyphosis
(side view)

Lordosis
(side view)

Scoliosis
(back view)

flat feet. General symptoms of postural problems in children include the following:

1. Head tilted forward, chin-in appearance
2. Exaggerated front-to-back spinal curves
3. Lateral spinal curves (scoliosis); one shoulder lower than the
   other
4. Flat-chestedness
5. Flat feet (no arch)
6. Cramped toes
7. Ptosis (protruding stomach); obesity
8. Unstable balance
9. Hand and shoulder joint forward of ears and hips

FIGURE 9-3.   *Correct body alignment.*

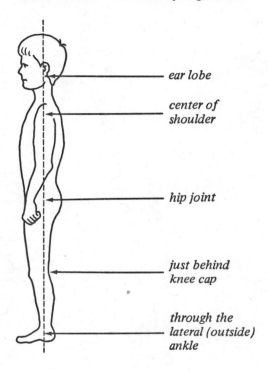

ear lobe

center of
shoulder

hip joint

just behind
knee cap

through the
lateral (outside)
ankle

Behavior of students with postural problems is also characteristic. A lack of energy or restlessness, clumsiness and lack of coordination, forward slouch, repeated shifts of sitting positions, a desire to go barefoot or take off shoes, and withdrawal from strenuous activity are behavioral symptoms of postural problems. Typical complaints revolve around sore feet, sore back, and fatigue.

What can teachers do to promote good posture? Start by paying good attention to the student's environment. A correctly lighted classroom helps by requiring students to make only minimal adjustments to see. Teach the students to use the backrests of chairs so that the buttocks and back are resting against the backrest. Have them practice a "head up–chest out" position. Elementary students need changes of activity so that they will not sit for long periods of time. Some of those activities should be large-muscle activities. Encourage coordination and graceful movements. Use teaching methods that produce good attitudes and motivation toward good posture. Help parents understand what good posture is so they can also encourage it.

SPINAL DEFORMITY IN ADOLESCENCE

Spinal deformity can be crippling, emotionally as well as physically. Surgery can correct or arrest a spinal deformity, but the most effective treatment is to arrest it early in its development, before it requires surgery.

The two most common spinal deformities are kyphosis and scoliosis. It is important to understand these as conditions, not disease entities. Scoliosis may be caused by leg-length difference, muscle spasms over a long period of time, and unilateral muscle weakness. In addition, heredity and congenital abnormalities may be causal factors. Neuromuscular diseases, such as polio paraplegia, cerebral palsy, and muscular dystrophy, can also lead to scoliosis.

In elementary school students, kyphosis most often is attributable to poor posture. The next most common cause is Scheuermann's disease (adolescent kyphosis). Other, less common causes include bone diseases, infections, and congenital problems.

Lordosis also develops most often from postural problems, but it can be a complication of kyphosis. Different neuromuscular problems can give rise to weak anterior abdominal muscles and, consequently, to lumbar lordosis. A child who experiences hip flexion contractures (inefficient hip movement) will develop a lumbar lordosis.

All spinal deformities are detectable long before they become grossly evident. Therefore the key to effective treatment is early detection. The following physical features are clues that a spinal deformity is developing:

1. The presence of unequal shoulder height (may be apparent in conditions other than shoulder height, such as unequal hip height).
2. Asymmetry of the tips of the scapulae (shoulder blades) in elevation and distance from the midline of the back.
3. Prominence of one scapula (or both).
4. A crooked plumb line of the spinous processes of the vertebrae.
5. Asymmetry of posterior chest wall when the student bends forward. Forward bending allows the shoulders to drop forward, unmasking the rib hump, which is concealed by the scapulae when the individual stands erect.
6. A difference in space between the arm and the lateral side of the thorax on the two sides of the body.

To receive an adequate postural evaluation, the student must be unclothed and in an upright position. The best way to detect scoliosis is with the student bending forward: facing the seated examiner, the student bends forward at the waist, knees straight, hands together fingertip to fingertip, and arms dangling straight down toward the floor. The teacher should then look for small differences in the rotational dimensions of the thorax. Usually the two sides will be absolutely symmetrical. Deviations from these normally symmetrical contours indicate a probable spinal deformity.

There are two types of kyphosis, structural and postural. To correct postural kyphosis, have students stand, straighten the back, pull in the stomach, and pull back the shoulder blades. If it is easy for the subject to follow these instructions, you can safely rule out the existence of spinal deformity. To check for structural kyphosis ask students to hyperextend the spine (extend beyond the usual range of motion) while in the prone position, put their hands behind their buttocks, and lift their heads and shoulders as well as the legs so they are rocking on their abdomens. Students whose spines come to full extension, or even hyperextend, may have structural kyphosis. This condition requires medical attention.

Evaluation for lordosis entails bending forward with the knees straight. Normally this position eliminates postural lumbar lordosis. Next, while the child is laying flat on the back, knees fully flexed, palpate the back by slipping your hands under each side of the lumbar arch. If the student does *not* have a lordosis, the lumbar spine comes flat against your hand. Otherwise, the student probably has structural lordosis.

Students are often very self-conscious about being seen undressed by parents, teachers or peers. For that reason, physical education teachers may be the most appropriate people to closely examine the spine for deformity. Suspected deformities require examination by the family physician, who can recommend appropriate orthopedic services.

In the early stages, spinal deformity is not a disease, and its progress is easy to arrest. If scoliosis or kyphosis has progressed to the point at which correction is necessary, nonsurgical methods often fail. Therefore, early detection is a must. The most effective and efficient way to detect spinal deformity early is to hold annual school screening clinics for ten- to thirteen-year-old children. Studies indicate that approximately 10 percent of schoolchildren in this age group show some slight abnormality of the spine. One to 2 percent have significant deformity requiring treatment. Periodical observation of the rest is advisable.

Treatment for patients with true spinal deformity is threefold:

1. Serial observation: A growing child with a mild spinal deformity needs careful monitoring by a physician. Severe spinal deformities can develop very quickly.
2. Brace treatment: The most common corrective brace is the Milwaukee brace.

3. Surgical correction and fusion: Serious spine curvatures require this treatment not only to straighten the spine, but also to weld the involved vertebrae into a solid unit that will resist the lateral forces pulling on it.

Without treatment the child will develop severe scoliosis, which usually leads to serious cardiovascular and arthritic problems.

Postural problems do not require surgery or braces. Most postural problems in children are self-resolving, especially when they become interested in how they look to peers. Constant nagging by parents and teachers usually has a negative effect, both on posture and on family relations. Building the child's self-concept, encouraging a good appearance, and giving constructive advice on how to look better will meet with more success.

EXERCISES FOR GOOD POSTURE

The following exercises are a guide to involving students in a quest for good posture. Student participation in these exercises may also allow teachers to detect skeletal and muscle deviations.

General Postural Exercises

1. Face the wall so that the toes and chest touch it. Then tuck in the stomach and pull the head away from the wall. The abdominal and spinal muscles contract holding the body erect (see Figure 9–4).

FIGURE 9-4. *With toes and chest touching the wall, tuck in the stomach and pull head away from the wall to strengthen abdominal and spinal muscles.*

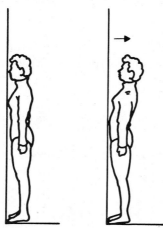

2. Walk sideways as if to get through a narrow space.
3. Standing with the back to the wall, reach both hands as high as possible. Stand on tiptoe and reach high. Lower feet and then arms, but keep back flat against the wall.
4. Play follow the leader with a book or object on the head.

Foot Exercises

1. Pick up marbles with toes and put them in a container.
2. Walk barefoot in the sand.
3. Wrinkle a towel with the toes.
4. Walk on the outside edges of the feet.

Leg Exercises

1. Run in place or around the track.
2. Lift a weight that is secured to the foot (see Figure 9–5).
3. Stand with back against the wall. Slide down the wall into a sitting position. Stay there for thirty seconds to a minute (see Figure 9–6).
4. Stand with back against the wall. Squat down, then slide backside up the wall *first,* straightening the knees (see Figure 9–7). You should feel stretch pains in the back of the legs.

Abdominal Exercises (Lordosis, Weak Abdominal Musculature)

1. Lie on the floor with the feet elevated against the wall for about five minutes. The buttocks should be against the wall also (see Figure 9–8).
2. On hands and knees, rock forward onto the hands and backwards onto the heels (see Figure 9–9).
3. To do the pelvic tilt lie on back, knees bent, and tilt the pelvis until the back is flat on the floor. This exercise may be done also in a standing position.

FIGURE 9-5. *Lift a weight that is securely attached to foot to improve muscle tone in legs.*

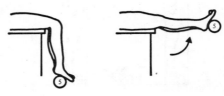

FIGURE 9-6. *Lower body to sitting position with back against the wall to condition legs.*

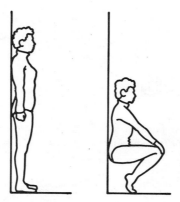

FIGURE 9-7. *To condition legs, squat with back against the wall and then slide backside up the wall as you straighten knees.*

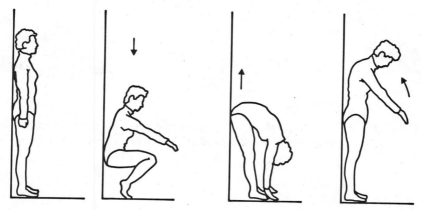

FIGURE 9-8. *Hold this position for five minutes to strengthen abdominal muscles.*

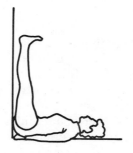

FIGURE 9-9. *To increase abdominal muscle tone, rock back and forth on hands and knees.*

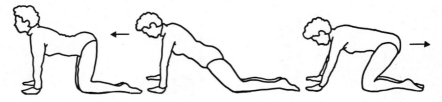

FIGURE 9-10. *Lie on back, knees bent. Tuck chin toward chest and roll to a sitting position to condition abdominal muscles.*

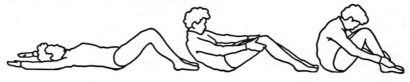

FIGURE 9-11. *Lying down as shown, rotate legs from side to side to exercise abdominal muscles.*

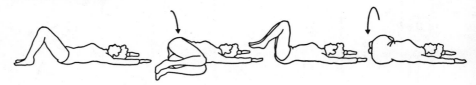

FIGURE 9-12. *To improve abdominal muscle tone, lie down as shown and, keeping knees bent, raise legs off floor and rotate them from side to side.*

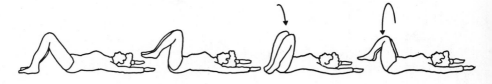

4. Lying on the back with the knees bent, tuck the chin into the shirt collar and *roll* to a sitting position (see Figure 9-10). Arms may be extended in front of the body or folded across the chest. The lower back must stay in a curled position.
5. Lying on the back with knees bent and arms raised beside head in bent position, rotate legs from side to side (see Figure 9-11). Hesitate when the legs come to neutral position so that the abdominal muscles have to work.
6. Lying on the back with knees bent and arms raised beside head in bent position, raise legs and, keeping knees bent, rotate legs from side to side. Keep the shoulders on the mat (see Figure 9-12).

FIGURE 9-13. *To achieve better control over abdominal muscles, lie down as shown, raise one leg and cross it over the other. Repeat with other leg.*

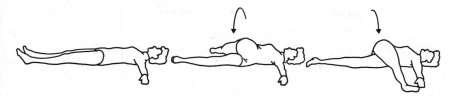

FIGURE 9-14. *Tone trunk muscles by lifting a towel overhead, behind back, and forward to starting position.*

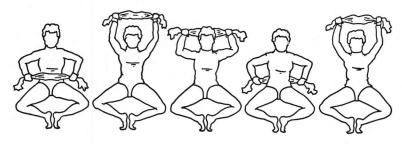

FIGURE 9-15. *To arrest lordosis, lie face down, as shown, and raise head and shoulders while keeping eyes on mat.*

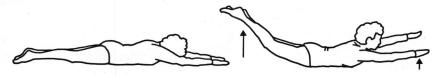

7. Lying on the back with legs extended and the arms next to the head, raise one leg and cross it over the other. Return the leg to starting position and repeat using the other leg (see Figure 9–13).

Trunk Exercises

1. Hang in the stall bars (an apparatus similar to parallel bars).
2. Sitting with legs crossed, grab both ends of a towel with hands. Reaching overhead, pass the towel behind the head and then forward to starting position (see Figure 9–14).
3. Lying on stomach, raise head and shoulders off the mat (see Figure 9–15). Keep eyes on the mat so that the head does not go any higher than the shoulders. This movement prevents the progress of lordosis.
4. Perform exercise 3 over the edge of a table if strong enough to

FIGURE 9-16. *With trunk extended over the edge of a table, raise head and shoulders.*

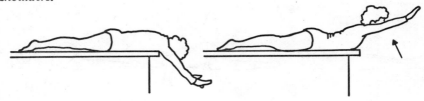

FIGURE 9-17. *Another trunk exercise involves rotating the body to the left and/or right while trunk is extended from the edge of a table.*

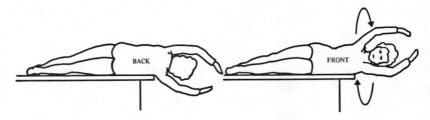

accomplish it (see Figure 9-16). A variation is to rotate the body either to the left or the right or both when fully extended (see Figure 9-17).

PREVENTION OF POSTURAL PROBLEMS

Postural problems usually originate during the early formative years and are most responsive to correction while children are in elementary school. Parents may not notice the subtle changes in a child's posture over a period of months. For this reason, elementary school teachers are the best candidates to watch for and discover postural deviations. Teachers should bring deviations to attention of the school nurse and advise the parents to seek professional consultation.

Elementary school teachers also have an excellent opportunity to effect good attitudes about posture and encourage habits of good posture. With the help of the activities discussed in this chapter, teachers should have no trouble carrying out this responsibility.

RESOURCES

Booklets

The Bad Back Booklet, The Simmons Company, Attention: John Capizzo, 1 Park Avenue, New York, N.Y. 10016. (Illustration of good posture, diet, exercise. Available individually or in classroom quantities.)

Bad Backs and the Mattress (1975), The Simmons Company, 2 Park Avenue, New York, N.Y. 10016.

W.W. Bauer. *Health for All.* Chicago: Scott, Foresman and Co., 1965.

Oliver E. Byrd. *Habits for Health.* Summit, N.Y.: Laidlaw Brothers, 1963. (New Road to Health Series.)

Leslie W. Irwin. *Growing Every Day.* Chicago: Lyons and Carnahan, 1965. (Dimensions in Health Series.)

Charles Lowman. *Postural Fitness–Significances and Variances.* Philadelphia: Lea and Febiger, 1960.

Posture Activity Book B-2, American Chiropractic Association, Sales and Services Department, 2200 Grand Avenue, Des Moines, Ia. 50312. (Coloring book and puzzle page. *One copy free,* extras 25¢ each. For lower grades. Teachers and librarians request on official stationery.)

Posture From the Ground Up, Metropolitan Life, 1 Madison Avenue, New York, N.Y.

Posture Growth Chart B-11, American Chiropractic Association, Sales and Services Department, 2200 Grand Avenue, Des Moines, Ia. 50312. (Norms on height and weight for ages 3–16. *Limit 10 copies free;* 15¢ each. Teachers and librarians request on official stationery.)

C.E. Turner, C. Morley Sellery, and Sara Louise Smith. *School Health and Health Education.* St. Louis: C.V. Mosby Co., 1966.

Maryhelene, Vannier. *Teaching Health in the Elementary Schools.* Philadelphia: Lea and Febiger, 1974.

George M. Wheatley. *Health Observation of School Children.* New York: McGraw-Hill Book Co., 1951.

Carl E. Willgoose. *Health Education in the Elementary School.* Philadelphia: W.B. Saunders Co., 1974.

Films

Our Aching Backs, Sandia Laboratories, Motion Picture Division 3153, P.O. Box 5800, Albuquerque, N.M. 87115. (16mm., sound, color, 14 min. *Free.* Allow 3 weeks for delivery.)

Posture, Encyclopedia Britannica, Inc., Chicago, Ill. 60011.

CHAPTER 10

Physical Fitness

Perhaps one time physical fitness could be taken for granted. It was the natural result of an agrarian life-style that more nearly matched caloric intake with caloric output. Today a life of physical ease has resulted in a sedentary life-style accompanied by a variety of correlated ills, among them obesity and cardiovascular disease. Physical activity, as a planned program and a way of life, is essential today. Physical educators, through their influence on children, have an excellent opportunity to instill habits and attitudes in the young that will ultimately enhance longevity and the quality of their lives.

School physical educators have multiple objectives. In addition to physical fitness, they endeavor to improve the personal-social relations of boys and girls and their recreational and sports competencies. Adequate physical fitness is a vital biological need, the neglect of which handicaps the total effectiveness of the individual. Exercise has an essential role in optimal healthful living. The need for vigorous developmental activities, of course, is greatest for boys and girls who lack basic physical-fitness components, but everyone needs a maintenance program.

PHYSICAL FITNESS VALUES

Physical educators should have a thorough grasp of the values of physical fitness for the following reasons:

1. All children have a basic need for physical fitness. Recognition of this need should stimulate a determination to formulate and conduct a sound and effective physical fitness program for them.
2. Orientation of all pupils to the values of physical fitness should follow. Once pupils have accepted the need for physical fitness in their own lives, they are much more likely to participate wholeheartedly in the exercise regimens planned for them and to exercise when they are not in school.
3. School administrators, boards of education, other teachers, parents, and the public at large should also recognize the need for proper exercise and other practices for the improvement and maintenance of physical fitness. Advantages of such an understanding include widespread support for the physical fitness program employed in physical education, parental encouragement for children to participate fully in the physical fitness activities planned for them, and recognition among parents and the public of their own exercise needs so that they will engage in physical fitness activities on a regular basis. Understanding the value of exercise is essential and powerful motivation for all concerned with the promotion of physical fitness.

Physical traits and physical activity greatly affect the continued well-being and the total effectiveness of all of us. Research demonstrates that an individual acts and reacts as an integral whole, rather than as separate physical, mental, psychological, and social entities. Further, exercise is necessary to maintain organic soundness, reduce body fat, and to sustain athletic competency. Of course, physical fitness alone does not guarantee the optimal functioning of all parts of an individual. Interests, motivation, opportunities, cultural and social backgrounds, economic status, parental influences, and peer mores are also influential factors. For example, a pupil's grades in school may be low because of mediocre intelligence and poor vitality; however, a brilliant mind and ample vitality will not produce high grades if a student lacks motivation and devotes time and energy to other pursuits. Or physically fit children may expend abundant energies toward outstanding leadership on the athletic field, whereby they exert dynamic influence directly upon teammates and indirectly upon the total school population; wrongly applied, however, the energies of physically fit youngsters could be a destructive force if they belonged to a gang devoted to disruptive acts.

Many studies relate physical fitness to various dimensions of the individual's life:

1. Mental achievement: More often than not, studies confirm positive relationships between physical and motor traits and mental achievements. Most of the ones that have played down or denied the existence of a relationship between physical and mental

measures were correlational in nature and ignored the intelligence of the subjects. By contrast, when intelligence is held constant, more studies show positive relationships when only pupils who scored low on physical fitness measures are compared with a control population, or when high and low groups on such tests are compared with each other. Based on available evidence we can conclude that *general learning potential for a given level of intelligence* increases or decreases in accordance with the degree of physical fitness.[1]

2. Personal-social status: According to psychological inventories, peer-status indicators, teacher's assessments, and self-concept instruments, physical and motor traits correspond to certain personal-social characteristics. Generally, boys—and to a smaller extent, girls—who score high on physical/motor tests tend to be extroverted, dominant, sociable, dependable, tolerant, active, and competitive. They are prone to be leaders and popular with their peers. Low scores on the same measures correspond to feelings of insecurity, inferiority, and inadequacy and predict difficulties in social relationships. Rebelliousness, emotional instability, defensiveness, and a negative self-concept also characterized low scorers. When asked to check adjectives that they considered applied to themselves, they chose such words as "sissy," "nervous," "cry-baby," "unhappy," "clumsy," "bossy," and "careless."[2]

3. Organic soundness: Kraus and Raab extensively researched the concept of *hypokinetic disease,* defined as the "whole spectrum of inactivity-induced somatic and mental derangements."[3] Relying on many sources, they maintain that coronary heart disease is twice as prevalent in the sedentary as in the active. Other diseases that are more common among sedentary adults than among active ones are diabetes, ulcers, and other internal conditions. Eighty percent of low back pain is due to lack of adequate physical activity. Lack of physical exercise parallels emotional difficulties. Physically active people show better adaptability to stress, less neuromuscular tension, and greater resistance to fatigue. Active persons age later, do not tend toward absolute or relative overweight, have lower blood pressure, are stronger and more flexible, and have greater breathing capacity.

An overwhelming majority of studies from several countries concur that the more physical activity a person gets, the smaller the risk of coronary heart disease. Regular physical activity does not necessarily prevent a heart attack, but it will make it less likely to occur, and in the event the individual suffers an attack, it lessens its severity and increases the likelihood of survival.[4]

The effects of fitness on blood cholesterol and other such factors are significant. Regimens that exercise the cardiorespiratory system, after a period of time, effect a reduction in serum cholesterol and triglyceride levels, development of collateral circulation around coronary artery restrictions, improvement in blood supply to the heart muscle, increases in number of red blood cells and blood volume, improved clot-dissolving capability, and reduction in blood pressure.[5]

4. Exercise and fat reduction: The internationally renowned nutritionist Jean Mayer has proved that physical inactivity is the single most important explanation for the increasing number of overweight people in modern Western societies. Intensive physical conditioning causes a depletion of excess fat and an increase in lean body weight. Although some studies have demonstrated no appreciable change in body weight, they indicate that body composition did change with a decrease in body fat and a balancing increase in muscular tissue. Obviously, diet and other factors are important in fat reduction, but proper exercise regimens are vital.[6]

5. Motor-athletic abilities: Little doubt exists that the appropriate kind and amount of exercise, consistently employed, will develop muscular strength and endurance, body flexibility, and cardio-respiratory endurance. In fact, properly directed exercise is the only means of acquiring the ability to engage in tasks demanding strong and sustained physical efforts.[7] Athletes in all sports, especially boys, engage in weight training to improve overall body strength and particularly to strengthen muscles that undergo the greatest amount of stress in their respective sports. An increasing number of female athletes are seeking the benefits of weight training. Fear of muscle-bound effects from weight training may be laid to rest: studies predominantly show that weight training enhances, rather than retards, speed of movement.

Physical fitness is not a panacea. Obviously, many other factors contribute significantly to performance. Other things being equal, however, evidence suggests that physical fitness positively affects students' performance.

DEFINITION OF PHYSICAL FITNESS

Before we can consider physical fitness practices and programs, we need a clear definition of physical fitness and a description of its essential components. *Physical fitness* is the ability to carry out daily tasks with vigor and alertness, without undue fatigue, and with ample energy to enjoy leisure-time pursuits and to cope with unusual situations and emergencies. Thus, physical fitness is the ability to last, to bear up, to withstand stress, and to persevere under difficult circumstances in which an unfit person would be ineffective or would quit. The definition implies that physical fitness is more than "not being sick" or merely "being well." It is a positive quality that extends on a continuum from death to abundant life. Thus, all living individuals have some degree of physical fitness. In the severely ill, it is minimal, and in the highly trained athlete, it is maximal. The degree of physical fitness varies considerably from person to person and in the same person from time to time.

Inasmuch as physical fitness is so variable, we can only measure it by breaking it down into measurable components. Assuming a body which is organically sound and free from disease, the basic components that concern physical educators are muscular strength, muscular endurance, and cardiorespiratory endurance. The broader concept of motor fitness includes muscular power, agility, and speed. Inadequate trunk-hip flexibility and marked postural deviations require corrective measures.

The components of physical fitness should determine what tests physical educators use to evaluate physical fitness and should form the basis for designing the curriculum and for the formulating of a physical fitness program for boys and girls in the schools.

APPROACH TO SCHOOL PHYSICAL FITNESS

Since 1961, a basic tenet of the President's Council on Physical Fitness and Sports has been to provide special programs for boys and girls who are "physically underdeveloped," interpreted here as those who fail to meet acceptable standards on the basic physical fitness components. The council has also urged that schools provide special programs for pupils with orthopedic disabilities, postural faults, obesity, malnutrition, perceptual motor difficulties, and other health-related problems. Its recommendations focus on the development of the three basic physical-fitness components (muscular strength, muscular endurance, and cardiorespiratory endurance) and stress the improvement of performance in children who prove to be deficient in one or more of these components. The procedure proposed for conducting physical fitness programs in schools are as follows:

1. Discover boys and girls who are deficient in the basic physical-fitness components by use of valid tests.
2. For those who demonstrate deficiencies, provide appropriate exercises.
3. Identify the cause or causes of the subfit condition among children who show unsatisfactory improvement on retests.
4. Enlist the help of other specialists, such as the physician, guidance personnel, and school nurse, when physical defects, organic le-

sions, personality maladjustments, or nutritional disturbances are evident.
5. Conduct maintenance physical fitness activities for students who meet physical fitness standards.
6. Check physical fitness status periodically in order to make individual program adjustments when indicated.

Physical Fitness Testing

Every teacher knows that in a typical group of elementary school-children the physical capabilities vary widely. Each classroom has a star athlete who seems to outperform the other children and an aesthetic little playground recluse who dreads recess time. Yet there are some norms that indicate whether the "outstanding" child is really fit or just at the head of a whole class of misfits.

Testing physical ability because it is fashionable to do so and then filing away the results is pointless. Test results should be the basis of an effective and efficiently run physical fitness program. The real value of testing is that it enables physical educators to serve children better than would otherwise be possible. To be sure, test results have other uses, for example, reports to administrators, boards of education, parents, and the public. Test results may also serve to convince pupils of their physical fitness status and to motivate those who are deficient in basic components to participate fully in programs planned for them.

Table 10–1 suggests some exercise tests for elementary school-children. If school physical educators accept muscular strength, muscular endurance, and cardiorespiratory endurance as basic physical-fitness components, then these are the components they should measure. The following paragraphs describe some of the tests that educators can use to evaluate these components.

Muscular Strength

If we define strength as the tension a muscle or muscle group can apply in a single maximum contraction, only one battery of strength tests is available—the Oregon Cable-tension Tests.[8] A cable-tension strength test consists of a maximal pull on a light cable while a tensionmeter records the tension applied. Three-item batteries with norms are available for boys and girls separately at the upper-elementary, junior high, senior high, and college levels. Two-battery measures are the Strength Composite, a gross strength score obtained by adding the individual strength scores, and the Strength Quotient, a relative strength score obtained by relating the Strength Composite to a norm. The purpose of using the Strength Quotient is to

TABLE 10-1. Fitness Tests for Elementary School Children

Name	Grade	Items	Source
AAHPER Youth Fitness Test	5-College	Pull-ups, Sit-ups Shuttle run Standing broad jump 50-yd. dash Softball throw 600-yd. run-walk	AAHPER Washington, D.C.
New York State Physical Fitness Test	4-12	Posture test Target throw Modified push-up Side-step 50-yd. dash Squat stand Treadmill	New York State Education Dept. Albany, N.Y.
North Carolina Fitness Test	4-12	Sit-ups Side stepping Standing broad jump Pull-ups Squat thrust	Dept. of Public Instruction Raleigh, N.C.
State of Washington Physical Fitness Test for Elementary School Children	Ages 6-12	Standing broad jump Bench push-ups Curl-ups Squat jump 30-yd. dash	State Office of Public Instruction Olympia, Wash.

Test	Grades/Ages	Items	Source
Tulsa Elementary Physical Fitness Test	4-6	25-50-yd. dash Pull-ups Zigzag run Sit and reach Sit-ups Standing broad jump Softball throw Side-step 300-600-yd. walk-run	Supervisor of Elementary Education in Public Schools Tulsa, Okla.
Glover Physical Fitness Items	Ages 6-9	Seal walk Shuttle run Standing broad jump Sit-ups	Barrow et al, *Measurement in Physical Education* (Philadelphia: Lea and Febiger, 1964)
Amateur Athletic Union Physical Fitness Proficiency Test	1-12	Sprint-walk-run Sit-ups Pull-ups Push-ups Standing broad jump Baseball throw Continuous hike for distance Running high jump	AAU 231 W. 58th St. New York, N.Y.
Modified Junior Fitness and Proficiency Test of the Amateur Athletic Union of the United States			AAU 233 Broadway New York, N.Y.

identify boys and girls who are muscularly weak for their sex, age, and weight.

Muscular Strength and Endurance

A test that has had considerable use in schools and colleges for evaluating muscular strength and endurance is Rogers' Physical Fitness Index (PFI). The PFI battery consists of four muscular strength tests (right and left grips, back and leg lifts), two muscular endurance tests (pull-ups, push-ups), and lung capacity. The Strength Index is a gross score obtained by adding all tests. The PFI is derived by dividing the achieved Strength Index by a norm based on sex, age, and weight. A score of 100 is considered average; scores of 85 and 115 mark the first and third quartiles, respectively.[9] The Oregon simplification reduces the number of test items;[10] by use of a formula, you can predict the full Strength Index and use the norms to predict the PFI.

Cardiorespiratory Endurance

In the research laboratory, very sophisticated tests of cardiorespiratory endurance are possible. These include maximum oxygen uptake, electromyography, blood sample analyses, and heartometer-tracing evaluations. In schools, where large numbers of subjects require examination, these tests are not practical for routine use. Therefore physical educators have based their cardiorespiratory evaluations on endurance running and bench stepping. Endurance runs are more prevalent. Commonly in use are timed runs for a given distance (e.g., 600-yard run-walk) and distance covered in a given time (twelve-minute run).[11] The 600-yard run-walk has been part of the AAHPER Youth Fitness Tests since they began; in the current version runs for nine and twelve minutes may be substituted.[12] Evidence indicates that the longer runs have greater aerobic involvement.

Motor Fitness Tests

Motor fitness tests measure several components, including muscular endurance, cardiorespiratory endurance, speed, agility, and muscular power. This is by far the most prevalent form of fitness testing in the schools, largely because teachers can administer them to large numbers of students in a short time with minimal equipment and testing expertise. Several states have produced such tests for use in their schools. Among the prominent state tests are the California Physical Performance Tests, the Indiana Motor Fitness Test, the New York State Physical Fitness Test, the North Carolina Fitness Test, the Oregon Motor Fitness Test, and the Washington Motor Fitness Test. In addition, several colleges have their own motor fitness tests, and the armed forces have used them since the time of World War II.

The motor fitness test most widely used in schools throughout the country is the AAHPER Youth Fitness Test, which originated in 1958 and was revised most recently in 1975.[13] The 1975 battery consists of six items:

1. Pull-ups for boys, bent-arm hang for girls
2. Bent-knee sit-ups for one minute
3. 40-yard shuttle run
4. Standing broad jump
5. 50-yard dash
6. 600-yard run or runs of 1 mile or nine minutes for ages 10–12 and 1.5 miles or twelve minutes for ages 13 and over

The President's Council on Physical Fitness and Sports has officially incorporated this test, which has national percentile norms, in its motivational and evaluative processes. The test items form the basis for the Presidential Physical Fitness Award, which over two million boys and girls have won since its inception in 1966. To earn an award, a child must score at or above 85 percentile on all tests.

At the beginning of the school year pupils should take a screening test. Each six weeks thereafter they should repeat the tests they failed until they can pass them. The tests should measure levels of cardiorespiratory endurance, muscular endurance, and agility. Three of four recommended tests are: pull-ups for boys and flexed-arm hang for girls, knee-bent sit-ups for one minute, and squat thrusts for ten seconds. The fourth item is a *Recovery Index Test,* which measures heart-rate recovery following stepping up and down on a bench thirty times per minute for four minutes; the height of the bench varies from fourteen to sixteen to twenty inches, depending on the height of the subjects.[14]

Another convenient test with norms appears in Appendix B. The test items given provide a good standard for individual and group comparisons and they are easy to use.

DEVELOPMENTAL PROGRAMS

As in the selection of tests, the choice of physical activities for the physical fitness program should center primarily on those that will improve students' muscular strength, muscular endurance, and cardiorespiratory endurance.

Muscular Strength and Endurance

To develop muscular strength and muscular endurance, physical activities should offer strong resistance to the muscles. Four categories of strength-development exercises are:

1. Resistance supplied by parts of the body, as in calisthenics, football "grass" drills, "guerilla" exercises, Danish drills, and the like
2. Resistance supplied by inanimate objects, as in weight training, log drills, relays and races carrying weights or another person, and so forth
3. Resistance applied by body weight, as in chinning, push-ups, use of traveling rings and peg boards, rope climbing, exercises on the horse, horizontal bar, and parallel bars, and others
4. Resistance applied by another individual, as in wrestling, tug-of-war, and various pulls and pushes, hand wrestling, and other contests

Several principles influence the effectiveness of exercise used to improve muscle strength and endurance. They are:

1. Developing the strength of the total musculature requires a systematic involvement of all large-muscle groups, since pronounced specificity of strength among the muscle groups of the body exists.
2. The isotonic form of muscular conditioning, which combines muscle interaction with movement of the body parts, is preferable to the isometric form, which produces muscle tension but involves no movement. Isotonic exercise is the better form for developing muscular strength and is superior at improving muscular endurance. Further, motivation is greater, because the participant can watch the procedure and explicit goals are easier to set.
3. The use of progressive resistance exercise (PRE), especially weight training, has much to commend it in the development of strength and endurance. Research supports the following PRE principles: for strength, use heavy weights with few repetitions; for endurance, use lighter weights with many repetitions.
4. In an experimental application of the overload principle to resistance exercises, Hellebrandt and Houtz concluded that: strength and endurance increase as a result of performing repetitive exercise against heavy resistance; mere repetition of contractions that place little stress on the neuromuscular system have little effect on the functional capacity of the skeletal muscle; and the amount of

work done per unit of time is the critical variable upon which extension of the limits of performance depend.[15]

5. Williams found that junior high school girls participating in a rope-climbing conditioning program improved significantly on four arm and shoulder girdle strength tests and that a group training with the bent-arm hand did nearly as well because they improved significantly on three of the strength tests. A push-up training group bettered scores on one strength test, but a control group showed no gains on any test.[16]

6. In a study by MacIntyre, college women who participated in progressive weight training improved their body contours—as indicated by reductions in five skin-fold and four girth measures—. much more than did women who performed calisthenic-type exercises.[17]

Cardiorespiratory Endurance

Cardiorespiratory endurance results from moderate contractions of muscle groups for relatively long periods of time, during which maximal adjustments of the cardiorespiratory system are necessary. This physical fitness component is most complex, as the number of elements of the cardiorespiratory systems affected by this form of exercise makes obvious. They include the heart and lungs, the vessels that supply blood to all parts of the body, the oxygen-carrying capacity of that blood, and the capillary system, which dispenses blood to the tissues. Other body systems that benefit from such exercise are the muscles, the digestion-absorption-elimination processes, the internal secretion glands, the bones, bone-marrow production of red blood corpuscles, and the brain.

The basic forms of exercise that help to develop cardiorespiratory endurance involve self-propulsion of the body over a distance. The propulsion should be sufficiently severe and prolonged to require a definite adjustment of the circulation and respiration. Particularly desirable for school use are running (including jogging) and swimming, since these exercises are reasonably easy to control. In other words, physical educators can specify distance, speed, and duration to accommodate the exercise tolerance of the individual; provide overload; and plan progression. Activities such as vigorous walking, rope skipping, skiing, and skating have similar values. Many sports have a high endurance potential, including soccer, basketball, handball, hockey, and other sports requiring sustained running. Sufficient skill in a sport is necessary to permit endurance development. For the *unfit* sports participant, some caution is advisable to insure that the competitive element does not lead to overexertion.

A few observations regarding cardiorespiratory training are noteworthy:

1. Continuous running, interval training, bicycle riding, walking, swimming, bench stepping, and Cureton's progressive rhythmical nonstop exercises combining jogging and calisthenics[18] provide effective cardiorespiratory training, when practiced properly.
2. As would be expected, the benefits of cardiorespiratory endurance exercise are dependent on their intensity, duration, and frequency. When these three factors are the same, a variety of training modes produce similar results.
   a. Pollack, Cureton, and Greninger formed two groups that participated in the same program of running, jogging, and walking with increased intensity as adaptation occurred. One group exercised twice a week and the other group trained four times a week.[19] The latter group experienced greater improvement in working capacity, cardiovascular fitness, and body composition. In a study by Franks, five days of training per week produced greater improvement on cardiorespiratory measures than did three days, as a result of participation in Cureton's low- and middle-gear exercise sessions.[20]
   b. In a duration study by Toshi, running regimens were the same for three groups, but the lengths of daily participation varied from 15 to 30 to 45 minutes.[21] The 15-minute group improved only in running time. The other groups improved not only in the same runs but also on several cardiovascular measures. Furthermore, the 45-minute group was the only one to significantly reduce serum cholesterol and body fat. In a bench-stepping study by Faria, subjects exercised with one of three groups, based on the length of time necessary to reach pulse rates per minute of 120–130, 140–150, and 160–170. The results showed that only training regimens requiring 140 beats per minute improved the efficiency of the oxygen transport system.[22]
3. In a study by Knuttgen et al., individual improvement proved to be inversely related to initial fitness (i.e., the lower the level at the start of training, the greater the increase in cardiorespiratory endurance for a given training program).[23]

It is apparent, then, that as little as 15 minutes of regular, appropriate exercise will produce minimal cardiorespiratory endurance benefits. Longer periods of 30 and 45 minutes are more beneficial, not only in terms of endurance but also in terms of desirable cardiovascular and body-composition changes and cholesterol reduction. The application of proper principles of exercise is essential for effective results.

PRINCIPLES OF EXERCISE

Although everyone should observe sensible principles of exercise, they are especially important for *sedentary* children, youth, and adults who embark on physical fitness programs. The following principles are applicable to both strength-building and cardiorespiratory activities.

1. *Exercise should be appropriate to the individual's exercise tolerance. Exercise tolerance* refers to the ability of an individual to execute a given exercise, series of exercises, or activities involving exercise at a specified level without undue discomfort or fatigue. An exercise regimen that is easy for the person falls short of exercise tolerance; on the other hand, an exercise that either is impossible to perform or leaves the individual in severe distress exceeds a reasonable interpretation of exercise tolerance.

2. *Overloading is essential to induce a higher level of performance.* In overloading, the individual's exercise increases in intensity or extends over a longer time than normally. *Overload* is a relative term: a slight overload exceeds usual activity to a small degree, whereas the greatest overload equals the person's exercise tolerance at the moment.

3. *The exercise plan should provide for progression.* Progression relates to the first two principles. The exercise plan starts with an understanding of the individual's exercise tolerance. Then, within this tolerance range, an exercise regimen begins by overloading the muscles to develop strength or increasing the demands on the cardiorespiratory system to improve endurance. If the exercise regimen stopped after the individual reached these initial goals, some improvement in fitness components would result, but there would be no further improvement once the body had adjusted to the new requirements in output; both normal and exercise tolerance levels have risen. Progression increases exercise in a logical way and thus keeps its demands ahead of the improvement made. Progression requires increasing the intensity and duration of exercise.

4. *Individuals must desire to improve.* The desire to be fit is an essential factor if students are to improve their fitness status. Every effort should be made to secure their full cooperation, for the effectiveness of any exercise regimen depends on the degree of the individual's voluntary participation in it. First on the list of essential steps in this process is to provide a thorough understanding of the importance of physical fitness in the person's daily and future life as suggested earlier in this chapter.

5. *Advance the unfit individual's psychological limits of effort.* Many who are unaccustomed to physical exertion may reach their

psychological tolerance for exercise well before attaining their physiological limits. Psychological limits may be attributable to habit, boredom, slight aches, breathlessness, and mental factors, such as anxiety and fear of physical harm. Such mildly distressful feelings halt exercise before appreciable overloading has occurred. Consequently, only minimal increases in strength and endurance result. Increasing psychological limits requires some judgment since certain associated factors also serve as safeguards in the prevention of excess strain. A progressive approach to exercise dosage will help individuals gradually to accept strenuous exercise and realize their true limits.

6. *Physical development should be tested and recorded.* A number of the exercise activities frequently included in physical fitness programs, such as sit-ups, push-ups, weightlifting, and cumulative-distance jogging, are self-testing. To formalize self-testing instructors can provide individual progress charts, upon which everyone can periodically record their performance. Individual progress charts may include physical/motor fitness measures to be repeated periodically. These charts can have excellent motivational values.

In some of the studies reviewed above, daily physical education in the schools proved to be superior to fewer days per week in improving basic physical fitness components. The cardiorespiratory endurance studies by Pollock, Cureton, and Grenninger[24] and Franks[25] demonstrated this advantage. Hanson[26] reported that the five-day-a-week program resulted in a significantly higher degree of physical fitness among children than did the three-day-a-week program on nearly all test items. During the school year 1969–70, a significant research project examined the effectiveness of daily physical education in developing physical fitness as contrasted with various methods of flexible scheduling in twelve California schools.[27] The results supported a daily physical education requirement. In all events except the mile run differences in performance were significant. Eighty-three percent of these differences favored the daily program.

FITNESS FOR UNFIT CHILDREN

It is desirable to improve the status of "underdeveloped" children, those whose performance falls below accepted standards in basic physical fitness components. Pupils at all levels of fitness need maintenance programs, but the needs of the unfit demand careful attention.

In the late 1920s the New York state director of physical education, Frederick Rand Rogers, proposed and promoted a program for physically unfit boys and girls that would use his Physical Fitness Index as the evaluative instrument. Since the implementation of this program variations have come into use across the United States, including Massachusetts, Oregon, and Washington. Based on the logical assumption that physical unfitness may be due to causes other than the lack of the proper kind and amount of exercise—although this is the most frequent cause—this program also acknowledges that physical fitness tests provide generalized indices and are not diagnostic. In this respect, they are comparable to clinical thermometer readings by a physician; a high thermometer reading indicates that the individual has a fever and thus tells the physician that something is wrong without revealing what that something is. In like manner, a low physical-fitness score calls attention to a deficient condition, but it does not specify what is causing that deficiency.

Like the patient with a fever, who needs medical diagnosis and prescription, the unfit require examination to determine the cause of the condition, especially if they fail to improve or do not improve appreciably after participating in an appropriate exercise regimen. One approach to the problems of physically underdeveloped boys and girls comes from Clarke and Clarke. The full realization of the program involves the following steps:*

1. Discover boys and girls with special deficiencies revealed by medical, nutritional, and psychological tests and examinations. An adequate health appraisal is needed for any physical fitness program.
2. Select those who are below predetermined standards of strength, stamina, and other basic physical fitness elements through the administration of valid tests available to the physical educator.
3. For the subfit group, conduct physical activities selected to improve their condition, especially related to muscular strength, muscular endurance, and circulatory-respiratory endurance. Apply proper principles of exercise in their conduct.
4. After six weeks, retest the subfit group in order to determine progress or lack of adequate progress. For students who improve at a satisfactory rate, their exercise regimens should continue with progressive increase in dosage until fitness standards are reached or, preferably, exceeded.
5. Identify the cause or causes of the subfit condition for those who do not improve scores satisfactorily on retests. These causes may be located by use of case-study procedures, living-habit surveys, personal interviews, and supplementary tests. Field experience has shown that approximately 10–15 percent of subfit students fall in this category.
6. Refer to other specialists, such as the physician, school nurse, or guidance

---

*H. Harrison Clarke, David H. Clarke, *Developmental and Adapted Physical Education,* 2nd edition, © 1978, pp. 168–169. Reprinted by permission of Prentice-Hall, Inc., Englewood Cliffs, N.J.

personnel, when physical defects, organic lesions, personality maladjustments, or nutritional disturbances are encountered or suspected as a
result of the case-study processes. Actually, case-study procedures should
be instituted after initial physical fitness tests in some instances, as in the
case of obese boys and girls or other easily recognized atypical conditions.

7. Provide individually planned physical fitness programs utilizing the following as appropriate in each case: Proper kind and amount of exercise,
   health guidance, relaxation procedures, methods and activities applied
   to improve social and psychological adjustment, and medical attention.

8. Relate all factors accumulated in the case study to the individual's soma-
   totype, mental aptitude, and scholastic success. These may be related, so
   an understanding of the configuration of the total person is desirable.

9. Repeat physical fitness tests at intervals of about six weeks in order to
   continue checking on the progress made by each subfit boy and girl.

10. Redirect programs in individual cases as found desirable in the light of
    retest and restudy results.

These procedures should not preclude the participation of unfit
children in the regular activities of physical education. Except
for those whose doctors have restricted exercise for medical reasons,
unfit individuals should participate in the regular physical education
program, for they need to learn the skills and to benefit from the
social opportunities of the full physical-education experience.
Emphasis on their physical fitness needs should be primary, however,
until their fitness status has adequately improved.

THE ROLE OF THE HOME IN PHYSICAL FITNESS

Ideally, the family setting will provide a good experience in physical
activity and will motivate children to be active in a variety of sports
and games. Homework assignments requiring the direct involvement
of family members in group activities may be as healthy for the
family unit as for the student. Survey families about leisure time
activities and parent opinion and publish the results. Bestowing
special awards and recognition to families (in PTA, newsnotes, etc.)
and children who successfully involve each other in fitness programs
is another effective way of securing family interest. Still another
is to conduct a parents' night so that students can demonstrate
their skills. Opening school facilities for a weekly family sports night
promotes awareness and appreciation for joint activity. Providing
fitness instruction for parents is another positive approach..

NOTES

1. *Physical Fitness Research Digest,* October 1971, pp. 1-2.
2. *Physical Fitness Research Digest,* January 1972, p. 5.

3. Hans Kraus and Wilhelm Raab, *Hypokinetic Disease* (Springfield, Ill.: Charles C. Thomas, 1961), p. 8.

4. *Physical Fitness Research Digest*, April 1972, p. 9.

5. *Physical Fitness Research Digest*, July 1972, p. 7, and October 1972, p. 1.

6. *Physical Fitness Research Digest*, April 1975, p. 4.

7. *Physical Fitness Research Digest*, October 1974, pp. 2–3.

8. H. Harrison Clarke and Richard A. Munroe, *Oregon Cable-tension Strength Test Batteries for Boys and Girls from Fourth Grade Through College* (Eugene, Ore.: Microform Publications, University of Oregon, 1970).

9. H. Harrison Clarke, *Application of Measurement to Health and Physical Education* (Englewood Cliffs, N.J.: Prentice-Hall, 1976), chap. 7. Donald K. Mathews, *Measurement in Physical Education* (Philadelphia: W.B. Saunders Co., 1973), chap. 4.

10. Clarke, p. 142.

11. Kenneth H. Cooper, *The New Aerobics* (New York: M. Evans and Co., 1970). Mildred Cooper and Kenneth H. Cooper *Aerobics for Woman* (New York: M. Evans and Co., 1972).

12. *AAHPER Youth Fitness Test Manual* (Washington, D.C.: American Alliance for Health, Physical Education, and Recreation, 1975).

13. Ibid.

14. President's Council on Physical Fitness and Sports, *Youth Physical Fitness: Suggestions for School Programs* (Washington, D.C.: U.S. Government Printing Office, 1973), p. 4.

15. F.A. Hellebrandt and Sara Jane Houtz, "Mechanisms of Muscle Training in Man: Experimental Demonstration of the Overload Principle," *Physical Therapy Review* 36 (June 1956): 371.

16. *Physical Fitness Research Digest*, April 1975.

17. Christine MacIntyre, "Effect of a Weight Training Program on Body Contours of Young Women 18-22," Master's thesis, University of California, Los Angeles, 1967.

18. Thomas K. Cureton and L.F. Sterling, "Factor Analysis of Cardiovascular Test Variables," *Journal of Sports Medicine and Physical Fitness* 4 (March 1964): 1.

19. Michael L. Pollack, Thomas K. Cureton, and Leonard Greninger, "Effects of Frequency of Training on Working Capacity, Cardiovascular Function, and Body Composition," *Medicine and Science in Sports* 1 (June 1969): 70.

20. Don B. Franks, "Effects of Different Types and Amounts of Training on Selected Fitness Measures," in *Exercise and Fitness–1969*, ed. B.D. Franks (Chicago: The Athletic Institute, 1969), p. 293.

21. *Physical Fitness Research Digest*, October 1972.

22. Irvin E. Faria, "Cardiovascular Response to Exercise as Influenced by Training of Various Intensities," *Research Quarterly* 41 (March 1970): 44.

23. H.G. Knuttgen et al., "Physical Conditioning Through Interval Training," *Medicine and Science in Sports* 5 (Winter 1973): 220.

24. *Physical Fitness Research Digest*, January 1972.

25. Franks, p. 293.

26. Margie Hanson, *A Comparison of the Effects of a Five-day-a-week Versus a Three-day-a-week Physical Education Program on Achievement Scores of Sixth Grade Children in the Youth Fitness Test Battery* (Margie Hanson 1964).

27. "California Proves Daily Physical Education Best," University of Oregon *Physical Fitness News Letter* 18 (November 1971): 1. "Flexible Scheduling Applied to Physical Education," University of Oregon *Physical Fitness News Letter* 18 (December 1971): 2. John J. Klumb and Stan LeProtti, *Evaluation of the Effects of Flexible Scheduling on Physical Education* (Sacramento, Calif.: California Bureau of Health Education, Physical Education, Athletics, and Recreation, 1971), p. 3. "More on California Scheduling Research," University of Oregon *Physical Fitness News Letter* 18 (December 1971): 1.

RESOURCES

Books and Pamphlets

American Association for Health, Physical Education, and Recreation. *Exercise and Fitness.* Washington, D.C.: American Association for HPER, 1972.

American Association for Health, Physical Education, and Recreation. *Special Fitness Test Manual.* Washington, D.C.: American Association for HPER, 1968.

American Association for Health, Physical Education, and Recreation. *Youth Fitness Test Manual.* Washington, D.C.: American Association for HPER, 1976.

C. Corbin et al., *Concept in Physical Education.* Dubuque, Iowa: William C. Brown and Co., 1970.

P. Metzger. *Elementary School Physical Education: A Book of Readings.* Dubuque, Iowa: William C. Brown and Co., 1972.

E.C. Olson. *Conditioning Fundamentals.* Columbus, O.: Charles E. Merrill Books, 1968.

The Editors of Time-Life Books. *The Healthy Life.* New York: Time, 1966.

E. Wallis and G. Logan. *Exercise for Children.* Englewood Cliffs, N.J.: Prentice-Hall, 1966.

President's Council on Physical Fitness. *Youth Physical Fitness.* Washington, D.C.: U.S. Government Printing Office, 1973. (Contains physical-fitness screening tests, conditioning exercises. Illustrated.)

Films

The Time of Our Lives (16mm., color, sound, 28 min.). Association Films, 600 Madison Avenue, New York, N.Y. 10022. (Free.)

Youth Physical Fitness: A Report to the Nation (16 mm., color, sound, 28 min.). Equitable Life Assurance Company, 1285 Avenue of the Americas, New York, N.Y. 10019. (Free.)

Youth Physical Fitness—A Basic School Program (16 mm., color or black and white, sound, 13 min.). President's Council on Physical Fitness, Washington, D.C.

Vigorous Physical Fitness Activities, President's Council on Physical Fitness, Washington, D.C. (16 mm., color or black and white, sound, 13 min.)

Your Child's Health and Fitness, American Association for Health, Physical Education, and Recreation, 1201 16th St. N.W., Washington, D.C. 20036. (16 min., color filmstrip, 33⅓ rpm record.)

Evaluating Physical Fitness. The Athletic Institute, Room 805, Merchandise Mart, Chicago, Ill.

CHAPTER 11
Childhood Nutrition

The purpose of this chapter is threefold. First, it provides background information about the essentials of good nutrition. Second, it explains what is now known about childhood undernutrition, learning, and behavior. Finally, this chapter will help teachers understand and deal with problems of overnutrition (obesity).

Even though elementary-age schoolchildren have had considerable experience with food before they enter school, going to school marks the beginning of their nutritional emancipation. Teachers are in a position to help students make wise decisions about their nutrition as well as develop habits that will result in a healthy life-style. A highly recommended reference for teachers is a nutrition teaching package entitled *Food—Your Choice,* an excellent learning system produced by the National Dairy Council. Although this chapter will introduce teachers to nutrition, the National Dairy Council's materials provide background information, visuals, class handouts, and so on for classroom use.

Dr. Jean Mayer, a world-famous nutritionist, summarizes some of the main nutritional needs of the elementary-age child in the following suggestions:

1. There is no special nutritional virtue in eating at particular times during the day. Children, however, should not be expected to play or study all

morning without food. If they will eat a good breakfast, give it to them. Otherwise, prepare a nutritious midmorning snack to eat at home or at school.

2. Children's physical activity varies widely from day to day, so expect that on some days youngsters will eat more than on others.

3. Don't force a child to finish everything on his or her plate. This may push him or her toward overweight. Teach children to take helpings small enough that they are sure to eat them. Seconds, if wanted, will be requested.

4. Give children some say in the planning of menus, but don't cater excessively to their whims. Allow them to replace foods they dislike with other foods in the same category. But don't let them force a lot of additional work on you. Try to develop their taste for a great variety of foods.

5. Don't let them pass up the nutritious main course and then gorge themselves on dessert. One way to prevent that is just not to serve high-calorie, low-nutrient desserts. Instead, use fruit as much as possible.

6. There is nothing wrong with snacks for children; just be sure that they're nutritious. A good sandwich is vastly preferable to a piece of cake; a glass of skim milk or fruit juice is always preferable to a soft drink. High-fat or high-sugar snack foods give very poor value, both from the viewpoint of your pocketbook and of child nutrition.

7. Children need ample vitamin D or they get rickets. They can obtain enough of it if they drink vitamin D-enriched milk or get plenty of sunshine or take a vitamin supplement.

8. The prevalence of overweight among children is increasing. It is linked much more closely to underexercising than to overeating. When overweight children are compared to those of normal weight, the extra calories going to fat come much more frequently from physical inactivity than from consuming too much food. Get your children to exercise every day. If possible, get them to walk to school. If not, perhaps they can walk part of the way. Get them to cultivate those sports such as hiking, tennis and swimming which they can take part in all their lives. Don't drive them to places they could reach by walking or bicycling. And make sure they get plenty of activity during the weekend.[1]

In brief, the rule for children's nutrition is: plenty of variety, whenever they're hungry—whether at breakfast, midmorning, midafternoon, or bedtime. While a child's appetite is still uncorrupted by social pressures, fads, weight consciousness, the eight-hour workday, and other forces, it is easy to take good nutritional advantage of it.[2]

BASIC NUTRITION[3]

Food is more than something to eat. In this land of plenty, millions of Americans are not eating wisely, not because they lack enough to eat, but because they eat too much of the wrong things or too little of the right ones. Food is what you eat, but nutrition is how the body uses food. Children whose diets do not meet body needs may be suffering from poor nutrition.

Few people have a basic understanding of nutrition. Literally, "You are what you eat." Protein, carbohydrates, fats, vitamins, minerals, and water are all essential to human life. They nourish the body. Not all foods contain these nutrients, and not all nutrients serve the same purpose in the body. It is important to remember that no one food does everything and no one food provides all of the nutrients we need. A variety of different types of foods is necessary for all the nutrients most of us need.

Protein

Next to water, proteins are the most abundant substance in body cells. They perform almost endless functions in the body and also account for the tough, fibrous nature of hair, nails, and ligaments, as well as the structure of muscles. They are components of hemoglobin, which transports oxygen in the blood; insulin, which regulates blood sugar; enzymes, which control the speed of chemical reactions in the body, including digestion; and hormones, which regulate growth. For building and maintaining body tissues proteins, or *amino acids,* are essential, and they help make up deoxyribonucleic acid (DNA), which controls the genetic code and thus all hereditary characteristics in body cells.

Eight of the many different amino acids are called *essential* since body tissues cannot manufacture them. The diet must supply them. Each protein has a unique essential amino acid content. Those proteins that contain a large amount of the essential amino acids are said to have a high nutritional value. Those that lack any of the essential amino acids or have insignificant amounts of one or more of them have a low, or poor, nutritional value. In general, foods of animal origin, including eggs, meats, fish, poultry, and milk, contain proteins of better nutritional value than foods of plant origin. But a diet that contains both animal and plant proteins is nutritionally acceptable and economically more practical. In fact, with careful planning, plants can provide proper protein intake.

The body's demand for proteins is greatest when the body is building new tissues rapidly, as it is during infancy and pregnancy and when a mother is nursing a child. A need for extra protein also follows excessive destruction or loss of body protein from hemorrhage, burns, surgery, infections, and so on. Contrary to popular belief, except for the small amount of protein necessary for developing muscles during conditioning, people engaged in sports and other strenuous physical activities do not need increased protein, provided their diets supply enough calories from carbohydrates and fats to meet their energy needs.

Common sources of protein, arranged in descending order of approximate nutritive value, are eggs, milk and cheese, meats, fish, poultry, soybeans, beans and peas, grains and cereals, and nuts. The last six foods mentioned (and vegetable proteins, in general) provide a better nutritive value when consumed in combination with animal proteins, for instance, cereal with milk, chili beans with meat, and macaroni with cheese. By consuming a mixture of foods that contain both animal and plant proteins at each meal, we are more likely to secure all the essential amino acids. See Table 11–1 for a list of the functions and food sources of the essential nutrients.

Carbohydrates

The major function of carbohydrates in the diet is to provide energy for the work of the body. They also enable the body to manufacture some of the B-complex vitamins and they contribute to the structure of many other biological compounds. In addition, carbohydrates add flavor to our food.

Carbohydrates are economical to produce in abundance, a characteristic that helps a majority of the people in the world to survive. In the United States and Canada, carbohydrates provide 40 to 50 percent of the total food intake; the entire population of the world obtains about 70 percent of its intake in the form of carbohydrates. The cereal grains (e.g., wheat, rice, corn, and oats), potatoes, many fruits and vegetables, peas, beans, taro, and sugar cane and sugar beets are major sources of the world's carbohydrates. Many processed foods, including breads and other baked goods, jams and jellies, candy, soft drinks, molasses, noodles, spaghetti, and dried fruits, are also rich in carbohydrates.

When the body receives more carbohydrates than it needs to function normally, it converts the excess into fat and stores it in fatty tissues. Thus, eating more starchy foods and sweets than are sufficient to supply the energy requirement for daily activities may lead to obesity. A regular diet that is high in refined sugar (candy, jam, etc.) may encourage the formation of cavities in the teeth of growing children.

Fats

The fats in our diet serve a variety of functions. We need to consume some fat to get linoleic acid, which is necessary for proper growth and healthy skin, but the amount necessary is quite small—about 1 to 2 percent of the total calories consumed. The unsaturated fatty acids that provide linoleic acid occur particularly in liquid vegetable oils such as corn, cottonseed, peanut, and soybean oil and in many

TABLE 11-1. Summary of Essential Nutrients

Essential Nutrients	Function in the Body	Food Sources	Comments
Protein	Required for growth, maintenance, and repair of body tissues. Helps to make hemoglobin, form antibodies to fight infection, and supply energy.	Meat, poultry, fish, eggs, milk, cheese, soybeans, beans, peas, grains, and nuts.	Foods of animal origin contain protein of better nutritional value than foods of plant origin.
Carbohydrates (starches, sugars, and celluloses)	Starches and sugars are major sources of energy for internal and external work and for maintenance of body temperature. Celluloses furnish bulk.	Grains (wheat, oats, corn, rice) and grain products (flour, bread, cereal, macaroni, etc.), sugar, jams and jellies, candy, soft drinks, honey, and most fruits and vegetables.	The body converts excess carbohydrates in diet into fat and stores them.
Fats	Concentrated source of energy. Carry fat-soluble vitamins and help body to use them. Also make up part of cell structure, cushion vital organs. Some contain linoleic acid, believed to be essential to health.	Butter, margarine, cooking and salad oils, cream, most cheeses, bacon, fatty meats and—to some extent—whole milk, eggs, chocolate, and most meat.	Unsaturated fat, or linoleic acid, is present in most vegetable oils. Poultry and fish oils contain more than other animal fats.
Vitamins Vitamin A	Important for skeletal growth and normal tooth structure. Necessary for healthy mucous membranes in mouth, nose, throat, and digestive and urinary tracts. Essential for night vision.	Fish-liver oils, liver, butter, cream, milk, cheese, egg yolk, dark green and yellow vegetables, yellow fruits, and fortified margarine.	Fat soluble. Destroyed by oxidation and very high temperatures.

Vitamin	Function	Sources	Properties
Vitamin B_1 (thiamine)	Necessary to convert sugar and starches into energy.	Pork, liver, heart, kidney, milk, yeast, whole-grain and enriched cereals and breads, soybeans, legumes, peanuts, and wheat germ.	Quickly destroyed by heat in neutral or alkaline solutions.
Vitamin B_2 (riboflavin)	Essential link in the body's use of protein, carbohydrates, and fats for energy.	Milk, powdered whey, liver, kidney, heart, meats, eggs, green leafy vegetables, dried yeast.	Decomposes quickly in light or in alkaline solutions.
Vitamin B_6 (pyridoxine, pyridoxal, pyridoxamine)	Important for the body's use of protein, carbohydrates, and fat. Aids in formation of hemoglobin.	Wheat germ, meat, liver, kidney, whole-grain cereals, soybeans, peanuts, corn. Some in milk and green vegetables.	Water soluble. Destroyed by ultraviolet light and heat.
Vitamin B_{12} (cobalamin)	Essential for formation of red blood cells. Helps form all cells in body and facilitates functioning of nervous system.	Milk, eggs, cheese, liver, kidney, muscle meats contain small amounts needed for normal body functioning.	Inactivated by air and light. Water soluble.
Folic acid	Needed for body's use of protein and for regeneration of blood cells.	Green leafy vegetables, liver, kidney, yeast, and small quantities in many foods.	Easily inactivated in sunlight and acid solutions.
Pantothenic acid	Necessary for body's use of carbohydrates, fats, and protein in conjunction with other substances.	Almost universally present in plant and animal tissue. Loss of 50 percent in milling of flour. Cooking meat destroys 33 percent.	Water soluble. Destroyed easily by dry heat and alkaline solutions.
Niacin	Active in normal functioning of tissues, particularly of skin, gastrointestinal tract, and nervous system. With other vitamins, converts carbohydrates into energy.	Lean meat, liver, kidney, whole-grain and enriched cereals and breads, green vegetables, peanuts, yeast.	Water soluble. Stable in heat, air, light.

(continued)

TABLE 11-1 (Continued)

Essential Nutrients	Function in the Body	Food Sources	Comments
Biotin	Essential for functioning of many body systems and use of food for energy.	Liver, kidney, molasses, milk, yeast, egg yolk, and green vegetables.	Water soluble. Quite stable in heat, air, and light.
Vitamin C (ascorbic acid)	Essential for formation of collagen, a protein which supports the body structures. Needed for the absorption of iron, some proteins, and folic acid.	Citrus fruits, strawberries, cantaloupe, tomatoes, cabbage, potatoes, green peppers, and broccoli.	Water soluble. Destroyed by heat, air, and light, as well as by age, drying, and copper contact.
Vitamin D	Promotes normal bone and tooth development. Necessary for absorption and stabilization of calcium and phosphorus.	Fish-liver oils, fortified milk, sunlight, and very small amounts in butter, liver, and egg yolks.	Fat soluble. Stable in heat and air.
Vitamin E (tocopherol)	Protects the body's store of vitamin A and tissue fat from destructive oxidation. Also prevents breakdown of red blood corpuscles.	Oils of wheat germ, rice germ, cottonseed, and the germs of other seeds. Green leafy vegetables, nuts, and legumes.	Fat soluble. Breaks down in presence of lead and iron salts, alkalies, and ultraviolet light.
Vitamin K	Essential for blood clotting.	Green leafy vegetables such as alfalfa, spinach, and cabbage, and liver.	Fat soluble. Unstable in light.
Minerals Calcium	Builds bones and teeth. Aids in proper functioning of muscles, heart, and nerves. Helps in blood coagulation.	Milk and hard cheese, kale, mustard, turnip and collard greens. Also some in oysters, shrimp, salmon, clams, and dairy products.	Calcium is the most abundant mineral in the body.
Iron	One of the constituents of hemoglobin, which carries oxygen to tissues via	All kinds of liver are the best source of iron. Meat, egg yolk, legumes,	Iron deficiency is most common in growing children,

	the blood. Iron is present in all body cells.	molasses, dark-green leafy vegetables, peaches, prunes, apricots, raisins, and food made with enriched flour or cereal.	adolescent girls, and pregnant or nursing women.
Phosphorus	Builds bones and teeth (with other minerals). Important in a number of body systems that use fats, carbohydrates, salts, and enzymes.	Milk, cheese, egg yolk, meat, fish, fowl, legumes, nuts, whole-grain cereals.	Some forms of phosphorus are not utilized if the vitamin D level in the diet is inadequate.
Iodine	Required to regulate the exchange of food for energy.	Iodized salt best source. Salt-water fish.	The need for iodine increases in adolescence and during pregnancy.
Potassium	Needed to maintain fluid balance within cells. Regulates muscle and nerve irritability. Necessary for regular heart rhythm.	Meat, fish, fowl, cereals, fruits, vegetables.	Dietary deficiency uncommon, but may occur in connection with some diseases.
Sodium	Protects body against excessive fluid loss. Regulates muscle and nerve irritability.	Table salt, meat, fish, fowl, milk, eggs, and sodium compounds.	Excessive salt intake dangerous for persons subject to hypertension and kidney disorders.
Fluorine	In small quantities, protects teeth against cavities. In larger quantities, fluorine causes mottling of the teeth.	Milk, eggs, and fish. Many communities add low concentrations of fluorine to drinking water.	Prolonged high intake of fluorine may cause skeletal abnormalities.

Other minerals which are considered essential for good health are: chlorine, sulfur, magnesium, manganese, copper, zinc, cobalt, and molybdenum. In most cases, diet provides adequate intake.

Water	Essential for life. Solvent for all products of digestion and medium of body fluids. Regulates body temperature.	Beverages and many solid foods (for example, potatoes contain 78 percent water).	One-half to two-thirds of the body is water.

fish oils. Other common sources of fat are fatty meats, butter, margarine, cream, most cheeses, whole milk, mayonnaise and salad dressings, egg yolks, nuts, and peanut butter.

Fats also carry fat-soluble vitamins into the body and aid in their absorption. In addition, fats serve as a concentrated source of energy, and because they slow digestion and the emptying of the stomach, they delay the onset of hunger. Fats also contribute to our enjoyment of foods because they add flavor and improve texture.

Fats are called a "concentrated source of energy" because they contain more than twice the energy value of carbohydrates and proteins; that is, one gram of fat provides nine calories, whereas one gram of protein or carbohydrate provides only four calories. Consequently, foods rich in fats add many calories to the diet, and all calories in excess of the body's demands are stored in fat deposits.

Many physicians and nutritionists believe that most Americans should lower their fat intake. The reason for this recommendation is an apparent relationship between dietary fats and atherosclerosis, a disease condition in which deposits of cholesterol and other fatty substances accumulate on the inner walls of arteries. Atherosclerosis is often linked to high blood pressure and heart disease. Saturated fats, which are present in animal fats, are responsible for increased cholesterol levels. Cholesterol is a normal constituent of blood and tissues, however, and the body synthesizes it. It is in excessive quantities that it is harmful.[4] Another principal reason for reducing the consumption of fat is to make room in the diet for more starches (vegetables, grains, and fruits), which generally carry higher levels of vitamins and minerals without the health complications of fat.[5]

Vitamins

Vitamins are organic compounds that are necessary in small amounts for the normal growth and maintenance of life of animals, including humans. They do not provide energy, nor do they construct or build any part of the body. Rather, their function is to transform foods into energy and to maintain a normal body. We need at least fifteen vitamins to protect us against deficiency diseases.

Vitamins are alike because they contain the same elements: carbon, hydrogen, oxygen, and sometimes nitrogen. (Vitamin B_{12} contains cobalt, an essential mineral.) They are different because their elements are arranged in different combinations, and each vitamin exclusively performs one or more functions in the body.

Getting enough vitamins is essential to life, but the body has no use for excess vitamins. Many people believe in insurance, however, so, fearful of not eating a well-balanced diet, they take extra vitamins. So-called "average," or normal, eaters probably never need supplemental vitamins, although many think they do. People whose diets are known to be deficient do require them, as do individuals recovering from a specific illness or from vitamin deficiencies that have been identified by a physician.

Vitamins occur in varying quantities in different foods. Most foods contain more than one vitamin, but no one food contains all of them in sufficient quantity to satisfy the human body's requirements. Ordinarily, a well-balanced diet will provide enough of all essential vitamins. The functions and sources of vitamins are innumerable. Table 11–1 lists the more important ones.

Minerals

Today's consumers are more aware of the existence of vitamins and minerals than any previous generation. The increasing sales of vitamin-mineral supplements and the considerable interest shown in new FDA regulations pertaining to them attest to this elevated awareness.

While vitamins usually take center stage in any discussion of dietary supplements, minerals, too, are essential for good health and growth. Without a certain level of minerals in our diets, we would suffer some type of nutritional deficiency. We need to consume relatively large amounts of the so-called macrominerals, namely, calcium, phosphorus, sodium chloride, potassium, magnesium, and sulfur. By "large" we mean dosages of between 100 milligrams and 1 gram. *Trace minerals* are necessary in smaller amounts. These elements include iron, manganese, copper, iodine, zinc, cobalt, fluorine, and selenium.

In general, mineral elements perform two body functions: building and regulating. They are essential for the growth and repair of the skeleton and all soft tissues. As regulatory agents they are vital to a wide variety of activities, including the beating of the heart, blood clotting, maintaining the internal pressure of body fluids, mediating nerve responses, and transporting oxygen from lungs to tissues.

Most of the hard tissues of the human body, for example, bones and teeth, consist, in part, of mineral elements. In the case of bones and teeth, relatively large amounts of calcium and phosphorus are necessary for structural soundness. But the body needs many other minerals, some in very minute quantities, to carry on life processes. For instance, in order to function properly, muscles, nerves, and the heart require constant nourishment from body fluids containing the correct proportion of sodium, potassium, calcium, and the like. Similarly, red blood cells cannot form or function properly if the body's iron supply is low. The consumption of small amounts of another mineral, fluorine, prevents excessive tooth decay.

Altogether, the body needs about fifteen different mineral elements, all of which must enter it in the form of food or drink. The minerals in which diets are most likely to be low, or deficient, are calcium, iron, iodine, and fluorine. A few minerals, including lead, mercury, and cadmium are regarded as harmful.

Dietary Fiber

Usually, when we talk of food in terms of nutritional qualities, we talk about protein, carbohydrate, fat, vitamin, and mineral content. Mention of the importance of the fiber, or roughage, that certain foods provide is less frequent, although its value in promoting bowel regularity has been evident throughout the ages.

The fiber in our diet comes only from plant sources (and does not include the tough, fibrous portions of some meats). It consists of complex carbohydrates, for example, cellulose, and other substances that constitute the cell walls and structural formations in plants. Salad greens, celery, wheat bran, and apple skins all contain large amounts of these materials.

Fiber stimulates the normal, waste-removing action of the intestinal tract. In addition to providing bulk, it absorbs many times its weight in water. Thus it softens stools and promotes regular elimination.

Many weight-reduction diets encourage the consumption of raw vegetables and fruits because these foods contain fair amounts of fiber and are generally low in calories. The increased bulk also contributes to a feeling of fullness.

Recent studies have suggested that dietary fiber may make yet another contribution to our well-being, probably as a result of the greater bulk and more rapid elimination. Some researchers feel that fiber may protect against many of the noninfectious diseases of the large intestine that are prevalent in our society. These conditions include cancer of the colon, hemorrhoids, appendicitis, colitis, and diverticulosis (pouchelike protuberances from the intestinal wall). The incidence of these diseases appears to be lower in less-developed societies where the normal diet contains larger amounts of dietary fiber. Some researchers have also associated increased dietary fiber with reduction in blood cholesterol levels and suggested that a relationship may exist between dietary fiber and freedom from atherosclerosis (fatty deposits on the inner walls of arteries). Based on these research reports, some health authorities believe that an increase in dietary fiber, particularly in cereal fiber, would be beneficial to the American diet.[6] Of course, we must recognize that dietary fiber is a popular nutritional topic at the present time and most of the recommendations concerning the health benefits of fiber are theories that the research literature has not totally substantiated.

Water

Water is second only to air in importance to life. You can get along for days, even weeks, without food, but only for a few days without water. Water is necessary for all the processes of digestion. It dissolves nutrients so they can pass through the intestinal wall and into the bloodstream for use throughout the body. Water carries waste out of the body and also helps to regulate body temperature.

The body's most obvious source of water is drinking water, but the body produces some by burning food for energy. The beverages we drink are mostly water. Soup is a water source, and so are many fruits and vegetables. Even meat can be up to 80 percent water. Insufficient intake of water may cause you to tire easily and make it hard to concentrate. Many people drink less water than the optimum for the best function of the body. The shipwrecked sailor who goes without water for much more than forty-eight hours will die.

Although water makes up more than half of body weight we are constantly losing it and must replace it. Not all this water leaves the body through urination. Perspiration and unseen, unfelt evaporation through the skin are other escape routes. Some water escapes through the lungs into the air (you can see this moisture by breathing on a mirror).

The need for liquids depends on body size and weight. As a general guide, adults should drink from one and a half to two quarts of fluid a day. Children, of course, need proportionately less. The amount of water consumed is very important. Too little may mean that the kidneys cannot completely flush excess salts and minerals from the system. If they remain in the kidneys they may form kidney stones. Also, many doctors believe that bacteria, which cause infections, can grow more easily when urine flow is low.

NUTRITION LABELING

As a result of public pressure, the Food and Drug Administration has established new regulations pertaining to the use of uniform and informative nutrition labeling. Manufacturers now must use nutrition labeling when they add any nutrient to packaged food or when they make some nutritional claim for a product on the label or in advertising. Diet foods also must exhibit complete nutritional information.

The term *enriched* applies to cereal products (flours, macaroni, noodles, etc.) that meet federally prescribed levels for four nutrients—thiamine, riboflavin, niacin, and iron. It does not mean that the manufacturer has replaced other nutrients lost in the milling process.

Fortified refers to the addition of nutrients above the natural level contained in the ingredients, including some not present in the original product. Examples include the addition of vitamin D to milk and iodine to salt. Also, many cereals today are fortified.

FDA regulations not only spell out what is to appear on nutrition labels (see Table 11-2), but they expressly forbid certain claims about nutrition and diet. Long concerned about misleading claims made to promote the sale of some foods and dietary supplements, the FDA considers foods misbranded if their labels violate the regulation. Thus, the FDA is trying to do two things with nutrition labeling regulation: provide more information about the nutrients in food and protect the public from misinformation.

The regulation prohibits a label from specifying or even implying any of the following:

1. That a food can prevent, cure, mitigate, or treat any disease or symptom
2. That a balanced diet of ordinary foods cannot supply adequate amounts of nutrients
3. That a lack of optimal nutritive quality of food, because of the

TABLE 11-2.   FDA Food Label Format

Nutrition Information (Per Serving)	
Serving size = 8 oz.	
Servings per container = 2	
Calories	560
Protein	23 g
Carbohydrate	43 g
Fat	33 g
(Percent of calories from fat = 53%)	
Polyunsaturated*	22 g
Saturated	9 g
Cholesterol* (20 mg/100 g)	40 mg
Sodium (365 mg/100 g)	810 mg

Percentage of U.S. Recommended Daily Allowances (U.S. RDA)			
Protein	35	Niacin	25
Vitamin A	35	Calcium	2
Vitamin C	10	Iron	25
Thiamine	15	Vitamin B_6	20
Riboflavin	15	Vitamin B_{12}	15

*Information on fat and cholesterol content is provided for individuals who, on the advice of a physician, are modifying their total dietary intake of fat and cholesterol.

soil on which that food was grown, is or may be responsible for an inadequacy or deficiency in the daily diet
4. That storage, transportation, processing, or cooking of a food is, or may be responsible for, an inadequacy or deficiency in the daily diet
5. That a natural vitamin is superior to an added or synthetic vitamin
6. That a food contains certain nutrients when such substances are of no known need or significant value in human nutrition

The FDA states that these prohibitions are intended to stop unsupported generalizations and fraudulent statements. A manufacturer who has adequate scientific data proving that a product has higher nutrient retention than a competitor's may make that claim. But the burden of proof rests with the manufacturer.

NUTRITIONAL QUACKERY

Despite efforts to promote nutrition education in the schools and among the public, much nutritional nonsense receives too much attention. The following fallacies are but a few of the common nutritional myths that many people believe:[7]

1. Claim: Our soil has lost its vitamins and minerals; thus our food crops have little nutritional value. Fact: Fertilizers replenish plant nutrients in the soil and produce contains the expected nutritional value.
2. Claim: You are what you eat. Fact: In one sense, that statement is true. But you are also a product of your heredity and environment.
3. Claim: Chemical fertilizers are poisoning our soil. Fact: Modern fertilizers are necessary to produce enough food for our population. There is no scientific evidence to indicate chemical fertilizers are poisoning us.
4. Claim: Natural, organic fertilizers not only are safer than chemical fertilizers but also produce healthier crops. Fact: Organic and chemical fertilizers produce crops of equal quality and are equally safe. Chemical fertilizers are easier to use than organic fertilizers, however, because plants cannot absorb organic fertilizers as such. Bacteria in the soil must first break down organic fertilizers into the same chemical elements—potassium, phosphorus, and nitrogen—that modern chemical fertilizers supply directly and more quickly.

5. Claim: Modern processing removes most vitamins and minerals from foods. Fact: Although any type of processing, including simple cooking, reduces the nutrient content or quality of foods to some extent, modern processing methods keep such losses as low as possible. Enrichment after processing restores some nutrients.

6. Claim: Pesticides are poisoning our nation. Fact: If pesticides leave a residue on food crops, FDA and the Environmental Protection Agency (EPA) make sure the amount will be safe for consumers. They set the permissible level as low as possible, even though a higher level might be safe.

7. Claim: Cooking with Teflon-coated utensils is dangerous. Fact: Careful testing of this commercial product has proved that there is no danger from normal kitchen use.

8. Claim: Aluminum cooking utensils are dangerous to health. Fact: Cooking in aluminum utensils is harmless. Aluminum is the second most abundant mineral element in the soil and therefore occurs naturally in many foods.

9. Claim: An ache or pain or feeling of fatigue probably means you are suffering from a vitamin deficiency. Fact: Most people feel tired or suffer aches and pains at one time or another. They may be symptoms of overwork, emotional stress, disease, or lack of sleep, as well as poor nutrition. If such symptoms persist, you should see your physician, for it is difficult for the average person to accurately diagnose their cause.

10. Claim: You have to eat special foods if you want to lose weight. Fact: Successful weight control depends primarily on self-control of one's total food intake while maintaining a reasonable level of physical activity. Your physician should prescribe a special diet if you need one.

11. Claim: Vitamins from natural sources are much better than synthetic vitamins. Fact: Vitamins are specific chemical compounds. The human body can use them equally well whether a chemist has synthesized them or whether nature has produced them.

12. Claim: Everyone should take vitamins, just to be safe. Fact: Most healthy individuals whose diet regularly includes even modest amounts of meat and eggs, milk products, fruits and vegetables, bread and other cereal products need not resort to dietary supplements. Some persons under a doctor's care or in institutions need dietary supplements because of special conditions that restrict their ability to eat a well-balanced diet. Generally, modest supplementation with certain vitamins is also recommended during infancy and pregnancy and while breast feeding. But if you eat a well-balanced diet, you probably do not need vitamin supplements.

TABLE 11-3. The National Dairy Council Guide to Good Eating

Use Daily:

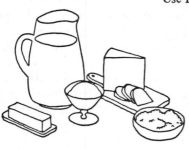

Milk Group — 3 or more glasses milk— children.
Smaller glasses for some children under 9.
4 or more glasses—teen-agers.
2 or more glasses—adults.
Cheese, ice cream, and other milk-made foods can supply part of the milk.

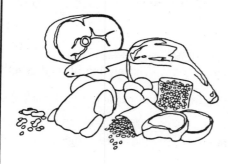

Meat Group — 2 or more servings.
Meat, fish, poultry, eggs, or cheese—with dry beans, peas, nuts as alternates.

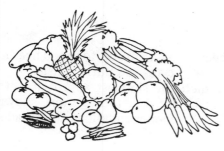

Vegetables and Fruit — 4 or more servings.
Include dark green or yellow vegetables and citrus fruit or tomatoes.

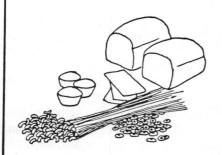

Bread and Cereals — 4 or more servings.
Enriched or whole grain and added milk improves nutritional values.

A GUIDE TO GOOD NUTRITION

You would have to spend years in intensive study to even begin to learn all that is known about nutrition, but you need not know everything to be able to plan a well-balanced diet that will help keep you healthy. To develop a sense of good nutrition you need only to study sound nutrition information.

Recently the U.S. Senate Select Committee on Nutrition and Human Needs reported: "In the view of doctors and nutritionists consulted by the Select Committee . . . changes in the diet amount to a wave of malnutrition—of both over- and underconsumption—that may be as profoundly damaging to the Nation's health as the widespread contagious diseases of the early part of the century." As a result of their investigation, the committee recommended the following dietary goals.

1. Increase consumption of fruits and vegetables and whole grains.
2. Decrease consumption of meat and increase consumption of poultry and fish.
3. Decrease consumption of foods high in fat and partially substitute polyunsaturated fat for saturated fat.
4. Substitute nonfat milk for whole milk.
5. Decrease consumption of butterfat, eggs, and other high-cholesterol sources.
6. Decrease consumption of sugar and foods high in sugar content.
7. Decrease consumption of salt and foods high in salt content.[8]

These recommendations are not necessarily a cure-all for good health, nor do they have the support of all physicians and nutritionists.

In planning a nutritious daily diet, the simplest approach is to consult the National Dairy Council's basic four food groups, shown in Table 11–3. This list provides good recommendations for an adequate diet.

MALNUTRITION, LEARNING, AND BEHAVIOR[9]

Malnutrition is a condition in which a prolonged lack of one or more nutrients retards physical development or causes specific clinical disorders, such as anemia, goiter, and rickets. Severe malnutrition generally produces clinical manifestations that may require hospital treatment. There are two basic types of severe malnutrition: *kwashiorkor,* caused by protein deficiency; and *marasmus,* brought about by an overall caloric deficit. Infantile marasmus most frequently results from early cessation of breast feeding, overdilution of bottle-fed formula, or gastrointestinal infection early in life. Symptoms of marasmus are wasting away of tissues and extreme growth retardation. Kwashiorkor generally occurs at or after weaning, when milk that is high in protein is replaced by a starchy staple food that does not provide sufficient protein for growth and development. Children with kwashiorkor, a condition that is rare in the United States, usually display stunted growth, edema (accumulation of water), skin sores, and discoloration of dark hair to red or blond.

While only 1 to 2 percent of the world's children suffer from severe malnutrition, up to half may suffer from moderate malnutrition or chronic undernutrition (the terms "moderate malnutrition" and "chronic undernutrition" are interchangeable for purposes of this chapter). *Undernutrition* refers to a deficit in the quantity of food intake, while *malnourished* refers to the quality of food intake.

What are the signs of undernourishment? Biochemical and clinical signs of malnutrition, although often used, are not very precise gauges of undernourishment, except in cases of extremely inadequate diets. Chronic, or long-term, undernutrition generally stunts growth, and often the degree of malnutrition is proportional to the degree that the child is subnormal in height or weight. Therefore, anthropometric measures (height, weight, and fatness) are the most commonly used indices of undernutrition.

There are two types of moderate malnutrition. One is atibutable to chronic food restriction (manifested by growth retardation), whereas the other results from vitamin or mineral deficiency and is accompanied by clinical problems such as rickets or pellegra. Deficiency malnutrition is most often associated with poverty. Determining its effects on a given individual is extremely difficult since many other factors influence human growth and behavioral development, including an individual's innate potential, health status, and environment.

The Prevalence of Malnutrition

Three extensive surveys of nutritional status in the United States conducted in recent years have reached similar conclusions: in the United States, marasmus and kwashiorkor are quite rare (despite frequent assertions to the contrary), but chronic undernutrition and iron deficiency are surprisingly common.[10] These studies provided a wealth of information concerning food habits. For instance, almost 20 percent of the children under six consumed less than the recommended daily intake of calories. For low-income families this figure increased to 30 percent. Children from some southern states and poor black and Hispano-American children were much more likely to have insufficient calorie intakes.

Contrary to the expectations of many, adults and children generally had enough protein in their diets. The study of preschool children found that less than 2 percent did not eat sufficient protein. The link between protein consumption and total calorie consumption was strong. Thus, children who were not eating enough protein tended to have low calorie intakes. In short, the problem appeared to involve the quantity rather than the nutritional quality of food.

Recommended daily allowances are only gross estimates of nutritional needs and, in fact, were not designed to assess an individual's nutritional status. A more accurate indication of whether a child is receiving sufficient nutrients is the child's growth record. The nationwide surveys consistently found a larger-than-expected percentage of children with very low height and weight for age, especially children from low socioeconomic classes. Many factors, including the mother's weight and nutritional status during pregnancy as well as the child's history of infection, contribute to the height and weight of a child. Nevertheless, the primary determinant is the adequacy of the child's diet. Consequently, the fact that a large number of children had extremely low anthropometric indices suggests that chronic undernutrition is a significant problem in this country.

Many studies have shown that iron deficiency is widespread in the United States. Iron is present in only trace amounts in milk and in most baby foods. Furthermore, the need for iron increases after an infection or blood loss. More than one-half of American children between one and five years old may have an inadequate iron intake, a deficiency does not afflict only lower socioeconomic classes. Anemia, the medical consequence of prolonged iron deficit, is common in this age group also; the incidence climbs to 30 percent in some low-income groups. Iron deficiency seems to recede in incidence at about age five, but it reappears as a major nutritional problem in adolescent boys and girls.

Finally, except for the iron deficiency, the national surveys found little dietary or clinical evidence of vitamin or mineral deficiencies among the children in this country. Once again research refutes a commonly held opinion.

To the extent that the poor in the United States live under unsatisfactory health conditions and are without access to medical care, malnutrition raises susceptibility to infection. Most malnourished children come from poor families that have many children closely spaced in age and do not participate fully in public health programs. They are more likely to come from one-parent households than to have two parents. Parents of malnourished children generally have low-status, unskilled jobs, which reflect their lack of education. In short, malnutrition usually exists where there is poverty. Many aspects of this environment, including malnutrition, affect learning.

Malnutrition and the Brain

The human brain approaches adult size, weight, and cell number by age two. From about the second trimester of pregnancy to six months of age, there is a *brain growth spurt,* when brain cells rapidly multiply and grow. This period of rapid brain growth continues, although at a more moderate pace, until eighteen to twenty-four months of age.

For the purposes of description, we can divide the brain growth spurt in two general stages. The first stage, concurrent in humans with the second trimester of pregnancy, involves increasing the number of neurons, the basic functional cell of the brain. The second stage extends from the third trimester of pregnancy through the normal period of breast feeding. Throughout this stage, the supporting cells of the nervous system (the glia) multiply and branches (dendrites) from already established neurons grow to form synaptic connections, which transmit nerve impulses between neurons. The two stages overlap considerably, and the number of neurons continues to multiply after birth. Of immediate interest is that the processes of dendritic growth and synapse formation, which occur mainly during the second stage, are probably more important to human mental performance than is neuronal cell number.

Superimposed on the two stages of the growth spurt are regional variations in brain development. Some sections of the brain develop earlier than others, and some develop quickly whereas others evolve relatively slowly.

Throughout the growth spurt, the brain needs adequate nutrients in order to grow. Research findings indicate that severe malnutrition in animals during this period can produce brain deficits that cannot be rectified nutritionally. Available evidence shows that the human brain, like those of other animals, is probably more vulnerable to malnutrition throughout the growth spurt than at other times. The fetal brain is most likely to suffer if the mother's body stores of nutrients are low due to a lifetime of undernutrition and an inadequate diet during pregnancy. The region of the brain that most needs nutrients is the one that is growing most rapidly at a given time. Since each region is responsible for specific brain and behavior functions, a deficit in one region caused by malnutrition might produce specific behavioral abnormalities.

Severe Malnutrition and Learning

Researchers have made many studies of humans and animals to determine if severe malnutrition (prolonged calorie or protein deprivation leading to gross clinical symptoms and frequently to hospitalization) results in permanent learning handicaps. These experiments have led to a number of important conclusions.

First of all severe malnutrition in infancy apparently does significantly alter human behavior. The impact on human behavior directly relates to the severity of malnutrition and its duration during the brain growth spurt. One investigator has suggested that any malnutrition severe enough to require hospitalization due to growth failure before two years of age will have irreversible adverse results. Another has postulated similar effects from any bout of extreme malnutrition lasting longer than four months during early life.

Second, recent research has shown that severe malnutrition may permanently affect motivation, attention span, and arousal. Children who were severely malnourished early in life seem to have short attention spans and consistently perform poorly on tests of concentration ability. On the other hand, malnutrition does not appear to impair long-term memory.

Third, severely malnourished babies tend to develop poor motor capabilities. Many have abnormal difficulty manipulating objects, owing to a lack of fine motor control.

Finally, children who were malnourished during infancy probably have some yet-undefined retardation in sensory integration. For example, in learning to read, such a child may have difficulty connecting the visual image of a word with the sound of a word. Obviously, impaired sensory integration would considerably retard learning, but we do not yet know what types of integration malnutrition restrains.

As might be expected, previously deprived children seem to do poorly in school. Their teachers tend to mark them as problem children, and usually they receive lower-than-average grades. In sum, very severe malnutrition in infancy, if it lasts a while and precedes a period of childhood undernutrition, produces irreversible effects on behavior, which, in turn, impair a child's ability to learn.

Chronic Undernutrition and Learning

Moderate, or chronic, undernutrition is more prevalent than severe malnutrition in the United States. Poor physical growth and anemia are signs that undernutrition is a problem here. Nevertheless, there are fewer reported studies on undernutrition, and the findings are more confusing. First, the effects, if any, are probably less serious and therefore harder to measure. Second and equally important, understanding moderate, or chronic, malnutrition requires knowledge of the context of the malnourished child's social and familial environment, many parts of which also shape behavioral development. Thus, the difficulties of designing and performing these studies, not to mention problems of interpretation, are discouraging to researchers.

Despite these problems, a number of studies have shown that chronically undernourished children tend to lag behind their well-nourished counterparts in behavioral development. This retardation probably lasts at least until adolescence. The primary deficits appear in motor-integrative performance, reading ability, concentration, and motivation. Even within the same family, children who were more poorly nourished did less well on behavioral tests and in school than did their better-nourished brothers and sisters. Of course, we cannot attribute all behavioral deficits to malnutrition. Socioeconomic factors contribute importantly to performance, as one study of physically comparable children from different social strata revealed.

The best way to determine nutritional status is to measure an individual's food intake over time. Studies recently undertaken are using this longitudinal approach.

Iron Deficiency and Learning

Iron deficiency, the most prevalent nutritional problem in the United States, is defined as the depletion of iron stores in the body. It can be measured in various ways. Usually a significant and prolonged deficit in iron intake will cause *anemia,* a condition in which either the hemoglobin concentration, or the volume of packed red-blood cells (hematocrit), is lower than normal. Many people are iron deficient but do not manifest iron-deficiency anemia. Since anemia constitutes the most frequent evidence of iron deficit, most published studies of iron-deficient conditions have used it as the primary variable.

Like other forms of malnutrition, anemia affects behavior according to its severity. Only very severe anemia appears to have any measurable impact on adult performance. Mild anemia, on the other hand, significantly influences the behavior of young children, probably due to the combined impact of anemia and rapid growth. No evidence yet suggests, however, that permanent neurological damage results from anemia during pregnancy or early childhood.

Childhood anemia does not seem to have any direct effect on intelligence, as measured by IQ tests. Rather, it appears to influence selected behaviors. For example, anemic children are less attentive and persistent but more irritable than other children. Unlike severe malnutrition, however, anemia during gestation or early infancy does not impair current performance. Chronic undernutrition in conjunction with anemia probably has a more deleterious effect on behavior than anemia alone.

The impact of iron deficiency on behavior is probably related to the anemia that so often accompanies it. Iron supplementation will quickly relieve adverse behavioral consequences. The physiological explanation for the effects of iron depletion are still unknown, although some have speculated that enzymes which require iron for activity are sensitive to iron levels in the body.

Whatever the physiological explanation, withdrawal from the environment as a result of iron deficiency will prevent a child from learning. And missing one step in the learning process makes it harder to master the next. Thus, prolonged iron deficiency, like chronic undernutrition, could irreparably impair intellectual development even if neurological structures remained essentially intact.

Hunger and Learning

 Up to one-fourth of American schoolchildren arrive at school without having eaten breakfast. Many others do not have lunch. Often such children are hungry.

Hunger and malnutrition are not identical. Whereas malnutrition applies to specific physiological symptoms caused by prolonged lack of food, hunger is a physiological and psychological state that occurs when immediate food needs are not met. Hunger can be relieved quickly by food, but recovery from malnutrition requires extended rehabilitation.

Hunger is nearly impossible to quantify. Consequently, despite numerous studies involving school breakfast, snack, or lunch programs (food intervention to relieve hunger), many of the questions about hunger's effects on behavior and growth remain unanswered. The varying results of school food programs, in terms of improved growth and nutritional status, undoubtedly reflect the varying degrees of undernutrition among the children in the programs.

The research consensus is that hunger affects behavior. It increases nervousness, irritability, and disinterest in a learning situation. Thus, although hunger probably has neither direct effects on learning nor permanent effects on behavior, it potentially disrupts the learning process. Disinterest and inability to concentrate tend to isolate a hungry child and negative responses to the child's behavior heightens feelings of isolation to create a vicious circle. The child fails to learn for social and psychological rather than biological reasons.

THE CYCLE OF MALNUTRITION

As is apparent from the previous sections, malnutrition and environment are intimately intertwined. Their interaction often creates a cycle wherein poor environment leads to malnutrition, which, in turn, shapes behavior to perpetuate poverty, intellectual disability, and malnutrition.

Women who have been undernourished throughout life differ from well-nourished women in at least three significant ways. First, they tend to give birth to babies who are undernourished and underweight. Second, if they are undernourished during pregnancy, they will produce less breast milk and the duration of breast feeding will be shorter, even though their undernourished condition probably will not affect the quality of their milk. Finally, undernourished mothers play less with their new children since they are considerably less active than normal mothers.

From birth until weaning, infants receive most of their nourishment and environmental stimulation from their mothers. Breast-fed children are probably fairly well fed throughout early life because their nutritional needs are low. By six months of age (or even earlier if the mother is very malnourished), however, the amount of maternal milk begins to affect growth. As infants' needs begin to surpass their undernourished mothers' ability to fulfill them, the infants tend to become less active in order to conserve food energy. The energy needs for physical growth take precedence over energy for activity and play.

Not surprisingly, at about six months of age, undernourished infants become visibly distinguishable from normal infants. According to a longitudinal study done in rural Mexico, undernourished infants sleep more and play and explore their environment considerably less. Less active, malnourished young children elicit less stimulation and attention from parents, siblings, and later from peers. Their mothers leave them in the cradle for longer periods of time. The net effect is that malnourished infants tend to develop into passive, apathetic children.

Furthermore, infants who are undernourished before weaning are apt to become more malnourished, because they are inactive and make few demands on their mothers. In addition, their sucking behavior may be both less effective and less frequent. Thus, these babies probably receive less milk because they are already undernourished. At weaning, infants more fully enter the outside world. During the postweaning period, the developmental deficits of malnourished children may multiply. Normally active infants play more with parents and brothers and sisters at this stage. Well-nourished children are spoken to more frequently; they are praised and rewarded more often. Undernourished infants, on the other hand, do not advance developmentally, probably because they are timid and passive, explore little, and demand little. Having become accustomed to meager food supplies, they assume a conservative mode of living consistent with available energy. They cannot develop satisfactorily because development requires physical activity, which, over the long run, they cannot afford.

The picture that emerges of chronically undernourished children shows them to be developmentally disadvantaged in many ways. What happens when these children interact with peers and go to school? By the time they enter school, children have developed a self-concept based on the way parents and others respond to them. Previously, malnourished children probably had great difficulty concentrating and were spoken to and praised infrequently. Most likely, they consider themselves less able than other children and their failures at learning tasks in school will contribute to this image. Because activity is harder for them and their concern for food often disrupts concentration, these children become discouraged. Their future prospects in school are gloomy at best.

The cycle that begins with early malnutrition, then, ends with learning difficulties. It is important to understand that a continuum exists between prolonged, severe malnutrition, which causes an infant to be very passive throughout early life, and a transitory episode of hunger, which may make an infant less active for a while. Obviously, the longer and more profound the passivity, the greater the effect on overall intellectual development.

THE OBESE CHILD

Obesity is probably the number-one nutrition problem among elementary-age children in the United States. Apart from the fact that untreated overweight children invariably become obese adults, childhood obesity is a source of concern also because it has grave physical, social, and psychological disadvantages. Although childhood obesity often starts in infancy, more commonly onset occurs during middle childhood. Studies have shown a correlation between obesity in the school-age child and obesity in later life.[11]

Obesity is a serious nutritional, behavioral, and metabolic disorder that affects between 15 and 25 percent of American children. It is also one of the most frustrating medical problems, because our current approaches to the management of childhood obesity have been almost completely unsuccessful and the cause of the disorder remains obscure.[12]

An estimated 3 to 20 percent of school-age children are obese, depending on the particular group examined and the examiners' definitions of obesity.[13] Four out of five overweight children become overweight adults, and studies within the past three years show that it is much more difficult to treat obese adults who were heavy as children.[14]

Perhaps the best definition of overweight children emphasizes the fat rather than the weight. In other words, overweight children carry more fat than they should. Another common definition of obesity is a condition in which the body weight exceeds by 20 percent the standard weight for a particular height and build, but more accurately, it is a condition characterized by excessive accumulation of body fat. It appears that the prognosis for eventual weight reduction by children who become obese before age ten is somber. Obviously, then, no one should lightly dismiss childhood obesity as baby fat.

It is apparent that Americans overeat. Twenty million of us are considered clinically obese and tens of millions more are grossly overweight. The rapid increase in the number of obese individuals during the past two or three decades worries public health officials. Some theories suggest that the growth in number of fat cells occurs predominantly in the first year of life and just before puberty. This is a result of *hyperplasia,* tissue growth accompanied by an increase in the number of fat cells. Normally, fat cells cease multiplying around fifteen years of age, so the early childhood years are vitally important because subsequent disproportionate increases in weight involve *hypertrophy,* an increase in fat-cell size, rather than increasing numbers of fat cells. Individuals who produced a greater number of fat cells during the childhood years appear to have a more difficult time controlling weight in the adult years. In any weight loss that occurs after fat cells have been deposited, the loss is a result of the reduction in the size of the fat cells rather than a decrease in their number.

Even though heredity may be partly responsible for the excess production of fat cells during childhood, overfeeding evidently can significantly increase hyperplasia.[15] A family's life-style significantly influences whether a genetic tendency toward overweight will make a child obese. Children tend to imitate their parents and once a pattern of overeating has been established, unfortunately it passes to the next generation.

Present-day environmental conditions also encourage overeating as well as a drop in physical activity. Studies have documented the extreme inactivity of the majority of obese children. In fact, some studies have shown that children invariably gain the most weight during the fall and winter months, their most inactive periods.[16] Other studies have shown that some overweight children may actually eat less than normal-weight children but are markedly less active.[17] It is vital to understand that exercise is probably the most important tool in preventing obesity and in treating overweight children. Overweight children should have at least an hour of exercise every weekday and two to three hours a day on weekends. The type of exercise is not as important as intensity and continuity.[18] It is important that the activity is enjoyable to these children so that they will continue to participate in it. Unfortunately, many obese children manage to drop out of physical education activities at school, and a number of schools have dropped many of the physical educations requirements for all students. A special effort to include the child in physical activities is essential. Teachers can easily work out daily errands and walking routes that will provide additional exercise for obese youngsters without embarrassing them.

Many have cited lack of exercise as the most important cause of increasing obesity in modern mechanized societies. Yet overweight is frequently blamed on other factors, such as glandular problems, body build, or heredity. Actually, obesity caused by endocrine gland disorders is exceptionally rare. Only 1 or 2 of every 100 children has a true metabolic problem. Also, familial obesity (obesity that runs in families) is more a matter of improper eating habits than one of heredity.

Lack of physical activity encourages the development of obesity in two ways. First, the absence of sufficient exercise means that an individual uses only a small proportion of generously consumed food calories to provide energy for physical exertion. The unused calories are converted into fat storage deposits in the body. Second, recent research has shown that the internal mechanisms that normally regulate appetite do not operate properly at low levels of physical exertion, which are so characteristic of many American children.[19] Obese children, as a result, are sometimes unable to perceive the internal signals that announce that they have consumed enough food to satisfy their bodies' needs, and they therefore continue to eat.

Psychological factors play a larger role in childhood obesity than in adult obesity. Poor adjustment to home, life, school, or other emotional problems can lead to an excessive, compensating interest in food. Early recognition of a child's tendency toward weight gain is an important factor in preventing what could become an irreversible condition. It appears likely that the psychological results of obesity, such as passivity and withdrawal tend to increase the physical inactivity of obese youngsters and thus make the obesity self-accelerating, or at least self-continuing.

Gratification of either conscious or unconscious emotional needs may underlie many cases of childhood obesity. Psychological obesity may be developmental, that is, involving the entire growing personality. Interestingly enough, some studies show that a specific event or situation often precipitates overeating behavior among the elementary-age group. For example, researchers have reported onset of obesity following surgery in children and during forced or prolonged periods of bed rest and after a move to a new neighborhood, loss of friends and a change of school. Other precipitating factors may be a mother starting work and family upset over the loss of another child, a job or an illness.[20] Eating and consequent obesity provide a refuge from insecurity, anxiety, and loneliness.

Some of the health problems that commonly plague obese children include clumsiness, shortness of breath during exertion, skin irritation due to friction and heat discomfort. These are frequent but minor complaints. The most devastating and serious of all the problems that face obese children are psychosocial. Unquestionably, many of these children have a poor self-image and express feelings of inferiority and rejection. Most of them encounter teasing, ridicule, and are often left out of games, activities, and athletics. Thus they become increasingly inactive (see Figure 11-1).[21]

An additional source of concern is the possible withdrawal of the obese child into antisocial behavior accompanied by deteriorating school performance. Confronted with rejection and possible self-imposed isolation, obese youngsters do not develop some of the social skills that would enable them to gain greater acceptance. It is interesting to note that the unusual and even bizarre eating patterns that afflict some obese persons are almost all found in those whose disorder began in childhood.[22]

Although not all obese persons experience health problems, it is well known that excessive weight can aggravate or precipitate high blood pressure, liver disease, arthritis, diabetes, and a host of other conditions that can shorten a normal life span. Most of these conditions are not prevalent in childhood, but the fact that many obese children become obese adults gives yet another reason for concern about childhood obesity.

Once educators have recognized that obesity in children is a true health hazard, they can mobilize the necessary support to carry out a preventive approach to the most prevalent nutritional problem in the United States—overweight.[23] Working closely with the child, family, and physicians, teachers can help to develop health and physical education programs for the elementary level that will facilitate the detection and prevention of this problem. More specifically, Sorochan and Bender suggest the following:

1. Become involved and interested in the overweight children as human beings.
2. Provide challenging alternatives to coping with problems of living.
3. Relate to the children's emotional needs, particularly some of those that may have been created as a result of their overweight.
4. Involve the children in a lot of physical activity and exercise; this should be done in a way that is not construed to be a penalty for a weight problem.
5. Discourage nibbling, snacks, and overeating; this should include elimination of vending machines in schools which provide easy access for candy bars and soda pop.

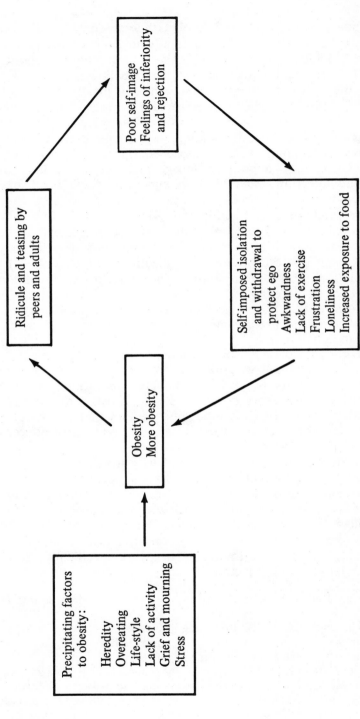

FIGURE 11-1. *Teachers can best break the vicious cycle of childhood obesity by taking a little extra time to help overweight youngsters realize that they are worthwhile and loved. Enhancing self-esteem will give them some of the courage they need to risk doing some of the things that are necessary to lose weight. (adapted from Jean Mayer, Overweight: Causes, Cost, and Control. Copyright © 1968, p. 129. Reprinted by permission of Prentice-Hall, Inc., Englewood Cliffs, New Jersey.)*

6. Help children to identify their own self-image; unfortunately, whatever the cause of obesity may be, children who are obese frequently develop psychological problems and sometimes deviant behavior because of ridicule by their own peers.
7. Allow for rest periods, but do not let rest become apathy.
8. Arrange social activities that are fun for everyone.
9. Help the children meet new friends.*

Teachers must always be careful to avoid making derogatory comments about a child's appearance—even in jest, because overweight youngsters usually have a low opinion of their bodies and personalties and are easily depressed. In addition, teachers should take every opportunity to reassure children that they are loved and esteemed.[24] Charlotte Young summarizes the teacher's role as follows:

> Perhaps teachers can help most by taking a personal interest in the child, not in his obesity; listening to his feelings and problems; sharing his confidences; accepting him as he is; giving him support in his efforts to be independent; and helping him to find personal recognition and success in assuming responsibilities and duties.
>
> Sometimes group activities engaged in with the help of a teacher or counselor are helpful to obese youngsters by providing an accepting climate in which they may socialize and concentrate on self-improvement rather than weight loss.[25]

Finally, one of the best preventive efforts that can take place in the elementary school is to teach children the essentials of proper nutrition and physical activity.

NOTES

1. Jean Mayer, *A Diet for Living* (New York: David McKay Co., 1975), pp. 172-3.
2. Johanna T. Dwyer, "The Seven Ages of Nutrition—Childhood," *Family Health*, July 1974, p. 32.
3. Adapted from *Food Is More than Just Something to Eat* (Washington, D.C.: U.S. Food and Drug Administration, 1975), and from Brent Q. Hafen, Alton Thygerson, and Ronald Rhodes, *Prescriptions for Health* (Provo, Utah: Brigham Young University Press, 1977), pp. 107–29.
4. G. Edward Damon, "A Primer on Four Nutrients: Proteins, Carbohydrates, Fats, and Fiber," *FDA Consumer*, February 1975, pp. 5–13.
5. Select Committee on Nutrition and Human Needs, U.S. Senate, *Dietary Goals for the United States* (Washington, D.C.: U.S. Government Printing Office, 1977), pp. 17–18.
6. Ibid.

*Sorochan/Bender, *Teaching Elementary Health Science*, 2nd ed., © 1979 Addison-Wesley Publishing Company, Inc. Page 81, "Suggestions for helping the child with a weight problem." Reprinted with permission.

7. "Nutrition Sense and Nonsense," *FDA Consumer,* May 1974, p. 5.
8. Select Committee on Nutrition and Human Needs, pp. 17–18.
9. Adapted from National Institute of Child Health and Human Development, *Malnutrition, Learning, and Behavior* (Washington, D.C.: U.S. Department of Health, Education, and Welfare, 1976).
10. George Owen and Gleen Lippman, "Nutritional Status of Infants and Young Children: U.S.A.," *Pediatric Clinics of North America,* February 1977, pp. 211–27.
11. Charlotte G. Neumann, "Obesity in Pediatric Practice: Obesity in the Preschool and School-age Child," *Pediatric Clinics of North America,* February 1977, pp. 117–22.
12. Robert H. A. Haslam and Peter J. Balleputti, *Medical Problems in the Classroom,* Baltimore, Md.: University Park Press, 1975), pp. 93–94.
13. Neumann, pp. 117–22.
14. Gurney Williams III, "Growing Up Fat," *Science Digest,* December 1974, pp. 61–65.
15. "What You Should Know About Obesity," *American Druggist,* 15 February 1974, pp. 57–59.
16. Mayer, pp. 115–28.
17. Ibid.
18. Ibid.
19. National Institutes of Health, *Facts About Obesity* (Washington, D.C.: U.S. Department of Health, Education, and Welfare, 1976).
20. Neumann, pp. 117–22.
21. Ibid.
22. Jean Mayer, ed., *U.S. Nutrition Policies in the Seventies* (San Francisco: W.H. Freeman and Co., 1978), p. 81.
23. Haslam and Balleputti, pp. 93–94.
24. Jean Mayer, "Thinning Down the Overweight Child," *Family Health,* December 1970, p. 27.
25. Charlotte M. Young, "The Fat Child," *Today's Education,* March 1971, p. 59.

RESOURCES

American Alliance for Health, Physical Education and Recreation, 1201 Sixteenth Street, N.W., Washington, D.C. 20036. (Materials: pamphlets, films, lists.)

American Association for Maternal and Child Health (AAMCH), P.O. Box 965, Los Altos, Calif. 94022.

American Cancer Society, Director of Public Education, 777 Third Avenue, New York, N.Y. 10017. (Materials: films, pamphlets, posters, etc.)

American Dental Association, Bureau of Dental Health Education, 211 E. Chicago Avenue, Chicago, Ill. 60611. (Materials: pamphlets, charts, posters, models.)

American Diabetes Association, 1 West 18th Street, New York, N.Y. 10020. (Materials: "A.D.A. Forecast" bimonthly magazine reprints, pamphlets.)

American Dietetic Association, 430 North Michigan Avenue, Chicago, Ill. 60611.
American Heart Association, 7320 Greenville Avenue, Dallas, Tex. 75231.
American Home Economics Association, 2010 Massachusetts Avenue, N.W., Washington, D.C. 20036. (Materials: pamphlets, reprints.)
American Medical Association, Bureau of Health Education, 535 North Dearborn Street, Chicago, Ill. 60610.
National Dairy Council, Rosemont, Ill. 60018.

CHAPTER 12

Dental Health

Children's dental health affects many aspects of their lives. For example, crooked teeth might cause a child to avoid smiling out of self-consciousness. This child's personality, personal appearance, and social adjustment may suffer as a result. In addition, inadequately treated dental disease and infection from the teeth and associated structures may spread to other areas of the body, precipitating disease in kidneys, heart, and other tissues and seriously threatening physical health.

Dental disease afflicts 98 percent of the American population. On the average, children have three decayed teeth when they enter elementary school and will have eleven caries by the time they reach 15 years of age. Twenty-five percent of children will have lost 1 or more teeth from decay before turning 15.[1] Unfortunately, the teeth that elementary children most often lose are the six-year molars, teeth that too many parents and teachers consider baby teeth rather than permanent ones. A further illustration of the poor oral health of children is the total absence of teeth in 1 percent of the 15–24 age group. One-third of people 46–64 years old are totally toothless, and the percentage increases to two-thirds among people over 75. These are rather sad statistics for structures that, given good personal and professional care, should last a lifetime.

Paradoxically, despite the nearly universal incidence of dental disorders Americans are pervasively apathetic toward dental health. Personal oral hygiene is poor despite continued, though often haphazard, attempts to correct the situation through education.

Decay is not the only dental problem of elementary schoolchildren. Fifty percent have periodontal disease. Most suffer from some degree of malocclusion (bad bite), and 30 percent of these cases are serious enough to warrant treatment.[2] Gingivitis, an inflammation of the gums that is almost exclusively the result of poor personal oral hygiene afflicts 90 percent of teenagers.

NORMAL TEETH DEVELOPMENT

We usually think of newborn babies as toothless. This notion is far from true. The deciduous teeth—commonly called "baby teeth"—are

FIGURE 12-1. *The structure of a permanent tooth. (Lon W. Moreey and Robert J. Nelson, eds.,* Dental Science Handbook *(Washington, D.C.: U.S. Department of Health, Education, and Welfare, 1970).)*

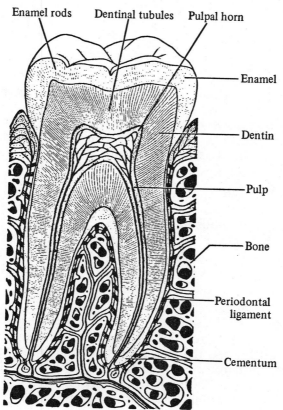

Enamel rods   Dentinal tubules   Pulpal horn

Enamel

Dentin

Pulp

Bone

Periodontal ligament

Cementum

well formed and lie just below the gum line awaiting the appropriate time to erupt. By the time these teeth have fully erupted, the permanent set are well on their way to making their first appearance when the child is about six years of age. The first permanent teeth do not replace any of the deciduous set, but rather erupt immediately behind the last deciduous molar. All of the other permanent teeth, with the exception of the second and third molars, replace the deciduous teeth.

Calcification, or hardening, of the permanent teeth has usually begun by the time of birth or begins shortly thereafter. As the crowns of the permanent teeth grow larger, deep in the bone tissue, the roots of the deciduous teeth dissolve, or resorb. By the time a permanent tooth is ready to erupt, the root of the deciduous tooth usually has completely resorbed and only the crown remains. The central incisors, usually the first deciduous teeth that a child loses, generally fall out at about six years of age. Before the child is twelve years old, permanent teeth will replace all of the deciduous teeth. By age twenty the permanent set of teeth will be complete. Figure 12–1 shows the structure of a normal tooth.

DENTAL DEFECTS

Dental Caries

Caries, or cavities, result from the colonization of teeth by certain bacteria called streptococci and perhaps other bacteria, followed by their utilization of dietary carbohydrates to produce a decay-inducing plaque on tooth surfaces. Analyzing this process suggests three ways to reduce the incidence of dental caries:

1. Eliminate the bacteria. This is not a practical procedure because the toxicity or caustic quality of bacteria-killing agents mediates against their continuous use.
2. Reduce dietary sugars. Good oral hygiene practices following eating have always been a part of the armament against caries.
3. Strengthening the tooth against the effects of plaque. (We will discuss the value of fluoride in this regard later.)

Dental caries are infectious and transmittable. Caries-free animals, fed a diet identical to a group of caries-active littermates, will develop dental caries only when the two groups of animals live together. Presumably, the initially microorganism-free mouth of the newborn human harbors a wide variety of microorganisms a few weeks later due to adult contact, primarily with the mother.

FIGURE 12-2. *Progress of decay. (a) The bacteria have penetrated the enamel and attacked the softer dentin. (b) The bacteria have penetrated the dentin and killed the pulp, causing an abscess to form at the apex of the root. This condition may often be treated successfully, or the tooth may have to be removed and replaced with an artificial tooth. (From* Dental Science Handbook *(Washington, D.C.: U.S. Department of Health, Education, and Welfare, 1970), p. 184.)*

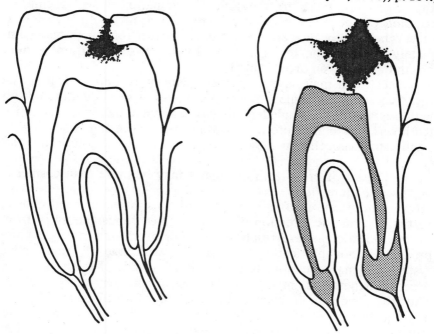

Streptococcus mutans is generally considered to be the bacterium that causes dental caries. It can exist only on hard surfaces. In the presence of colonies of these organisms, the decay process proceeds in accordance with the type and amount of dietary sugars, the frequency of their intake, and the age of the plaque. An important consideration that offers a good rationale for frequent cleaning is the fact that the older the plaque, the greater the acidity produced when sugar is present.

The potential hazards of dental caries are considerable. As Figure 12-2 indicates, the decay process may lead to root abcesses and subsequently spread via the blood stream to various areas of the body. Long-term abcess activity can erode and weaken the jawbones and predispose them to fractures. It is patently irresponsible to regard caries as a normal and acceptable hazard of living. Even the toothache is an experience that we can readily avoid. The decay process takes nearly two years to reach the point of producing pain, so parents can easily spare their children the discomfort of a toothache.

Malocclusion

Malocclusion is an irregularity in tooth position and *occlusion,* the coming together of the teeth when the jaws are closed. At least 50 percent of children in any age group probably have malocclusion. It is least likely to be present in the deciduous teeth and develops while the permanent teeth are erupting. Crowding, excessive spacing, or rotation of the teeth may be present. The front teeth may fail to meet when the back teeth are occluded, or the front teeth may completely overbite the lower teeth. Any of these conditions should prompt a visit to an orthodontist.

Malocclusion may have a significant emotional impact. If it is true that "an attractive smile is a person's greatest asset," then the person with severely maloccluded teeth has a distinct liability. Attractive teeth certainly contribute to a pleasing appearance and children with significant malocclusion may experience feelings of inferiority and insecurity.

The impact of poor teeth alignment may be more than cosmetic, however. Failure of the teeth to meet properly can interfere with efficient mastication of some foods and thus influence food choice, particularly in the direction of highly refined foods and away from fibrous selections. As a result, the child's nutritional status is compromised. Poor mastication increases the work load of the digestive system and may occasionally incite a mild episode of gastrointestinal upset. Furthermore, maloccluded teeth are harder to keep clean. Thus the condition aggravates the problems of tooth decay and periodontal disease. Some orthodontists and teachers are even able to detect articulation problems that are directly attributable to crooked teeth.

The major causes of malocclusion are heredity and neglect. Jaw and tooth size are genetically determined and frequently poorly matched, so that large teeth must often crowd into jawbones too small to receive them. The result is poor positioning of the teeth in the jaw and malocclusion.

Hereditary factors account for about 50 percent of malocclusion problems. The remainder are the result of parental or personal neglect. Thumb sucking is a normal practice in children under two years of age and it may persist as a normal nighttime or tension-reducing activity to age three or four. Allowed to continue beyond this age, it may affect the position of the incoming permanent teeth and the shape of the jawbone. Parents should contact the family dentist when such habits persist abnormally.

Another parental mistake is what some dentists call "nursing-bottle mouth." Putting a child to bed with a bottle means that the teeth tend to be bathed in the contained fluids all night long—an optimal condition for decay if the bottle contains anything but water. All but the lower front teeth, which the tongue and bottle nipple tend to protect, will undergo a continuous decay process leading to serious damage. If restoration of the affected teeth proves impossible, a very premature deciduous loss and severe malocclusion may occur in later years.

Whenever teeth fall out, the remaining teeth tend to fill in the gap. Thus, the premature loss of the last deciduous molar to decay may cause the six-year molar to come in too far forward and decrease the space available for eruption of the other permanent teeth. When deciduous teeth fall out too early, it is advisable to insert space maintainers to prevent occlusal problems later on. Even the loss of a permanent tooth will allow the remaining teeth to migrate and produce occlusal problems.

Periodontal Disease

Periodontics is the study and treatment of diseases involving the supporting structures of the teeth, namely, the *gingiva,* or gum tissue; cementum; periodontal ligament; and the *alveolar bone,* which supports the teeth. Most of the diseases that attack these tissues derive from initiating, extrinsic factors such as poor oral hygiene, malocclusion, improper dental treatment, and lack of preventive care.

Inflammation of any of the support structures, called *periodontitis,* usually begins with mild to severe involvement of the tissues surrounding the neck of the tooth (see Figure 12–3). This initial stage is

FIGURE 12-3. *Progress of periodontal infection. (a) Food and calcium deposits have irritated the gingiva, causing it to withdraw from the teeth. (b) Further destruction, including the beginning of a periodontal pocket. (c) The infection has destroyed most of the tissues around one tooth and weakened the other. (d) One tooth is lost, the other weakened. (From Lon W. Morrey and Robert J. Nelson, eds.,* Dental Science Handbook *(Washington, D.C.: U.S. Department of Health, Education, and Welfare, 1970), p. 205.)*

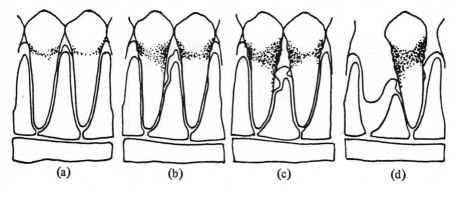

(a)   (b)   (c)   (d)

called *gingivitis* and will usually be evident as a slight bleeding or "pink toothbrush" on flossing or brushing the teeth. The inflammation is believed to be the result of tissue reaction to plaque material left in the groove between the teeth and gingiva due to poor oral hygiene. Gradually, the infection attacks the periodontal tissue that surrounds the root of the tooth. If the condition is not corrected through the adoption of more effective oral-hygiene techniques, it will deteriorate and a periodontal pocket will develop along the root. Food particles and bacteria enter the pocket to produce irritation and thus aggravate the condition. As the process becomes chronic, all of the supporting tissues may be lost in addition to the serious consequences that such continuing infections pose for general health. Eventually, in the absence of timely intervention, it will be necessary to remove the teeth.

Oral Injuries

Injuries to the teeth are common in children and should receive prompt professional attention. Chipped or broken teeth may suffer a rapid deterioration of deeper tooth substance or may seriously traumatize adjacent tissues if sharp or rough edges are present. They should be repaired or removed and replaced. Repositioning a tooth that has been completely knocked out is sometimes possible. Back in the socket, it may remain functional for several years. If such an accident occurs, wrapping the tooth in a damp cloth or placing it in water will keep it safe during the trip to the dentist for possible reinsertion.

ORAL HEALTH AND THE SCHOOL

Dental health is important to every schoolchild. Unlike many other kinds of disease and disorder, successful treatment of dental problems seldom requires only professional care. An hour with the dentist once every six months simply cannot compensate for consistent neglect by the patient through the remainder of the year. Proper habits of preventive care must be a daily routine for the maintenance of dental health. For the sake of their children, parents should have made considerable progress in teaching good oral hygiene before they enter school. Adjunctively, teachers can play a significant and important role in formulating such habits and thereby influence children's dental health for years to come. Dental health education should promote understanding in two important facets of dental health maintenance: diet and oral hygiene.

Diet

Heredity plays a very important role in dental health and, unfortunately, the effects may be somewhat less than desired. But whatever the hereditary potential, dental health depends greatly on the diet during the critical periods when the teeth are developing. To be sound and caries-resistant, teeth must be as well formed as heredity will allow. To insure that the teeth will be as perfect as possible, it is necessary to see that a child's daily nutritional intake includes the essential elements of good teeth formation in optimum quantities.

Properly developed tooth enamel must contain *fluorapetite,* a chemical compound made up of fluoride, calcium, and some other elements. These elements must be available in proper quantities throughout the dental formative period (before birth to about ten or twelve years of age) if the teeth are to be highly resistant to dental caries. A well-balanced and varied diet that promotes good general health will provide the necessary ingredients for good teeth, as does a diet based on the four food groups described in Table 11–3. The major source of dietary calcium is the dairy products group (excluding butter), which growing children require in abundance. Dietary fluoride is scarce in most food commodities. What is present in our food comes from the water and soil used in food production, although pesticides may contribute small amounts. By far the greatest source of dietary fluoride is generally the fluoride salts found in the supply of drinking water, but many of our supplies are substantially deficient in this element whereas others may contain toxic levels. Excessive concentrations of fluorides may produce tooth mottling, or discoloration, ranging from a loss of luster to a dark brown stain (mottling may also result from high fever and the use of certain antibiotics during the tooth-forming period). Concentrations of one part per million (1 ppm) or one part of fluoride for every million parts of water affords maximum protection against dental caries. Higher levels offer no known nutritional benefit with respect to dental health.

Fluoridation is the addition of fluoride to drinking water supplies to raise the level to 1 ppm. Fluoridation programs constitute a distinctly praiseworthy community effort to improve the nutrition of the populace and coincidentally its dental health. Children raised in such communities experience a 65 percent lower decay rate than children raised on fluoride-deficient water (see Figure 12–4).

Indirectly, fluoridation contributes in other ways to good dental health. Because much malocclusion is due to premature tooth loss, a caries-related event, adequate fluoride nutrition reduces orthodontic needs. In addition, a body of accumulating evidence suggests that fluoride in the diet throughout life acts as a deterrent to osteoporosis, a brittleness of the bones associated with aging that particularly strikes women.

FIGURE 12-4. *Effects of fluoridation in one community compared to non-fluoridation in another community. (Based on data from Lon W. Morrey and Robert J. Nelson, eds.,* Dental Science Handbook *(Washington, D.C.: U.S. Department of Health, Education, and Welfare, 1970).)*

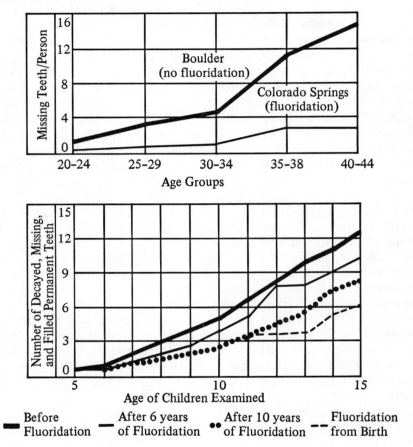

Finally, we should note that other approaches to fluoride nutrition, such as drops and pills, are practically unreliable, even though they are theoretically sound. Failure to continue using pills or drops is the reason. The use of fluoride toothpastes and topical application of fluoride by the dentist are helpful, but they are effective only on a small scale and are not cost effective.[3]

Along with consideration of what foods are critical to dental health, we must be aware of the items that can undermine dental health. Minimizing dental caries requires eliminating snacks that are high in sugar from the diet and limiting intake of sweets at regular mealtimes. In schools where vending machines reap daily revenues, it is necessary to carefully regulate the canteen fare for the health of the children. Rewarding good behavior with sweets is a particularly insidious threat to dental health and other health concerns and should never be a part of the operating procedures in any school.

Oral Hygiene

An effective dental-health education program in the school includes instruction designed to promote good personal oral-hygiene techniques. Even without the benefits of fluoridation, most tooth decay and gingival diseases are preventable through a consistently applied program of plaque removal with dental floss and a toothbrush. Because children's eating habits and other behavior render them susceptible to decay, they should learn to clean their teeth after each meal and at least rinse their mouths after snacks. Classroom activities can do much to encourage these procedures.

Teachers can check children's teeth for plaque by giving them disclosing tablets to chew. Available at local pharmacies, these tablets stain the plaque red. The child is taught how to brush the teeth in such a way that all of the red stain will be removed. When the red is gone, the teeth are clean. After children have learned plaque-removal techniques, continue dispensing disclosing tablets on a regular basis so that they can evaluate their own oral hygiene.

Toothbrushing is a technique that preschool children find difficult to learn. Even school-age youngsters require supervision for this task. An important part of toothbrushing is brushing the gums. Holding the toothbrush at a 45° angle to the gum line allows the bristles to reach into the grooves around the tooth to remove plaque and food material (see Figure 12-5).

Children should use straight-handled toothbrushes that have a flat brushing surface and soft bristles rounded on the ends. Small brushes provide greater mobility so that the child can do a thorough job. Soft, small toothbrushes in the hands of inexperienced children tend to wear out faster than adult models. Therefore efficient brushers will require new toothbrushes often.

The only way to remove plaque from between the teeth is by correctly using dental floss. Children may find it easier to hold floss if you tie the two ends together to form a circle about ten inches in diameter. The floss should be guided gently against the side of the tooth into the space between two teeth until resistance is felt (see Figure 12-6). It should then be wrapped in a "U" shape around the tooth and scraped up toward the crown of the tooth. Care must be taken not to pull the floss into the groove too forcefully or tissue damage will occur. Careful supervision is important.

FIGURE 12-5. *Acceptable toothbrushing method: Hold the jaws slightly apart. Brush each area of the teeth surfaces—inside, outside, and chewing—at least ten times. (a) Place the bristles of the brush pointing toward the roots of the teeth. Rotate the brush so that the bristles sweep down over the gingiva and teeth in the direction of the biting or grinding surfaces. Brush the outer surfaces of all the teeth, upper and lower. (b) Brush the upper teeth with a downward motion; the inside surfaces of the back teeth, upper and lower. (c) Brush the lower teeth with an upward stroke on the front teeth. (d) Brush the chewing surfaces of all teeth. Rinse the mouth thoroughly with warm water after brushing to remove the loose food particles and to help keep the mouth free from odors. (From Lon W. Morrey and Robert J. Nelson, eds.,* Dental Science Handbook *(Washington, D.C.: U.S. Department of Health, Education, and Welfare, 1970), p. 177.)*

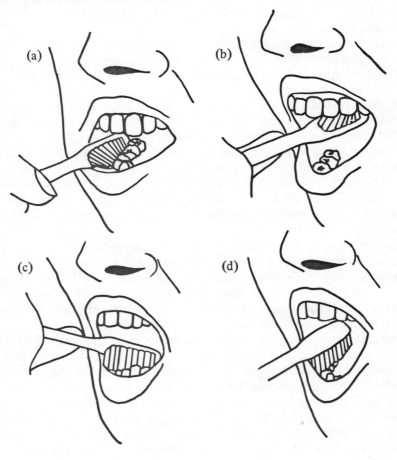

FIGURE 12-6. *The correct way to floss away dental plaque.*

(a) Floss position for upper teeth

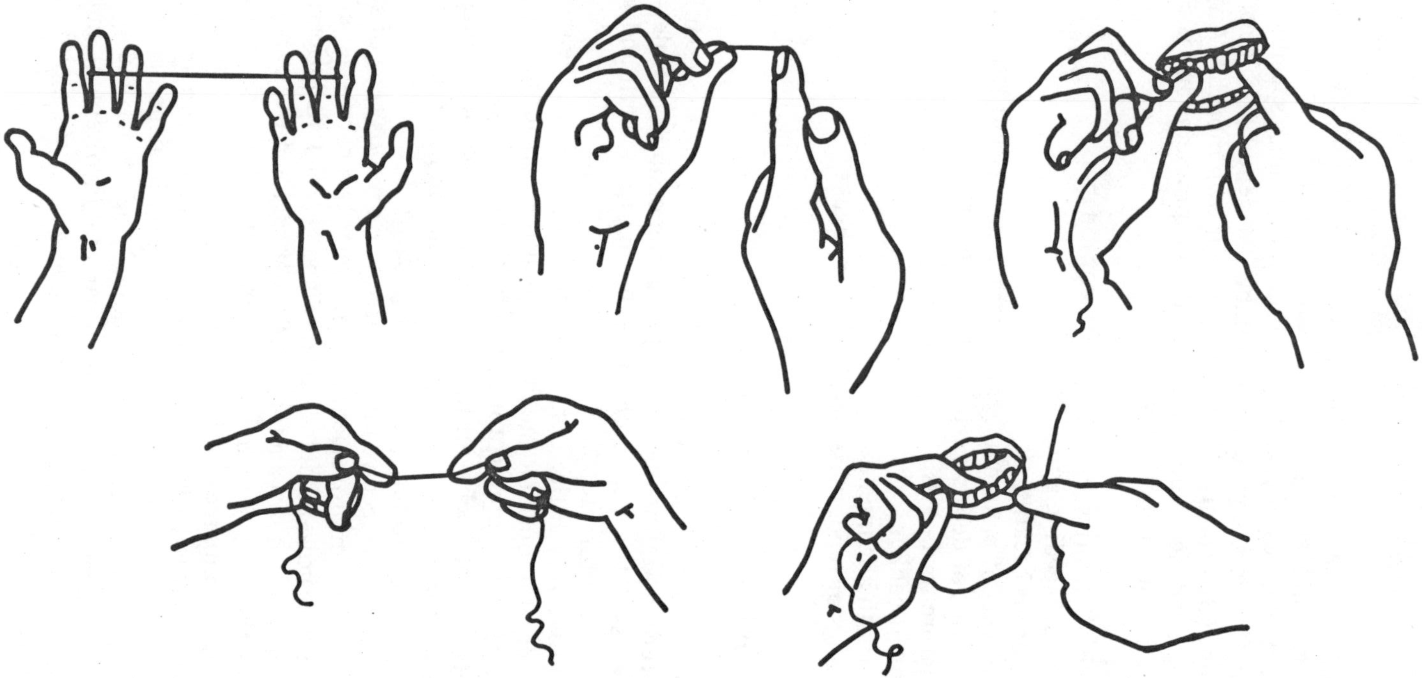

(b) Floss position for lower teeth

Teacher Observation

Children who are conscientious about dental health brush after every meal, floss once each day, avoid caries-promoting snacks, and visit the dentist twice each year. Try to find one of those specimens. What you will find is a considerable number of dental problems in your classroom. (How many of them are in your own mouth?) Any of the following conditions might indicate dental problems and is cause for closer examination and follow-up:

1. Speech difficulties, especially with consonants
2. Inflamed, bleeding gums
3. Malodorous breath
4. Complaints of pains and aches in oral and adjacent structures
5. Collections of debris on and between teeth
6. Premature tooth loss
7. Frequent canker sores
8. Poor tooth alignment
9. Swellings or tenderness around lips or cheeks

The Involvement of The Home

Preschool children lack the manual dexterity to successfully brush their teeth and flossing is a hopeless impossibility. Unless parents actively assist their children in caring for their teeth and gums the dental picture for preschool and elementary-age children will probably improve very little. Dental hygiene education in the school does not change the outlook much, although the classroom program may provide effective support for instruction in the home.

Experimental behavior-modification approaches initiated and guided by the school but implemented in the home have been most effective in controlling plaque and gingivitis.[4] Furthermore students whose classmates received home instruction in this type of study also experienced an improvement in oral hygiene—a carry-over effect. Parents learned how to detect plaque and learned to properly reward their children for satisfactory performance. Each week they reported back to the school to indicate their continuing participation in the program. Compared with self-teaching and teacher- and dental-hygienist-instructed students, the home-taught group demonstrated a statistically significant improvement in oral hygiene habits. Teachers who genuinely try to change children's behaviors will probably be more successful if they can obtain parental involvement and cooperation in implementing the preventive care program described in Table 12-1.

TABLE 12-1. Preventive Dental Program

Methods	Objectives	Means
Oral hygiene	Removal of food debris and calcium deposits Rinsing and stimulating tissues between the teeth	Personal care—cleansing the mouth immediately after meals and snacks by means of a toothbrush, dentifrice, and tepid water; dental tape, interdental stimulators; devices that irrigate the mouth with controlled force of water Professional care—prophylactic treatment by dentist or dental hygienist
Diet and nutrition	Optimal nutrition Reduced retention of fermentable carbohydrate foodstuffs on tooth surface Stimulation of soft supporting tissues	Nutritional guidance of patient Inclusion in the diet of an optimal amount of raw fruits, raw vegetables, whole-grain breads and cereals Inclusion in the diet of a minimal amount of sweets
Fluoride	Increased resistance to caries	Systemic addition—community water fluoridation; oral administration of fluoride Topical application—in dental office Home application—with dentifrice
Protective devices	Prevent dental damage in contact sports Prevent destruction of teeth and supporting structures through habits such as grinding the teeth	Mouth guards Night-guard prostheses Space maintainers

Source: *Dental Science Handbook* (Washington, D.C.: U.S. Department of Health, Education, and Welfare, 1970), p. 175.

NOTES

1. J.C. Green, "Dental Health Needs of the Nation," *Journal of American Dental Association* 84 (1972): 1073-75.
2. *A Supplemental Dental Health Guide for the Teachers of Utah* (Salt Lake City: Utah State Division of Health, 1974), p. 3.
3. F.A. Arnold, Jr., F.J. McClure, and C.L. White, "Sodium Fluoride Tablets for

Children," *Dental Progress* 1 (October 1960); *Your Child's Teeth,* (Chicago: American Dental Association, 1973), p. 8.
4. Jerrold S. Greenberg, "An Analysis of Various Teaching Modes in Dental Health Education," *Journal of School Health,* January 1977, p. 26.

RESOURCES

American Dental Association (or local association), Bureau of Dental Health Education, 211 East Chicago Avenue, Chicago, Ill. 60611. (Materials: pamphlets, catalog of literature, audiovisual aids, etc.)

Colgate-Palmolive Company, 300 Park Avenue, New York, N.Y. 10010. (Materials on skin care and dental health.)

Dental Digest, Inc., 1005 Liberty Avenue, Pittsburgh, Pa.

Lever Brothers, Co., Public Relations Div., Consumer Education Department, 390 Park Avenue, New York, N.Y. 10022. (Materials on dental health.)

Oral Hygiene Publications, 1005 Library Avenue, Pittsburgh, Pa. 15234. (Materials on dental health.)

CHAPTER 13
Visual Problems

Good vision is an essential learning tool in the typical classroom. Children who see poorly not only will find it very difficult to keep up with their classmates, but will likely suffer severe emotional setbacks as well. Poor performance fosters feelings of inadequacy and discouragement and is a common correlate of behavioral problems. The visually handicapped child is at a disadvantage in many ways. For example, it's hard to catch a football that you cannot see. Failure to recognize friends and appropriately greet them may leave people with an impression of aloofness or even conceit, which can endanger the establishment of healthy interpersonal relationships. Aware of the potential problems of the poorly sighted, teachers can be constantly vigilant for signs of visual difficulties in their students.

THE VISUAL APPARATUS

Figure 13-1 shows the parts of the human eye and Table 13-1 describes their functions. The outermost layer of the eye, the *sclera,* is a tough, elastic tissue modified in front to form the *cornea,* or window, through which light passes into the eye. The middle layer, the *choroid,* is heavily pigmented to prevent light from scat-

FIGURE 13-1. *Parts of the human eye. (Courtesy of the National Society to Prevent Blindness.)*

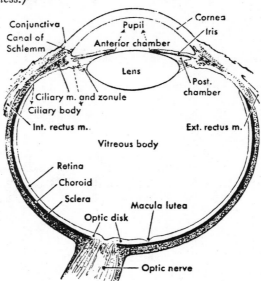

THE HUMAN EYE (RIGHT)

tering inside the eye and serves an important nutritional function for other structures of the eye. In front, the modified choroid forms the *iris* and *ciliary body.* The iris, which gives color to the eye, regulates the amount of light entering the eye and forms the *pupil,* a hole at the center. Behind the iris lies the *crystalline lens,* which changes shape under the influence of the ciliary muscle (another modification of the choroid) to accommodate near and far vision.

Secretory tissues located near the crystalline lens produce a fluid called the *aqueous humor,* which fills the chambers in front of the lens and may also filter into the posterior area of the eye where the *vitreous body* is. The aqueous humor maintains pressure within the eye, supports the metabolism of the lens, and provides nourishment for the cornea.

The innermost layer of the eye is the *retina,* an extension of nervous tissue into the eyeball. When light hits receptive cells in the retina, a photochemical change converts the light rays into nerve impulses that travel to the brain by way of the *optic nerve.* In the brain, the nerve impulses pattern and elicit nervous activity in other brain centers to form a perceptual experience.

The *conjunctiva* is the membrane that lines the underside of the eyelids and the anterior surface of the eyeball. Normally, the conjunctiva is transparent, but occasionally small blood vessels are visible over the scleral surface of the eye.

The *lens* of the eye is a pliable structure that can undergo modifi-

TABLE 13-1.   Parts of the Eye

Anterior chamber	Space in the front of the eye, bounded in front by the cornea and behind by the iris; filled with aqueous humor
Aqueous humor	Clear, watery fluid that fills the anterior and posterior chambers within the front part of the eye
Canal of Schlemm	A circular canal situated at the juncture of the sclera and cornea through which the aqueous humor drains after it has circulated between the lens and the iris and between the iris and the cornea
Choroid	The vascular, intermediate coat that furnishes nourishment to the other parts of the eyeball
Ciliary body	Portion of the vascular coat between the iris and the choroid consisting of ciliary processes and the ciliary muscle
Conjunctiva	Mucous membrane that lines the inner side of the eyelids and covers the front part of the eyeball
Cornea	Clear, transparent portion of the outer coat of eyeball forming front of aqueous chamber
Crystalline lens	A transparent, colorless body suspended in the front of the eyeball, between the aqueous humor and the vitreous body, the function of which is to bring the rays of light to a focus on the retina
Fovea	Small depression in the retina at the back of the eye; the part of the macula adapted for most acute vision
Iris	Colored, circular membrane suspended behind the cornea and immediately in front of the lens. The iris regulates the amount of light entering the eye by changing the size of the pupil
Macula lutea	The small area of the retina that surrounds the fovea and with the fovea comprises the area of distinct vision (synonym: *yellow spot*)
Optic disk	Head of the optic nerve in the eyeball
Optic nerve	The special nerve of the sense of sight that carries messages from the retina to the brain
Posterior chamber	Space between the back of the iris and the front of the lens filled with aqueous
Pupil	The contractile opening at the center of the iris for the transmission of light
Retina	Innermost coat of the eye formed of sensitive nerve fibers and connected with the optic nerve
Sclera	The white part of the eye—a tough covering that, with the cornea, forms the external, protective coat of the eye
Suspensory ligaments	A complex structure of multiple bands of tissue that hold the crystalline lens in place
Vitreous body	Transparent, colorless mass of soft, gelatinous material filling the eyeball behind the lens

cations in shape as a result of the action of the ciliary muscle and suspensory ligament. In order to minimize blur and distortion of an image falling upon the retina the nervous system sends nerve impulses to the ciliary muscle to adjust the shape of the lens for near or far objects. When this mechanism allows the eye to focus the image through the full range of vision (a few inches to twenty feet from the eye), the eye is normal, or *emmetropic.* More specifically, the eye is emmetropic if objects twenty feet away and beyond focus on the retina with the ciliary muscle completely relaxed. A *refractive error* exists when the shape of the eyeball, the characteristics of the lens, or the properties of any other medium through which the light must pass on its way to the retina are such that a focus does not occur.

DISEASES OF THE EYE

Table 13-2 lists several signs or symptoms that might alert teachers to possible visual problems. Although the majority of these problems will stem from refractive errors, children sometimes develop conjunctivitis, blepharitis, and sties.

Conjunctivitis

Bacterial invasions of the conjunctiva may cause *conjunctivitis,* or pinkeye, as it is commonly called. The conjunctiva is more susceptible to microbial invasion than other parts of the eye, in part, because of its constant exposure to air. Periodic rubbing of the eyes enhances the possibilities of infection.

During infection, the vessels of the conjunctiva dilate and the tissue becomes inflamed. Itching, burning, and pus formation are

TABLE 13-2.   Behavioral Indicators of Visual Problems

Rubbing eyes
Continual blinking
Squinting
Holding book as far away as possible
Reads only for brief periods
Reads with nose in the book
Headaches
Frequent accidents
Cranes neck to see distant objects
General inattention

other symptoms. The secretion and accumulation of pus may cause the eyelids to seal together overnight. The cornea may appear cloudy due to the secretions adhering to its surface. Corneal ulcers may occur, but they are not common and they heal quickly.

Conjunctivitis may strike only one eye, but frequent rubbing of the eyes to relieve itching can readily spread the disease via the hands to the other eye and to other persons. Teachers who can successfully train students to keep their hands away from their eyes will have done much to prevent the spread of conjuntivitis as well as certain other diseases of the eyes.

Fomites (objects which can harbor or transmit infectious material, e.g., pencils, table tops, handkerchiefs, etc.) may be the mode by which transmission occurs. Although it is correct to encourage children to always use only their own articles of clothing and personal hygiene, the desirability of this practice increases in the presence of a communicable disease.

A form of conjunctivitis called *trachoma* is potentially blinding. Although trachoma attacks the conjuntiva first, the virus ultimately will invade the cornea and tear glands and destroy them. Permanent blindness may occur without proper treatment, particularly if bacterial infection complicates the viral invasion. This disease thrives in hot, dry areas where water is scarce and hygiene poor. Among the Indian population of the southwestern United States, the infection is relatively common, but it is nearly universal among children.[1]

Personal cleanliness is very important as a preventive measure against trachoma, as it is against pinkeye. In arid locations it is possible to decrease the incidence of trachoma simply by providing sufficient water to promote frequent hand washing. Fly control is a good supplement to other preventive approaches.

Inflammation of the conjunctiva may also be the result of an allergic reaction. Occasionally the conjunctiva may become swollen without redness in response to an allergen and give the appearance of a gelatinous material on the scleral surface. Itching, tearing, and redness are the most common manifestations of allergic reactions, however, and these symptoms usually abate temporarily when the individual takes antihistamines. Discovery and removal of the causative agent will eliminate the symptoms entirely. Cosmetics, perfumes, and hair dressings are a few of the items that aggravate an existing allergy, so it is probably best to avoid them during periods of heightened allergic response.

Blepharitis

An eye infection that is common among children involves the margins of the eyelids. It causes itching, burning, and redness and makes the lids swell and the eyelashes fall out. In addition, scales or crusts that leave a bleeding surface when pulled away frequently cover the eyelids and lashes. Occasionally, the condition is ulcerative and causes permanent loss of eyelashes and, less frequently, ulceration of the cornea. The condition is somewhat resistant to treatment, and is frequently recurrent. Teachers should be alert for signs of this problem and encourage care by a physician.

Sty

A sty is an infection of the eyelash follicle, usually by staphylococcus bacterium. Localized swelling, redness, and pain are characteristic of the lesion, which is often associated with blepharitis. Recurrence is common and may be predisposed by visual problems, poor general health, and infection elsewhere in the body.

EYE TRAUMA

Foreign Body

When dirt and other small bodies come in contact with the conjunctiva, they produce considerable irritation. If they remain in the eye, and, in particular, if the eye is rubbed, they may imbed into the eye tissues and the conjunctiva, cornea, or sclera may suffer significant damage. If the object has been in the eye for only a short time, the nurse or the teacher may remove it safely by following the procedure outlined in Table 13–3. It is important that the child not touch his or her eyes. Usually the object will adhere to a moistened cotton swab lightly dabbed against the eye tissue. If not or if the object has been in the eye for some time, a physician should be consulted. Never touch the cornea.

TABLE 13–3.   Procedure for Removing Unimbedded Objects from the Surface of the Eye

1. Try to locate the object in the eye.

2. Have the child close the eye and roll the eyeball around.

3. Reopen the eye. If the object is in a different position, it has not lodged in the tissue and you can safely remove it.

4. Have the child close the eye and roll the eyeball. This action will usually cause the object to move into the margins of the sclera for easy removal.

Hematoma

Usually a blow to the eye is more frightening than serious. The brows and cheekbones provide good protection for the eyeball, but blood from ruptured vessels may seep into the soft orbital tissues surrounding the eyeball and produce a black eye. To reduce the degree of blackening, quickly place cold compresses on the eye and replace or recool them every fifteen to thirty seconds. Also the blood will reabsorb more rapidly and the blackness will disappear more quickly if hot compresses are regularly applied to the eye the following day.

A blow to the eye may damage the eyeball itself. Two guidelines will help to minimize damage and restore calm:

1. Penetrating wounds require immediate care by a physician only. Enroute to the doctor, it is advisable to cover both eyes to keep eye movement to a minimum.
2. Detachment of the retina from the choroid layer, if not properly treated, will lead to blindness. Any complaint of visual blurring or a "veil" being drawn across the eye should prompt immediate professional attention.

Preventive Measures

Constant vigilance of behavior is the only way to prevent eye injuries and disease. Teaching children to keep their hands away from their own and other's eyes will help to prevent infection as well as injury. Throwing or shooting objects at others, by whatever means, is intolerable behavior. Children who do not know how to hold, manipulate, or safely handle sharp or pointed objects, such as pencils and scissors, are distinct hazards to themselves and others. When introducing students to such objects, instruct them to use them safely and watch closely until they have acquired proper safety habits.

REFRACTIVE ERRORS

Light rays bend each time they pass from one medium to another having a different density. If the eyeball is not shaped properly or if the refractive components of the eye are irregular, the eye's ability to refract light may be subnormal. Consequently the image on the retina will be blurred or distorted. Such losses in visual acuity are referred to as *refractive errors*. In general, the three types of refractive errors are: nearsightedness (myopia), farsightedness (hyperopia), and astigmatism.

Myopia

Myopia is uncommon in children under six years of age, but the incidence grows from that age forward. Myopia is the most frequently encountered refractive error requiring glasses. Like other refractive errors, myopia is a genetically transmitted structural defect. In myopic individuals, the lens is too thick, the cornea too protuberant, or the eyeball is too long from front to back, a problem that causes the light rays to focus in front of the retina (see Figure 13-2) when distant objects are the object of attention. If the condition is progressive, the eye may be unable to properly discern even objects that are fairly close to the eye.

One of the characteristics of myopia is its typically insidious development, particularly in children. Since the condition produces no discomfort, myopic children may assume that their vision is normal when, in fact, it is quite poor. Unable to see distant objects clearly, they tend to ignore objects and activities beyond their visual horizon and become preoccupied with what is closest to them. Under the circumstances, they may be rather oblivious to instruction taking place in the front of the classroom and thereby perform their schoolwork poorly. Yet their myopic view of the situation may cause them to believe that they are short of intelligence rather than short of vision.

Although myopia produces no discomfort, the condition may produce some symptoms. Myopic individuals frequently learn that squinting improves their vision. Squinting reduces the amount of light entering the eye such that rays pass only through the very center of the lens. Restricting the entrance of light reduces distortion and the object of interest comes into better focus. Some myopic persons may become habitual squinters who continue to squint even after the visual problem has been corrected with glasses.

Myopia in children is likely to progress until the late teenage years. Thus the condition necessitates frequent examination and adjustment of glasses to maintain adequate vision. It is generally desirable to check myopic youngsters every six months.

Hyperopia

Hyperopia, or farsightedness, is a very common refractive error in children. Usually the condition is mild and well tolerated without the aid of glasses as long as reading does not continue for a long time (see Figure 13-2). The shorter the eyeball, however, the greater the strain on the muscles that must hold the shape of the lens and, hence, the more quickly visual blurring and headaches will occur. Educationally, it is desirable not to discourage a child's desire to

FIGURE 13-2. *(a) Nearsightedness and (b) farsightedness.*

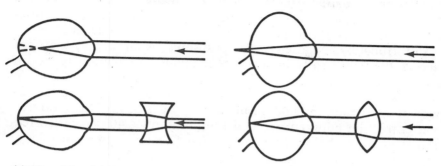

(a) Nearsightedness, or myopia, can be corrected by a biconcave lens.

(b) Farsightedness, or hyperopia, can be corrected by a convex lens.

read, and teachers should be sensitive to the possibility that the child who puts down a book may be experiencing discomfort rather than disinterest.

Astigmatism

Astigmatism is a blurring of vision due to irregularities in the curvature of the cornea or lens. The light rays spread out or scatter in such a way that there is no focus on the retina and vision of both near and distant objects is distorted.

NEUROMUSCULAR DISORDERS

Occasionally teachers encounter visual problems resulting from an imbalance of the muscles that control the movement of the eyes. Normally the so-called *extraocular muscles* move the eyeballs in complete coordination so that the images from both eyes fuse into a single perceptual experience. In *strabismus,* a muscle imbalance causes misalignment of the eyes. As a result, the eyes cannot fixate on a single object and double vision, which produces considerable visual discomfort, occurs. Most people, including infants, quickly overcome this handicap by suppressing the visual signals from the retina of the deviated eye. Although they may thereby regain visual comfort, they lose the advantages of binocular vision, or *stereopsis.* The visual field narrows greatly and depth perception disappears.

If the malalignment is not corrected and suppression of signals continues, a permanent visual block or loss will develop in the suppressed eye. This condition is called *amblyopia,* more popularly known as *lazy eye.* Amblyopia, which occurs in 2 percent of the population, has other causes besides muscular imbalance. Congenital disorders such as cataracts, retinal disease, and corneal abnormalities may distort vision to the point that image suppression occurs.

Unfortunately, children with strabismus or amblyopia may not receive treatment early enough for maximum correction to occur. To prevent permanent disability corrective measures should begin immediately upon detection. Proper treatment will produce an 80 percent correction in children up to two years of age and a 60 percent correction between two and four, but only a 40 percent correction is likely to be possible in children five to seven years of age. After age eight, the condition is probably not at all correctable.

It would take a concerted community effort to detect amblyopia early, but it is possible to give a Snellen test to preschool children. If vision in one eye is two Snellen lines better than in the other eye, amblyopia may be present.

Treatment for strabismus may require glasses, bifocals, chemicals, exercise, or surgery or some combination of these. Correction of visual suppression frequently can be accomplished by wearing a patch over the good eye to force the bad eye to see. Following removal of the patch, double vision returns, but fusion may yet occur. After age eight, the potential for learning fusion approaches zero and amblyopia is likely to become a permanent disability. Obviously, it is desirable to detect the condition early. A child with strabismus not only will see poorly but also is likely to be the object of some ridicule by his classmates. The resultant psychic trauma may be considerable. Surgical correction of strabismus after age eight certainly has value, if only for cosmetic considerations.

SCREENING FOR VISUAL PROBLEMS

The behavioral signs presented in Table 13–2 should alert teachers to visual problems in children. Watching children use their eyes will provide valuable indicators that may go unnoticed in casual home situations. Knowing the crucial interdependence of learning and vision, teachers should regularly watch each child with this question in mind: "Is he seeing well?"

Visual problems may deteriorate rapidly. A child who entered school in September with normal vision may experience significant refractive loss by January or February. Children with existing visual problems should receive regular checkups every six months to be sure that prescription lenses are still providing adequate correction. In the school a regular program of observation and screening is essential to ensure that children do not suffer needless decrements in this most important sense. Visual screening procedures that are applicable by teachers are included in Chapter 21.

DYSLEXIA

Dyslexia, though originally used to designate reading problems of neurological origin, now applies to all kinds of reading disabilities. An estimated 5 to 10 percent of children have severe reading disabilities; boys outnumber girls by as much as three to one.[2]

The majority of children acquire primary reading skills by the time they reach third grade. Persistent deficiencies frequently exist concomitantly with difficulties in speech and language skills. Many children with reading inadequacies, however, possess otherwise adequate communicative skills, so problems in one area do not necessarily lead to problems in the other.

The causes of dyslexia are legion. Neurological abnormalities, such as the inability to relate visual and auditory sensations, may be a factor. Sometimes auditory defects prevent normal establishment of neural hookups that are essential to the development of visual perception. This explanation gains support from the fact that some dyslexic individuals retain their disability into later life.

Educational causes are another possibility. Instruction that fails to provide related experience may be insufficient to produce the desired visual association. Early environmental conditions, such as the absence of good communicative models in the home, may also contribute negatively to development of communication skills, among them reading.

Whatever the causes, teachers should realize the importance of an early, thorough investigation of the problem. A physician should examine the child to rule out the possibility of an organic basis for the disorder. The school counselor will provide a psychological evaluation to discover any emotional factors that may be causing the child to reject or withdraw from particular or collective educational experiences.

Once specialists have discovered or eliminated causative or contributing factors, they may be able to suggest what types of experiences and approaches will best meet the needs of the dyslexic child.

THE VISUALLY HANDICAPPED CHILD

The term *visually handicapped,* as used in this section, applies to children who either have no vision or whose visual limitations after correction still leave them educationally handicapped unless special provisions are made. Some of the principles discussed here apply to the handicapped in general and not just to children with visual losses.

Most handicapped children have demonstrated that they are like children with normal vision in more ways than they are different from them. They have the same basic physical, intellectual, and emotional needs as all children. In addition, they have some special needs due to their particular impairments. Most of them can become mature, independent, contributing members of society as long as they have competent care, a good environment, and a suitable education. How well we meet the needs of these children and provide equal educational opportunities for them will determine whether the country is to have the benefit of their talents.

The number of handicapped children enrolled in the nation's schools has risen sharply in recent years. Enrollments of special residential schools have also mounted steadily. Not only have programs been expanded, but new philosophies and different types of programs have also evolved. The increased number of very young handicapped children and the fact that more of these children than ever are remaining at home to receive their education in local school programs have led to a growing concern for the effects of adverse parental attitudes and reactions.

The Visually Handicapped at Home

Parents of handicapped children face many problems. Authorities planning school programs for these children should recognize that some of the parents will require professional assistance if they are to develop satisfactory relationships with their children. Unless resolved, their problems may have lasting effects on their children's success in school and on their total life adjustment.

Handicapped children need the love and care of their parents just as normal brothers and sisters do. In fact, they may have even greater need for affection and understanding if they are to make a healthy adjustment to their defects. Many parents develop realistic attitudes toward their children and their handicaps. When told by the specialist that the handicap is permanent, they begin to study the impact on and possibilities for care and education. Such parents are able to make constructive plans. Their objective reaction to the handicap often contributes to their children's self-confidence and favorable progress.

Other parents find the task more difficult. In looking forward to the arrival of a baby, they think of one who is normal and not handicapped. All parents are saddened and somewhat bewildered when they discover that their baby is handicapped or that such a condition has developed in an older child. They may not recognize the basic similarities of all children and consequently may feel that they cannot share experiences with parents who have normal children. The only handicapped person some parents have known well may be an elderly man or woman sitting dejectedly at home or in a special institution. These thoughts, along with fear of doing the wrong thing for a child they cannot understand, may interfere with the normal parent-child relationship. Other parents may resent having a handicapped child and blame themselves or their families for the child they look upon as defective. Without help, these parents may be unable to see the potential within each child to become an active, happy, and responsible person filled with youthful zest for living.

Although parents may not openly state their feelings, their ability to cope with the fact that their child is limited often shows in their behavior. Some continue to anticipate these children's every need, dressing and feeding them long after they are old enough to learn such skills. Others shower their children with material things but are unable to give them affection. Handicapped children who are deprived of contact with warm, accepting parents are perhaps more prone than normal children to withdraw into a restricted world of their own in search of substitute satisfactions. Undesirable behavior patterns may arrest development at a low level. While the degree of satisfaction derived from such behavior is generally very limited, when combined with fear of reaching out for more normal personal relations, it may cause a child to resist professional help at a later date. It is a common observation that parents of handicapped children, in general, and particularly parents whose children have visual handicaps have special needs: (1) assistance should be readily accessible to these parents and (2) the parents should be aware of the availability and sources of counseling as soon as possible after handicaps have been diagnosed.

School-Home Relations

Parents can be especially effective in supplementing the school's efforts to provide well-rounded educational experiences for both normal and handicapped children. For children with visual problems, parents can best provide many of the detailed explanations and firsthand experiences they need to develop a meaningful understanding of the world in the home during leisure-time activities. Reading aloud not only is a pleasant experience for both parents and children, but may do much to motivate the development of independent reading skills as well. Through questions and discussions of material read aloud, children may reveal their limited understanding of words and concepts used. Alert parents, in cooperation with school personnel, can utilize home, family, and community resources to extend understanding and reinforce learning. Routine trips to stores and rides in buses, trains, and airplanes are rich in educational potential for visually handicapped children. Traveling with an understanding adult who is willing to grant time and freedom to explore the many curiosities aroused by such trips is particularly valuable. Farms, dairies, and bakeries will usually arrange visits, and trips to such public facilities as police and fire departments, libraries, museums, and zoos are good enrichment experiences. Recreational opportunites can be important to handicapped children and their parents and are readily available in many communities. These frequently include opportunities for lessons in swimming, rollerskating, music, and dancing, and membership in youth organizations.

Parents can be helpful also by presenting positive attitudes toward school. The degree of interest parents express in school activities may greatly affect their child's progress. It is particularly important for parents of children attending residential schools to take advantage of every opportunity to convey their interest both in their children and in their schooling through letters and visits and in conversations with them when they are at home.

Identification and Placement in School

The development of systematic statewide programs for early identification and referral of infants and preschool children who may be visually handicapped is receiving increased emphasis. State departments of education and other public and private agencies and organizations serving youth are coordinating their programs by establishing joint committees and procedures for the routine referral to education specialists of children with visual limitations. These procedures bring together parents who desire assistance and specialized personnel before the handicapped children have acquired undesirable behavior patterns. Sharing of information by agencies serving children also aids in the compilation of accurate statistics on the number and location of handicapped children, which is especially important in long-range planning of school programs.

Once children have enrolled in school, school officials must assume much of the responsibility of identifying those children who require special instruction because of defective vision. Because of the obvious nature of their disability, blind school-age children usually do not escape the attention of school authorities. Identification by the school of children often classified as "partially seeing" is sometimes more difficult. Partially seeing children are those whose limited vision constitutes an educational handicap but who have sufficient residual vision to be able to read print. Their visual impairment is not always as obvious as that of the blind child, and schools that have developed systematic procedures to identify and refer them have found such procedures very helpful.

In part, the basis of early school programs for visually handicapped children was the belief that children with limited vision would damage their eyes if they used them to full extent in school. Placed in separate rooms, they were not permitted to use their eyes any more than was absolutely necessary. Placement in special programs for blind and partially seeing children depended primarily on the nature and extent of visual limitations. Frequently only minor attention was given to the educational implications these visual impairments had for each child involved.

Special education of visually handicapped children entered a new era when it became apparent that use of vision rarely results in damage. Sight *utilization* rather than conservation came to be stressed as a result of the discovery that, under proper conditions, children learn to make good use of even slight amounts of residual vision. It became evident that children who formerly attended separate classes to "save their eyes" not only *could* but also *should* return to regular classrooms for all or part of their education. In addition, evidence has shown that individual children react quite differently to similar visual limitations. The decision to place a child in a special program now depends essentially on the extent to which the child's visual impairment represents an *educational handicap* rather than on the extent of visual loss. Information about the amount of visual acuity as an indication of loss is still useful to educators because it provides a gross, general guideline for preliminary referral—*not* for placement.

Educators of visually handicapped children are giving more attention to selection of criteria. They are making an increased effort to determine whether the learning problems exhibited by some children with impaired vision may have other causes, such as low ability or other physical disabilities. When this is the case, placement in school programs designed for children with these other types of disabilities may be more appropriate than placement in programs for the visually handicapped. Multiple-handicapped children require the services of several specialists, but before placing these children in classes for the visually handicapped, it should be clear that their visual problems are in some way responsible for their school problems. Otherwise the importance of limited vision in the learning process may assume greater significance than it should. Regular teachers and the children themselves may become overly concerned about a visual impairment that actually is not interfering with the child's schooling. In some cases, children may be able to profit more from the general school program than from unnecessary specialized instruction.

THE ROLE OF THE CLASSROOM TEACHER

Under current practices many persons assist in locating and referring visually handicapped children to education specialists: school and public health nurses, eye specialists, parents, and others. The role of the classroom teacher in identifying these children has grown in recent years due to the growing emphasis on selecting for special instruction only those children whose vision problems are directly responsible for their learning problems. Often, identification of partially seeing children occurs first at the primary level, where they come under close daily observation of classroom teachers. These teachers, of course, are the first to know that a child is having difficulty learning. If they know what type of assistance is available, they can refer potential candidates to programs designed to meet the particular needs of the visually handicapped.

In order for teachers to succeed in their efforts to identify and help partially seeing children, however, they must have access to specialized resources. Periodic consultations between specialists and classroom teachers and routine distribution of information describing what to look for in the school setting are helpful. For example, the following checklist itemizes behavior characteristics of children with vision problems that will help a specialist evaluate a referral:

The child who may be in need of special instruction because of limited vision, which cannot be brought up to normal or near normal with glasses or treatment by an eye specialist, frequently exhibits several of the following characteristics in school. Please check those which apply in the case of the child being referred.

— Progresses at a rate below that which might be considered appropriate for children of approximately the same age, grade, and intelligence test scores.
— Fails to complete long reading assignments or other school tasks involving extensive eye use, especially when time is limited.
— Understands the basic principles involved in certain areas of study such as long division, but makes errors in the comparatively easier procedures such as addition, particularly when working with long columns of figures.
— Remembers and understands material read to him/her better than that which he/she reads himself/herself.
— Confuses letters and words which look somewhat alike.
— Covers or shields one eye habitually while reading.
— Holds reading material at an unusual distance or angle.
— Skips letters, words, or lines while reading.
— Has difficulty copying from textbooks, workbooks, or chalkboards.
— Tires quickly or is easily distracted while working at his/her desk.
— Is confused by details such as those appearing on maps, charts, or diagrams.

— Writes unusually small, large, or very poorly.
— Appears clumsy or awkward on the playground.
— Has poor eye-hand coordination.
— Rubs or brushes eyes frequently.
— Thrusts head forward or squints when looking at near or far objects.
— Stumbles or trips often.

Specialists carefully study visually limited children before recommending them for special education. On many areas local and regional review teams assist in this process. Group recommendations from qualified people aid school administrators in placing partially seeing children in programs that best suit their needs. These teams assist also with the reappraisal and reassignment of children who are already participating in special programs. Members of these teams generally include:

1. The child's regular classroom teacher
2. The director, consultant, or supervisor of special education
3. The special teacher of visually handicapped children
4. The school principal
5. A school or public health nurse
6. A social worker or special parent counselor
7. A school psychologist or qualified psychological examiner

Early detection and assessment of all types of visual problems are critical to the prevention of developmental and instructional handicaps. Equally important is the prompt establishment of an effective educational program that meets the individual needs of the handicapped child.

NOTES

1. "Eye Care," *American Druggist,* March 1976, p. 47.
2. H.S. Lillywhite, N.B. Young, and R.W. Olstead, *Pediatrician's Handbook of Communication Disorders* (Philadelphia: Lea and Febiger, 1970), p. 102.

RESOURCES

American Foundation for the Blind, 15 West 16th Street, New York, N.Y. 10011.
American Optometric Association, Inc., Department of Public Information, 7000 Chippewa Street, St. Louis, Mo. 63119.

CHAPTER **14**
Hearing Disorders

A discussion of hearing problems attracts too few listeners. Yet, in the average school classroom of thirty students, one child has significant hearing loss. In other words 3.5 to 5 percent of school-age children are so afflicted.[1] The importance of such statistics to the elementary school teacher stems from the fact that 85 percent of hearing problems have developed by the third grade. Left undetected, hearing disorders put youngsters at an educational disadvantage. In too many instances they are considered mentally retarded until appropriate tests reveal hearing loss to be the problem. Elementary teachers should be alert for possible problems in their classes and render encouragement to make necessary corrections.

THE HEARING APPARATUS

The ear (see Figures 14–1 and 14–2) converts sound waves into nerve impulses. When sound reaches the outer ear, it passes through the *auditory canal* where the waves become vibrations in the *tympanum*, or eardrum. The *ossicles* (malleus, incus, and stapes), set in motion by the eardrum, transmit the sound waves to the *cochlea,* thereby producing vibrations of the *endolymph,* or cochlear fluid. The vibrating fluid stimulates *hair cells* on the *basilar membrane.* In turn, the

FIGURE 14-1. *Diagram of the human ear lying in place in the skull.*

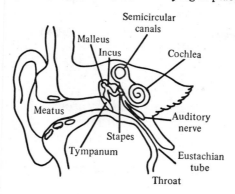

FIGURE 14-2. *Cross section of the cochlear canal.*

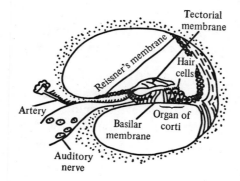

hair cells produce impulses in the *auditory nerve* that travel to the brain for interpretation. Half of the nerve impulses from each ear travel to one side of the brain and half go to the opposite side, an important factor in the ability to locate the source of sounds.

Thus, sound changes quantitatively as it passes from the outer ear into the cochlea. The movement of the ossicles amplifies the sound by 60 percent. Within the cochlea, however, a qualitative change takes place as the mechanical sound waves are converted into nerve impulses. Therefore, abnormalities in the outer ear and middle ear affect primarily the quantity, or loudness, of sound whereas cochlear disorders may alter the intelligibility, or qualitative dimensions of hearing.

DIMENSION OF SOUND

We perceive sounds as loud or soft and high or low. These psychological dimensions have important physical correlates:

1. Intensity: The loudness of a sound essentially depends on the amount of force associated with the sound wave. Loudness is measured in units called *decibels*.
2. Pitch: The highness or lowness of sound is a function of the rate at which the sound source is vibrating. The vibration is given in cycles per second (cps) and is called *frequency*. For example, A above middle C on the piano vibrates at 440 cps; middle C vibrates at 256 cps. The range of human hearing is between about 20 to 20,000 cps, but the usual speech range is between about 100 and 8000 with vowels at the lower frequency and consonants at the upper one. Most hearing impairment in children is around 3000–4000 cps. Consonants suffer the greatest loss.

HEARING AND SPEECH

Understandably the hard-of-hearing child may have speech problems. From the early months of life, we mimic the sound we hear. A hearing disability during this early developmental period inevitably will affect subsequent speech patterns. Much as amblyopia may prevent a child from learning fusion after the early critical years of life, so a severe hearing disability may deprive a young child of normal educational, social, and emotional development.

Vowels and consonants have different sound frequencies, vowels being low tones and consonants occupying the higher frequencies. Loss of frequencies in the range of 4000 cps, which is common, prevents hearing certain of the consonants correctly. Is it any wonder that a hearing-disabled child will pronounce those consonants incorrectly or perhaps drop them altogether and therefore fail to develop necessary communicative skills?

FACTORS PRODUCING HEARING LOSS

Ear Infections

Earache is a common childhood complaint. Too many parents and teachers fail to realize that earache is symptomatic of a variety of disorders, none of which is safe to ignore. Even a minor ache may represent a threat to hearing if not properly treated.

The most frequent cause of earache is middle-ear infection, or *otitis media,* which is usually a secondary infection of the nose, throat, or tonsils. Teachers can expect one in four students to experience this problem. If unattended, the condition may produce severe hearing loss. Severe middle ear infections can produce sufficient pressure to rupture the eardrum. In addition, they sometimes spread to the *mastoid bone,* a honey-combed area at the base of the skull behind the ear. Without adequate medical attention, mastoid infections may cause serious hearing loss, and in the days before antibiotics such damage was common. About one-third of all brain abscesses are due to middle-ear infections and mastoiditis.

Secretory otitis media is a condition in which a yellowish fluid accumulates in the middle ear, often despite the fact that the eustachian tube is open. The cause is unknown and treatment frequently is ineffective. In general, the disorder is self-limiting, but it usually impairs hearing until the fluid disappears. The incidence of secretory otitis media is increasing.

Occasionally the eardrum itself becomes infected (myringitis). The symptoms of this condition are pus accumulation, pressure, and pain. As in other cases of middle-ear infections, a physician may decide to cut the eardrum to relieve the pressure and pain and allow the pus to drain from the ear. Since the eardrum heals quickly, this procedure is of little consequence, and it greatly decreases discomfort.

The external ear may also be involved in hearing loss. Although the primary function of the auditory canal is to direct sound waves into the ear, the inventive youngster may find it to be a suitable storage area for beans, gum, marbles, and other small objects. Wax occasionally will accumulate to the point of impairing hearing. Since the skin of the canal is very delicate and easily injured, it is preferable to have a physician remove the wax accumulation. Certainly children should learn to keep all objects out of the ear.

Disorders of the Internal Ear

Abnormalities in the cochlea or associated nerves may produce sensorineural hearing loss. Occasionally such losses are attributable to hereditary factors, maternal measles in early pregnancy, or other congenital causes. More commonly, however, impairment follows a case of mumps, careless use of certain antibiotics, exposure to intense noise, or cochlear trauma caused by a head blow.

Hearing loss due to loud sound exposure is an interesting hazard. Electronic amplification has turned a lot of otherwise benign music into a distinct health threat. As Table 14–1 shows, sound levels commonly experienced by children often exceed 100 decibels, a level at which trauma to the organ of Corti is known to occur. Musicians risk this kind of damage most frequently, but their young devotees too commonly dance or sit right in front of the speakers to get the full effect. Wesley Bradley of the National Institute of Health maintains that various home appliances, including lawn mowers, garbage disposals, chain saws, vacuum cleaners, and blenders, also may produce enough noise to effect neurosensory loss.[2] Unfor-

TABLE 14-1. Sound Levels and Human Response

	Noise Level (db)	Response	Conversational Relationships
	150		
Carrier deck jet operation	140		
		Painfully loud	
	130	Limit amplified	
		Speech	
Jet takeoff (200 feet) Discotheque Auto horn (3 feet)	120	Maximum vocal effort	
Riveting machine Jet takeoff (2000 feet)	110		Shouting in ear
Garbage truck N.Y. subway station	100	Very annoying	
Heavy truck (50 feet)	90	Hearing damage	Shouting at 2 feet
Pneumatic drill (50 feet)		(8 hours)	Very loud conversation (2 feet)
Alarm clock Freight train (50 feet)	80	Annoying	
		Telephone use	Loud conversation (2 feet)
→ Freeway traffic (50 feet)	70	Difficult Intrusive	Loud conversation (4 feet)
Air conditioning unit (20 feet)	60		
Light auto traffic (100 feet)	50	Quiet	Normal conversation (12 feet)
Living room Bedroom	40		
Library		Very quiet	
Soft whisper (15 feet)	30		
Broadcasting studio	20		
	10	Just audible	
	0	Threshold of hearing	

(left margin, vertical: Contribution to Hearing Loss Begins)

Source: *Utah Environmental News,* August 1976, p. 4.

tunately, there is no way to repair or replace damaged or destroyed cells in neurosensory loss, so preventive measures are essential. Early diagnosis and treatment of infections have significantly prevented serious hearing loss. Coupled with better control of noise, these precautions should save the hearing of many children who might otherwise become badly handicapped.

DETECTION AND TREATMENT OF HEARING LOSS

The child who has trouble hearing may show various behavioral peculiarities. Teachers can easily spot some of the symptoms if they are attentive and know what to look for. Because teachers have a close association with students and because satisfactory classroom performance depends on hearing ability, teachers are more likely to notice hearing loss than other school personnel and even parents. Some common indicators of hearing problems are:

1. Inattention and irregularity in fulfilling assignments
2. Poor oral performance in comparison with written work
3. Abnormal speech, absence of consonants, distortion of words or sounds
4. Turning the head to favor one ear
5. Thrusting the head forward to get closer to the sound
6. Complaints involving the ears—aching, sensitive to touch, continuous sound, ringing in the ears
7. Constant use of "huh" or "what" when spoken to

These behaviors are not always hearing related, but they should certainly arouse teachers' suspicions.

Ideally, each schoolchild will receive an annual screening test by a trained audiologist. The test instrument, an *audiometer,* is the only satisfactory device that reliably detects hearing problems in schoolchildren. In recognition of the desirability of such testing, many states require regular audiometry screening procedures in their school systems. Good audiometry screening requires special training. Therefore, unless no audiologist is available teachers should not administer the test.

Two types of audiometers are available: the pure tone audiometer and the speech audiometer. The *pure tone audiometer* produces single tones of different frequencies and intensities in one ear at a time. Thus they detect hearing losses at specific frequencies and indicate the extent to which the loss would impair speech comprehension. Pure tone audiometers do not approximate the complexities of sound associated with the spoken word, however. A *speech audiometer test* is somewhat more discriminating. This test requires the subject to respond to words believed to represent all of the sounds in the language. The machine delivers the words at varying intensities. At the conclusion of speech audiometry, the trained audiologist knows the degree to which a child will have problems in normal conversational and classroom verbal experiences.

Although professionals usually should perform these tests, elementary teachers can administer the pure tone audiometer test. At 25 decibels and frequencies of 250, 500, 1000, 2000, 4000, and 8000 cps, the child who fails to hear two or more tones should undergo further testing by a specialist.

Conductive hearing loss is most amenable to treatment. Usually complete correction is possible. If not, treatment at least can considerably alleviate the problem. Clearing auditory canals, repairing eardrums, and repairing or replacing damaged ossicles are typical treatments for conductive hearing loss. On the other hand, sensorineural losses are generally untreatable. In these cases the abnormality is in the cochlea, nerves, or brain tissue. Most hearing loss in children is sensorineural, so it is important to determine the amount of serviceable hearing left in order to design an appropriate rehabilitation program.

Despite all attempts to correct the cause of hearing loss, many children will still be incapable of communicating and understanding. Table 14–2 indicates the types of problems that varying degrees of hearing disability produce. Children who have more than a thirty decibel loss (in the better ear) after treatment should receive special instruction and rehabilitation to improve their communicative skills and to afford the greatest utilization of what hearing remains.

Hearing aids may be emotionally repugnant to both parents and children, but a hearing aid may be the only satisfactory recourse in severe hearing loss. Generally the sooner children start wearing hearing aids, the better they adjust to them. Nevertheless adjustment to a hearing aid may take time and effort. Not all hearing aids are the same and the consumer must be wary of unprofessional sales promotion and shoddy products. A physician should always provide guidance in obtaining the proper equipment, and parents and teachers need to continually evaluate students' progress in using hearing aids effectively and assessing their suitability for a particular problem.

Although conductive losses respond well to hearing aids, sensorineural losses produce a sound distortion that is not treatable with amplification alone. Children with sensorineural losses must learn lipreading techniques to augment hearing perception. Usually they will pick up a great deal by observing facial expressions and movements of the mouth, but they benefit considerably from instruction on how to be more observant of the finer nuances of body and facial language associated with communication.

TABLE 14-2. Difficulty Experienced by Schoolchildren with Flat Hearing Losses

Average Hearing Loss (500, 1000, 2000 hz)		Degree of Difficulty
ASA-1951	ISO-1964	
Up to 10 db	Up to 21 db	No difficulty. Hearing sensitivity within normal limits.
10-15	21-26	Virtually no difficulty. Normally undetectable by patient and others.
15-25	26-36	Slight problem limited to failure to understand faint speech or speech heard in difficult listening situations.
25-35	36-46	Loss begins to produce significant handicap in most children. Child has difficulty with spelling and arithmetic in particular. Child frequently does not recognize loss, and others think child is slow or inattentive, or both. Hearing aid may be indicated.
35-45	46-56	Child has considerable difficulty with most schoolwork. He still may be mistaken for a slow, inattentive child. Hearing aid is usually indicated.
45-55	56-66	Most serious loss. Child is usually recognized to have a hearing loss but occasionally the problem goes unnoticed. Hearing aid and therapeutic help are essential.

Source: Reproduced from Gerald A. Studebaker, "Hearing Problems in School Children," *Postgraduate Medicine,* vol. 43, no. 1 (January 1968), p. 192. Copyright © McGraw-Hill, Inc.

THINGS THE TEACHER CAN DO

Above all, the hard-of-hearing child is a person. This reminder is not meant to be insulting, but it is all too easy to forget that we are dealing with an individual rather than a hearing problem. Psychologists can help parents and teachers to understand the emotional complexities associated with an inability to hear well. Hearing loss can produce a feeling of isolation and loneliness, which may drastically affect interpersonal relationships. Aversion and rejection by the nondeaf is all too common, and they lead to feelings of denial and suspicion on the part of the afflicted individual. Feelings of self-worth and acceptance may fail to develop, particularly in a school situation in which other children are insensitive to the hearing-disabled child's deep need for love and a sense of belonging.

Hearing-impaired students hear. The deaf do not. The deaf child has a peculiar set of communication problems that require a special type of communication:

One-to-one Communication

1. It is important to have the student's attention before speaking. The deaf student cannot hear the usual call to attention. He may need a tap on the shoulder, a wave, or other signals to catch his eye.
2. Speak slowly and clearly, enunciating each word, but without exaggerating or overpronouncing. Although it is necessary to speak slowly and clearly, exaggeration and overemphasis distorts lip movements, making lipreading more difficult. Try to enunciate each word, but without force or tension. Short sentences are easier to understand than long sentences.
3. Try to maintain eye contact with the student. Deaf students, like most students, prefer the feeling of direct communications. Eye contact establishes this feeling. Even in the presence of an interpreter, try to communicate to him. The student can then turn to the interpreter as he feels the need.
4. Try to rephrase a thought rather than repeating the same words. Sometimes particular combinations of lip movements are very difficult for a student to lip-read. If he is not understanding you, try to rephrase the sentence.

Classroom Situations

1. The student should be seated to his best advantage. Generally this is up to the student. It is very helpful if the instructor will assist the student to select an appropriate seat if he fails to do so.
2. Try to avoid standing with your back to a window or other light sources. Looking at someone standing in front of a light source practically blinds the deaf student. Lipreading is difficult if not impossible since the speaker's face is left in shadow.
3. Notify an interpreter in advance when you plan to use materials that require special lighting. Since it is impossible to lipread in the dark, the interpreter must have advance notice so necessary lighting can be provided.
4. A brief outline would aid an interpreter and the student to follow the lecture. It is very helpful to a deaf student to know in advance what will be studied next. He will then have a chance to read ahead and study vocabulary. After the lecture, he can better organize his notes.
5. Try to present new vocabulary in advance. If this is impossible, try to write new vocabulary on the chalkboard or overhead projector since it is difficult, if not impossible, to lip-read or finger-spell the unfamiliar.
6. Visual aids are a tremendous help to deaf students. Since vision is a deaf person's primary channel to receive information, a teaching aid that he can see may help him assimilate this information. Make full use of chalkboards, overhead projectors, films, diagrams, charts, etc.
7. Try to avoid unnecessary pacing and speaking while writing on the chalk-

board. It is difficult to lip-read a person in motion and impossible to read from behind. It is preferable to write or draw on the chalkborad, then face the class and explain the work. The overhead projector adapts readily to this type of situation.

8. Slowing the pace of communication often helps to facilitate comprehension. Speakers tend to quicken their pace when familiar with the material. In addition, there is an unavoidable time lag in the presentation when an interpreter is involved. Try to allow a little extra time for the student to ask or answer questions, since he has less time to assimilate the material and to respond.

9. When vital information is presented, try to make sure the deaf student isn't left out. Write on the chalkboard any changes in class time, examination dates, speèial assignments, additional instructions, etc. In lab or studio situation, allow extra time when pointing out the location of materials, referring to manuals or texts, etc., since the deaf student must look then return his attention for further instruction.

10. In the absence of an interpreter, questions or statements from the back of the room should be repeated. Deaf students are cut off from whatever happens that is not in their visual area. Since it is often necessary to know the question in order to fully understand the answer, questions or statements from the back of the room should be repeated.[3]

NOTES

1. Alexander Graham Bell Association for the Deaf, *News*, 1 November 1965.
2. Raymond E. Jordan, "Hearing Loss: Ways to Avoid It—or Live with It," *U.S. News and World Report*, 21 January 1974, p. 48.
3. National Technical Institute for the Deaf, *Information for Instructors with Deaf Students in Their Classes* (Rochester, N.Y.: Rochester Institute of Technology, n.d.).

RESOURCES

Consumer Survival Kit, Maryland Center for Public Broadcasting, Owings Mills, Md. 21117.

Do's and Don'ts for Parents of Pre-school Deaf and Hard of Hearing Children by Jean Utley Lehman (A–217), National Easter Seal Society for Crippled Children and Adults, 2033 West Ogden Avenue, Chicago, Ill. 60612. (Also available in Spanish (A–248). Send 15¢ plus stamped, self-addressed #10 envelope for this two-page booklet published in 1961.)

Where Hearing Losses Occur, Maico Hearing Instruments, 7375 Bush Lake Road, Minneapolis, Minn. 55435. (Cutaway illustration, 11 X 8½". Available to professional staff only upon receipt of request on official stationery. Limit 25 copies.)

Which Sounds Do You Fail to Hear?, Maico Hearing Instruments, 7375 Bush Lake Road, Minneapolis, Minn. 55435. (Available to professional staff only upon receipt of request on official stationery. Limit 5 copies.)

CHAPTER 15
Gastrointestinal Disorders

Where is the teacher who has not had a child look pleadingly upward and whimper, "Teacher, I've got a tummy ache"? The frequency of this experience is suggested by these observations: digestive tract diseases rank second only to cardiovascular diseases in number of physician visits in the United States[1] and nausea and vomiting episodes are more common in children than adults. Americans go to the hospital more often for digestive tract problems than for any other group of disorders, and schools must often send children home for gastrointestinal complaints.[2]

Teachers confronted with a nauseous child justifiably have difficulty deciding what action to take. Nausea, vomiting, and abdominal pain may portend grave disease problems or simply represent some minor, transient, and innocuous upset without significant consequences. Unfortunately, teachers are not in a position to decide which condition exists and therefore must shift the responsibility of investigating the problem to others. In the final analysis, qualified physicians are the only individuals who can decide the seriousness of the disturbance and even they often have trouble making a diagnosis. Teachers' immediate recourse should be to place sick children in the care of their parents, the school nurse, or a school administrator who will insure that they receive proper attention. Under conditions of duress, when such recourse is unavailable, teachers may need to advise the parents or decide whether direct and prompt medical aid is essential.

Adults entrusted with the care of children should have some knowledge of commonly occurring gastrointestinal disorders and be able to recognize potential hazards and implications for the classroom situation. Nausea and vomiting are symptomatic of problems in the digestive tract and/or the central nervous system control centers, which organize the nausea and vomiting reflexes. Irritation or distention of the digestive tract and direct irritation or stimulation of the brain centers are sufficient to produce the symptoms. Tables 15–1 and 15–2 list common causes of gastrointestinal distress. Some are potentially serious conditions.

Although teaching responsibilities do not include illness diagnosis there are certain danger signs that suggest a need for treatment without delay. Teachers should encourage prompt medical attention for any of these symptoms:

1. Abdominal pain: Many of the more serious gastrointestinal disorders present pain with nausea and vomiting. Intestinal obstruction, appendicitis, and a multitude of other problems demanding prompt surgical intervention may be present.
2. Regular occurrence: When gastrointestinal distress occurs frequently or at regular intervals (such as shortly after eating), it may indicate ulcers, gall bladder disease, and other significant disorders.
3. Bleeding: Bleeding in the digestive tract is always serious but may present itself in several ways.
   a. Bright red in vomitus; easily recognizable.
   b. Brown in vomitus; looking very much like coffee grounds.
   c. Black; in a tarlike, sticky stool.
4. Diarrhea: When continuous and present with nausea and vomiting, diarrhea may cause the loss of large amounts of fluid and dehydration, for which hospitalization may be necessary.

Because of the frequent and serious nature of peptic ulcers and appendicitis, teachers should be familiar with their characteristics. It may be up to them to help prevent and recognize them or even to assist children in the management of them.

The popular notion that ulcers are exclusively an adult affliction is erroneous. The factors that seem to promote them, namely, hereditary predisposition and psychological stress, occur (along with the ulcers) in children as well.

The usual symptom of a peptic ulcer is the onset of pain in the upper abdomen between one and three hours after eating. Although abdominal pain frequently has no relationship to any discoverable problem in children, all such episodes warrant investigation. Ulcer

TABLE 15–1. Causes of Nausea and Vomiting

Immediate Factor	Cause	Preventive or Control Measure
Irritation		
Infections	Viruses, bacteria, protozoa.	Eliminate case contacts, poor personal hygiene, contamination of food and water.
Injudicious eating	Sudden increases in dietary roughage or fiber. High spice or irritant content in food.	Better education and control of dietary intake.
"Food poisoning"	(See Table 15–2)	(See Table 15–2)
Distention		
Gas	Aerophagia (swallowing air); certain foods (broccoli, beans, cabbage, cauliflower, onions, peppers, radishes, turnips).	Change eating behaviors. Foods generally not a problem in otherwise healthy individuals.
Obstruction	Strangulating hernia. Intussusception (telescoping of the bowel). Volvulus (twisting of the bowel). Tumors. Adhesions caused by abdominal surgery, inflammation in abdominal cavity Bowel paralysis caused by infections, renal disease, and other painful conditions of the chest and lumbar area.	
Neurogenic (factors influencing the brain control center for vomiting)		
Emotional factors	Excitement, worry, fear, frustration.	
Motion sickness	Various conveyances producing up and down movements. Visual stimuli involving eyeball oscillations.	Preferential seating in front of conveyance; fresh air, fixing gaze on distant objects, medications.
Chemicals	Certain drugs, morning sickness, certain diseases that alter blood chemistry.	

FIGURE 15-1. *The digestive tract.*

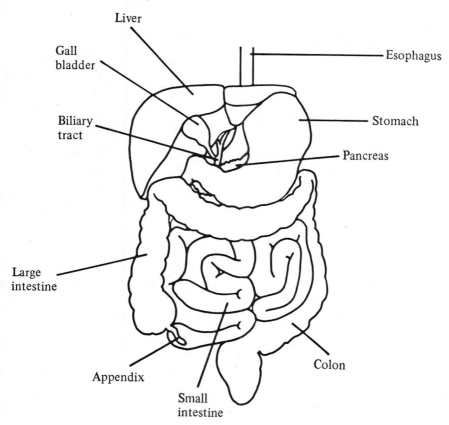

treatment generally includes milk or antacids, frequent bland snacks, and drugs to suppress secretions in the stomach. Owing to the stress component of this disorder, teachers should evaluate the classroom program to discover stress factors that they might be able to reduce or eliminate to promote healing. Schoolwork that is too demanding, threats or teasing by other children, and a variety of conflicts between a child's peculiar needs and existing classroom procedures are all possible sources of stress that teachers can modify. Frequently, however, the stress is at home and counseling is advisable for both parents and child.

The appendix is a blind pouch at the base of the large intestine (see Figure 15-1) that has no scientifically established function. Appendicitis reaches its maximum incidence in the second and third decades of life. It is rare before age two.[3] The predominant complaint is lower abdominal pain, the severity and location of which vary. When the appendix becomes inflamed, its blood supply diminishes. In the absence of treatment, gangrene and rupture (perfora-

TABLE 15-2. "Food Poisoning"

Name of Illness	What Causes It	Symptoms	Characteristics of Illness	Control Measures
Salmonellosis	*Salmonellae.* Bacteria widespread in nature, live and grow in intestinal tracts of human beings and animals. About 1200 species are known; one species causes typhoid fever. Bacteria grow and multiply at temperatures between 44° and 115°F. Poultry is a common source.	Severe headache, followed by vomiting, diarrhea, abdominal cramps, and fever. Infants, elderly, and persons with low resistance are most susceptible. Severe infections cause high fever and may even cause death.	Transmitted by eating contaminated food or by contact with infected persons or carriers of the infection. Also transmitted by insects, rodents, and pets. Onset: Usually within 12 to 36 hours. Duration: 2 to 7 days.	*Salmonellae* in food succumb to a temperature of 140°F maintained for 10 minutes or to higher temperatures for less time. Refrigeration at 45° inhibits the increase of *Salmonellae,* but they remain alive in the refrigerator or freezer, and even in dried foods.
Perfringens poisoning	*Clostridium perfringens.* Spore-forming bacteria that grow in the absence of oxygen. Spores can withstand temperatures usually reached in cooking most foods. Surviving bacteria continue to grow in cooked meats, gravies, and meat dishes held without proper refrigeration.	Nausea without vomiting, diarrhea, acute inflammation of stomach and intestines.	Transmitted by food contaminated with abnormally large numbers of the bacteria. Onset: Usually within 3 to 24 hours. Duration: May persist for 24 hours.	To control growth of surviving bacteria on cooked meats that are to be eaten later, cool meats rapidly and refrigerate promptly at 40°F or below.

	Organism	Symptoms	Transmission	Prevention
Staphylococcal poisoning (frequently called staph)	*Staphylococcus aureus.* Bacteria fairly resistant to heat. Bacteria grow profusely with production of toxin at temperatures between 44° and 115°F. Usual source: skin wounds and upper respiratory tract.	Vomiting, diarrhea, prostration, abdominal cramps. Generally mild and often attributed to other causes.	Transmitted by food handlers who carry the bacteria and by eating food containing the toxin. Onset: Usually within 3 to 8 hours. Duration: 1 or 2 days.	Growth of bacteria that produce toxin is inhibited by keeping hot foods above 140°F and cold foods at or below 40°F. Toxin is destroyed by boiling for several hours or heating the food in pressure cooker at 240°F for 30 minutes.
Botulism	*Clostridium botulinum.* Spore-forming organisms that grow and produce toxin in the absence of oxygen, such as in a sealed container. The bacteria can produce a toxin in low-acid foods that have been held in the refrigerator for 2 weeks or longer.	Weakness, unsteadiness, double vision, inability to swallow, speech difficulty, progressive respiratory paralysis. Fatality rate is high in the U.S., about 65 percent.	Transmitted by eating food containing the toxin. Onset: Usually within 12 to 36 hours or longer. Duration: 3 to 6 weeks	Bacterial spores in food succumb at high temperature obtained only in the pressure canner (212°F) for more than 6 hours. The toxin is destroyed by boiling for 10 to 20 minutes; time required depends on kind of food.

tion) occur, followed by peritonitis. Nausea and vomiting may or may not be present, but pain usually precedes these upsets. Appendicitis requires immediate attention.

Chronic infections, allergies, certain metabolic disorders, ulcers, and other gastrointestinal disorders may require consistent medical supervision and in-class management. Teachers can encourage proper and faithful use of medications; motivate changes in food preparation, storage and eating habits; modify the emotional environment; and improve coping skills to alleviate stress-induced gastrointestinal upsets.

Anything that will encourage intestinal activity or produce pressure in the abdominal cavity may be hazardous to children suffering from gastrointestinal disorders. In the event of an upset at school, adult supervisors should follow these rules:

1. Nothing should be given by mouth. It is all right to allow the child to sip water to moisten a dry mouth, but only in very small quantities.
2. Keep the child lying down and as quiet as possible.
3. Do not touch or probe abdomen in any way.
4. Call the child's parents or a physician immediately so that you can shift the care of the child to the proper individuals as soon as possible.

Teachers should also be observant. Shy, retiring children may be reluctant to complain of their discomforts until they are in extreme pain and an in-class incident is unavoidable. A pale and distressed appearance is usually an early warning signal that gives enough time to act before the situation becomes more difficult to manage.

NOTES

1. National Institute of Arthritis, Metabolism, and Digestive Diseases, *Digestive Diseases* (Washington, D.C.: Department of Health, Education, and Welfare, 1976).
2. Ibid.
3. Paul B. Beeson and Walsh McDermott, *Textbook of Medicine* (Philadelphia: W.B. Saunders, 1975), p. 1274.

CHAPTER 16
Communicable Diseases

Historically, the communicable diseases have occupied a prominent position in the lives of the world's people. Even political futures have been shaped by the lowly microbe, which certainly played as much of a role in the "winning of the West" as did the white man's militia. Much of our present longevity is due to the control of previously devastating acute infections by the sciences of epidemiology, immunology, and pharmacology. Right now the communicable diseases seem to be more of a nuisance than a life threat, although sporadic carelessness may still carry lethal consequences, and occasionally a mutant virus with highly communicable and virulent qualities confronts medical science.

Communicable diseases are illnesses that are attributable to a "specific infectious agent or its toxic products, which arises through transmission of that agent or its byproducts from reservoir to susceptible host, either directly or from an infected person or animal, or indirectly through the agency of an intermediate plant or animal host, a vector, or the inanimate environment."[1] The more common varieties, including influenza, colds, and even the venereal diseases, excite limited concern among the public who seem to accept these maladies as the inevitable hazards of life. Such apathy is not without its consequences as seen in such unfortunate episodes as the diphtheria, measles, and polio outbreaks of the early 1970s.[2] Certainly teachers, as well as parents, need to approach the subject of communicable disease control a bit more realistically.

School personnel have a moral obligation to help control the spread of health problems in the school and certainly a financial interest in doing so. Reducing the problem to a crude dollars-and-cents consideration, the school district officials must certainly see the advantage of minimizing absenteeism when they calculate budgets on the basis of average daily attendance. More altruistically speaking, classroom teachers should have enough personal concern for students to maintain a healthful classroom environment and give appropriate aid to unhealthy children.

THE INFECTION PROCESS

Control of communicable diseases in the classroom requires a basic understanding of the essential components of the infection process. These components fit together much like links in a chain; the breaking of any one of them will abort the spread of the disease (see Figure 16–1).

A Causative Agent

The causative agent of infectious disease is the invading organism, or *pathogen*. It is an agent that lives and reproduces at the expense of and detriment to the host. Several major groups of microorganisms are responsible for infection and disease in humans. These include

FIGURE 16-1. *Breaking any one of these links in the infectious disease chain will halt the spread of disease.*

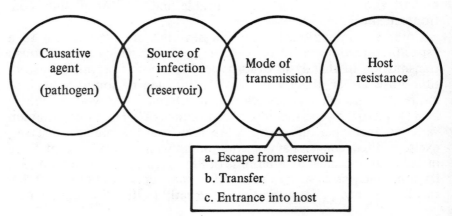

viruses, rickettsiae, bacteria, protozoa, fungi, and metazoa (see Figure 16–2).

1. *Viruses* are an ultramicroscopic form of life. Unlike bacteria, they invade living cells and multiply within them. The diseases they cause are distinguishable from bacterial diseases. Common viral diseases are mumps, smallpox, measles, rabies, and influenza.
2. Smaller than true bacteria, *rickettsiae* live within the cells of the host and require living cells for growth and multiplication. The organisms responsible for typhus, Rocky Mountain spotted fever, and rickettsial pox are of this type.
3. *Bacteria* are single-celled organisms that multiply by simple cellular

FIGURE 16–2. *Infectious organisms.*

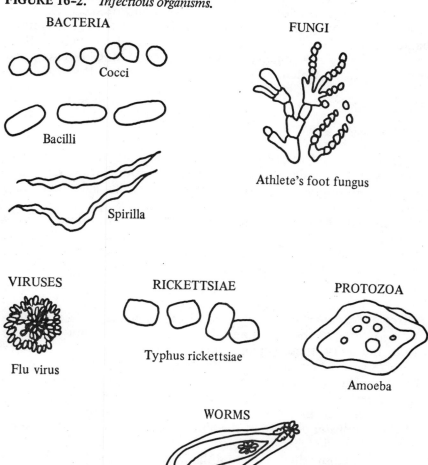

BACTERIA

Cocci

Bacilli

Spirilla

FUNGI

Athlete's foot fungus

VIRUSES

Flu virus

RICKETTSIAE

Typhus rickettsiae

PROTOZOA

Amoeba

WORMS

Liver fluke

division and are capable of growth outside living tissue. Within tissue, they do not invade the cells but rather grow on the surfaces of or between cells and thus attack the cells from without. Examples are cocci, bacilli, and spirilla.

4. Some *fungi* cause infections of the skin, such as ringworm and athlete's foot, and infections of other parts of the body.
5. *Protozoa* are one-celled animal forms such as amoeba, trypanosomes, and plasmodiae. They give rise to malaria, African sleeping sickness, and amoebic dysentery.
6. Various *metazoa* (worm) infestations, including trichinella, pinworms, flukes, hookworms, and tapeworms occur in children.

Invading pathogenic organisms may afflict the host either through direct invasion or through the production of *toxins,* or poison. *Disease* refers to the development of symptoms and/or signs related to invasions with an agent. The development of disease depends on the characteristics of the agent: the number of organisms present, their virulence (i. e., pathogenicity, or the ability to induce disease), and their invasiveness, which is measured by the extent of tissue damage.

A Source of Infection

The term *reservoir* refers to the natural habitat of the organism, that is, where it resides and multiplies. Some organisms have specific, known reservoirs. Knowing their reservoirs aids in disease investigation.

The most important reservoir of the diseases that infect children are children themselves. The majority of these diseases are specific for humans, so new infections come from infected persons. People serve as reservoirs in a variety of ways, which serve as a basis for classification:

1. *Cases* are persons who are obviously ill with the disease in question. As long as the infecting organisms have an avenue of escape from the body, these persons can transmit their infection to other persons with whom they are associated.
2. *Subclinical cases* are persons in whom the symptoms are so vague and apparently so insignificant that the patient fails to seek medical attention or in whom the physician overlooks the true nature of the condition because of the absence of evidence usually associated with the disease.[3]
3. *Carriers* are individuals in whom the microorganism does not cause any symptoms. Consequently, unless the infection shows up in laboratory tests, these individuals do not know of their infection.

They circulate freely in the community and thus they are effective spreaders of disease.

The second largest reservoir of organisms capable of infecting humans is the remainder of the animal kingdom. Although the number of other animal species is huge, only a few species harbor pathogens that are harmful to humans; others harbor organisms that could invade humans only under unusual circumstances. The principal animal reservoirs are domestic animals and rodents.[4] Consequently teachers must be very cautious about allowing animals in the classroom. The only animals in class should be domestic and well controlled (caged or chained preferably).

Any time an animal bites a child, it is imperative to have a physician examine the child. Catching the animal and retaining it for observation is helpful, but leave the task of catching dogs to dogcatchers.

Escape of Organisms from a Reservoir

The mere existence of a reservoir of infection is not sufficient to bring about the spread of infectious diseases. Before they can attack a new host, the organisms must find an avenue of escape. The respiratory tract is the most common and, at the same time, the most dangerous channel of escape from the standpoint of ease of spread. Whenever we speak, cough, sneeze, or even exhale, we could be expelling droplets containing infecting organisms. With a cough or a sneeze, we could drive the droplets many feet away from the body and possibly air currents will carry them even farther. The act of normal conversation drives the droplets several feet.[5]

The principal avenue of escape of infected material from the intestinal tract is through fecal discharge. Escape via the urinary tract is another possibility, although urine less frequently carries pathogenic organisms than do the feces.[6]

Another mode of organism escape is mechanical. This is the liberation of organisms by means of some external force from the tissues in which they are living. Generally some biting or sucking insect draws out the infected blood and thus becomes capable of transmitting the infection to others. Organisms may also escape through discharges from draining lesions, the urethra, and the vagina.

Transfer of Infections from Source to Host

The majority of diseases are spread by direct contact with a patient suffering from the disease or a carrier who either has recovered from the disease but still harbors the active infective organism or has never had the disease and is immune to it but is able to transmit the disease to susceptible persons because the organism is virulent to others.

Direct contact through sneezing, coughing, and other respiratory discharge constitutes so-called *droplet infection.* Transmission by indirect contact varies with the disease, but it is not uncommon. Thus, disease may be spread by contaminated hands and by means of articles of clothing, bed linen, feeding utensils, books, or playthings. Food—especially milk—and water transmit certain organisms. Some diseases can be transmitted by insects (vector-borne), such as the mosquito or louse. Whether transmission by air takes place has never been definitely settled, but quite probably it does, especially in the case of measles, smallpox, chicken pox, and rabies under conditions (e.g., bat caves) in which the concentration of viruses may be very high.

Entry of Organisms into Host

The portals of entry of organisms are principally four: the respiratory tract, the gastrointestinal tract, the urogenital tract, and skin. Entry through the respiratory tract occurs when the new host inhales fine droplets exhaled by infected persons. Once the organism has entered the respiratory passages, it attempts to invade the mucous membranes, but the mucous secretions that cover the membranes and the action of *cilia,* microscopic hairs that line the surfaces of the cells of the respiratory tract thwart the invasion. When the mucous membranes are diseased, invasion is easier. Organisms that we may inhale through the mouth or nose we may swallow; conversely, organisms that enter the mouth with food or drink may gain access to the respiratory passages.[7]

Infection that enters the body through the gastrointestinal system usually arrives through the mouth, principally with food or drink. Although saliva has the power to kill a few bacteria, the duration of stay in the mouth is so short that little real destruction occurs. In the stomach, the organisms encounter destructive forces in the form of digestive enzymes and hydrochloric acid. Entry of organisms into the digestive tract is not always followed by infection. Once the organism is in the digestive tract, it must survive other body defenses, such as vomiting and diarrhea. With these mechanisms, the body rids itself of a large number of pathogenic organisms.

The healthy skin is generally an effective barrier against invasion by pathogenic organisms. Pathogenic bacteria may exist on the surface of the skin and cause no disease. If a break occurs in the skin, however, invasion ensues. Insect-borne diseases are transmitted through the skin. The direct invasion of urogenital mucous membranes occurs with syphilis, gonorrhea, and similar diseases. Because these mucous membranes have little defense against invasion, these diseases spread easily.[8]

Resistance of Host

Nature has endowed individuals with certain mechanical and chemical mechanisms that enable them to resist invasion by pathogens. These mechanisms include external as well as nonspecific and specific internal defenses.

Mechanical Defenses

Skin and its secretions are a most important barrier, as the increased frequency of infection after burns or abrasions best illustrates. Mucous membranes have a similar function, to which the flow of secretions and the mechanical action of cilia at certain sites (e.g., the upper respiratory tract) contribute.[9] In addition, normal body secretions, such as the lacrimal fluid that bathes the eyes, perspiration, and vaginal and gastric secretions, kill many pathogens before they can produce disease.

A number of physiological factors influence the susceptibility of an individual to disease. Studies have shown, for example, that malnutrition resulting from insufficient or inadequate food, along with extreme fatigue and exhaustion, may decrease individual resistance and render a person more susceptible to diseases such as pneumonia or tuberculosis.[10] Although fever definitely eliminates certain infections (e.g., central nervous system syphilis), and elevated temperature inhibits the growth of some less virulent polio viruses, research has yet to establish the role of fever as a true defense mechanism.

Nonspecific Defenses

Our understanding of nonspecific defenses is less sophisticated. Evidence indicates that the blood and other body fluids offer limited resistance to pathogenic organisms.

Phagocytosis is one of the body's important nonspecific internal defense mechnisms. This defense hinges on the ability of white blood cells (leukocytes) to migrate to a point of cellular injury and engulf debris and microorganisms involved in the disease process.

The state of a person's health bears a positive relationship to the degree of resistance to communicable disease. For example, studies have shown that individuals with leukemia, cancer, diabetes, and uremia have increased susceptibility to infectious diseases. In addition, children who are ill with one infectious disease are very susceptible to additional infections.[11]

Immunity

Immunity to a disease may be defined as a lack of susceptibility to an infecting organism or its toxin. Immunity to a specific disease—such as that conferred by vaccines or by natural infection—depends primarily on the interaction of antigens and antibodies.

The exact mechanisms by which the body is able to resist infection are not all clearly understood. Body cells are capable of producing immune substances, or *antibodies,* against substances known as *antigens,* which include microorganisms and their products. An antigen may be defined as any substance that stimulates the production of antibodies in the body tissues or fluids. Antibodies are remarkably specific; that is, they defend the body only against the particular antigens that cause their production. A child who has had rubella (German measles) will not be immune to rubeola (another type of measles).

Whether an antigen is introduced into the body intentionally, as in immunization for the prevention of disease, or unintentionally, as in infection, some of it is trapped by phagocytic cells called *macrophages,* which have the capacity to break down or digest the antigen. A portion of the antigen remains on the surface of these cells. In this location, the antigen comes in contact with a type of small white blood cell called a *plasma cell,* which begins to manufacture antibodies. The antibodies thus produced enter into the blood stream to become part of the so-called *gamma globulin fraction.* If the antigen ever invades the body again, the antibody will combine with it in such a way as to render it ineffective in producing the disease.

Some children are born with or develop an inability to manufacture sufficient antibodies. Without adequate gamma globulin, they are highly susceptible to infection. Periodic gamma globulin shots are moderately effective in lowering susceptibility, but the condition increases the responsibility of the teacher to control the spread of communicable disease in the classroom.

Natural Immunity

Natural immunity is ours simply because we belong to the human race. It makes us immune to hoof and mouth, canine distemper, canine hepatitis, and other animal diseases. We may also inherit natural immunity through the gene pool of our ancestors. This type is known as *natural racial immunity.*

Natural immunity to certain diseases is present at birth. Since maternal antibodies can and do cross the placenta, a child usually has the same antibodies as its mother. This immunity does not last long, however. It usually has disappeared by the end of the first year of life.[12]

Acquired Immunity

Acquired immunity may be one of two kinds, active or passive. *Active immunity* is long-lasting and we may acquire it three ways: (1) by having had and recovered from the disease; (2) by having had a series of subclinical infections, which build up immunity; and (3) through inoculation or vaccination with products that produce active immunity, such as toxoids and vaccines made from inactivated (killed) organisms or living but attenuated (weakened) organisms.[13]

Passive immunity we acquire by the injection of serum or antitoxin containing antibodies from another source (animal or human), that is, as a gamma globulin shot. This immunity is immediate but weaker in effect than active immunity and of very short duration.

THE PROGRESS OF COMMUNICABLE DISEASES

Communicable diseases pass through four stages between the time the disease agent enters the body and recovery. They are incubation, prodrome, fastigium, and convalescence.

The *incubation stage* covers the time between the introduction of the causative agent into the body and the first signs or symptoms. Its length varies for different diseases and at times widely fluctuates from one case of a single disease to another. Apparently the duration depends on the time required for the multiplication and distribution of the causative organism and its products. The incubation period may last only a few hours, or it may last as long as several months. Most diseases, however, have an incubation period that ranges from several days to several weeks, during which time the disease organisms rapidly multiply until they are in sufficient number to overcome the body's defenses. Most infectious diseases are not contagious during the early part of the incubation stage but become highly contagious toward the end, just before symptoms occur. Nevertheless, some of the diseases that commonly affect the classroom, such as influenza and chicken pox, are communicable during the incubation stage.

The *prodromal period* is the interval of time that elapses between the earliest appearance of generalized symptoms and signs and the occurrence of the specific symptoms and signs that characterize the disease. This stage may last only a few hours or up to several days. Typical symptoms include headaches, aching muscles and/or joints, fever, scratchy throat, runny nose, coughing and sneezing, and other nonspecific symptoms. These constitute the earliest observable signs of infection and should prompt parents to keep children home and should alert the teacher to remove a child from the classroom. Most communicable diseases are very contagious during this stage.

During *fastigium* the clinical picture that is typical of the disease manifests itself. For example, measles cases will develop a rash and the lumps that characterize mumps will appear. The disease usually remains highly communicable during this stage.

As the disease begins to wane and the symptoms abate, the patient enters the *convalescence stage*. During this time, the disease-causing organisms are still in the body and treatment must continue to prevent relapse.

COMMUNICABLE DISEASE CONTROL

Although the number of measures used to control communicable diseases is large, all of them fall into one of three categories: (1) preventing spread, (2) increasing the resistance of the new host, and (3) minimizing the ill effects of actual cases. Each of these measures complements the other two, and an intelligent combination of them constitutes the usual effort to control a specific disease.[14]

Preventing Spread

The most desirable and permanently successful form of infectious disease control is to eliminate the reservoir of infection, for without it, spread cannot occur. In essence, this method entails successfully treating people.

The development of drugs that have the capacity to kill microorganisms within the body without seriously damaging the individual has opened the way for elimination of reservoirs of infection. The sulfa drugs and antibiotics such as penicillin and the tetracyclines are highly specific for certain bacteria. Drugs are not an immediate disease cure, but adequate treatment by the nurse or family physician may keep patients from spreading infection. As previously mentioned, keeping infected children away from school is essential to prevent escaping organisms from reaching other persons.

Environmental sanitation seeks to prevent spread by regulating those objects that transmit pathogens from a reservoir to a new host. These measures aim either at killing the organisms themselves or at destroying or controlling the carrier. Disinfection, control of insect vectors (destruction of insects, prevention of breeding), protection and purification of water supplies, milk sanitation, and disinfection of air (ultraviolet light, disinfectant mists, etc.) are common methods of environmental sanitation.[15]

Increasing Resistance of New Host

Immunization has become probably the most fundamental practice in contemporary medicine. Throughout the world, immunization programs focus on approximately twenty-five human diseases. About one-half of the toxoids and vaccines are in regular use as part of the so-called *basic series* of immunization for infants and children. Preschool immunization clinics and the public-school immunization programs still constitute the major means of maintaining immunity levels in a community.

During the past few years, however, immunization levels in preschool-age children against polio, measles, rubella, pertussis, diphtheria, tetanus, and mumps have declined alarmingly. National surveys indicate that approximately one-third of the nearly 14 million one- to four-year old preschool children have no protection against these diseases (see Table 16–1).[16] One cause is a lack of uniformity in state immunization. laws. Combined with a high degree of mobility among the population, this situation increases the risk of disease outbreaks. As Table 16–2 shows, several states have no laws requiring preschool immunization and experienced a diphtheria outbreak in the early 1970s.

According to some public health and school authorities parents will be sufficiently concerned about immunization to insure that their children are adequately protected without being legally required to do so. But parents are not adequately concerned for various reasons:

1. Today's mothers may never have seen, or at least do not remember, some of the diseases that used to be so common. So they become lax about immunizing their children. Fortunately, the one-third or so of preschoolers who have not been immunized are not repeatedly exposed to sick children, so even they have benefited from immunization. Yet failure to vaccinate susceptible children

TABLE 16-1. Immunization Status of Children One to Four Years Old

| Year | Percent Immunized | | | | |
	Rubella	Measles	DTP*	Polio*	Mumps
1970	37.2	57.2	76.1	65.9	—
1971	51.2	61.0	78.7	67.3	—
1972	56.9	62.2	75.6	62.9	—
1973	55.6	61.2	72.6	60.4	34.7
1974	59.8	64.5	73.9	63.1	39.4
1975	61.9	65.5	75.2	64.8	44.4
1976	61.7†	65.9†	71.4†	61.6†	48.3†

Source: 1975 United States immunization survey, Center for Disease Control, Atlanta, June 1976.
*Three doses.
†Preliminary estimate.

TABLE 16-2. Immunization Requirements Prior to School Entry, September 1977

State	Type of legislation			If no state law at present, are there plans pending for proposing such a law?		If yes, before September 1978?	Immunizations required for specific diseases							
	Mandatory	Permissive	None	Yes	No		Diphtheria	Pertussis	Tetanus	Measles	Mumps	Polio	Rubella	Smallpox
Alabama	X						X	X	X	X		X	X	
Alaska	X						X	X	X	X		X		
Arizona†			X†		X									
Arkansas	X						X	X	X	X		X	X	
California	X						X	X	X	X		X		
Colorado	X						X	X	X			X	X	
Connecticut*	X	X								X		X	X	
Delaware	X						X	X	X	X		X	X	
District of Columbia	X						X	X	X	X		X	X	
Florida	X						X	X	X	X	X	X	X	
Georgia	X						X	X	X	X		X	X	
Hawaii	X						X	X	X	X		X	X	
Idaho			X	X										
Illinois	X						X	X	X	X		X	X	
Indiana	X						X	X	X	X		X	X	
Iowa§	X§						X	X	X	X		X	X	
Kansas	X						X		X	X		X		
Kentucky	X						X		X	X		X		
Louisiana	X						X	X	X	X		X		
Maine		X					X	X	X	X	X	X	X	
Maryland	X						X	X	X	X		X	X	
Massachusetts	X						X	X	X	X		X		
Michigan	X						X	X	X	X		X	X	
Minnesota	X									X			X	
Mississippi		X					X	X	X	X		X	X	
Missouri	X						X			X		X	X	
Montana		X		X			X	X	X	X		X	X	
Nebraska	X						X	X	X	X		X	X	
Nevada	X						X	X	X	X		X	X	
New Hampshire	X						X	X	X	X		X	X	
New Jersey	X						X	X	X	X		X	X	
New Mexico	X						X	X	X	X		X	X	
New York	X						X		X	X	X	X	X	
North Carolina	X						X	X		X		X		
North Dakota	X						X	X	X	X	X	X	X	
Ohio	X						X	X	X	X		X	X	
Oklahoma	X						X	X	X	X		X	X	
Oregon	X						X	X	X	X		X		
Pennsylvania	X						X		X	X		X	X	
Rhode Island	X						X		X	X		X	X	
South Carolina	X						X	X	X	X		X	X	
South Dakota	X						X	X	X	X		X	X	
Tennessee	X						X	X	X	X		X	X	
Texas	X						X	X	X	X		X	X	
Utah	X						X	X	X	X	X	X	X	
Vermont‡			X‡		X									
Virginia	X						X	X	X	X		X	X	
Washington†			X†	X		Yes								
West Virginia	X						X	X	X	X		X	X	
Wisconsin	X						X	X	X	X		X	X	
Wyoming			X		X									
Guam†			X†		X									
Puerto Rico	X													
Virgin Islands	X						X	X	X	X		X	X	
Total	48*		6	3	4	1	45	38	43	47	5	46	42	0

*Connecticut: rubella and measles are mandatory; polio is permissive.
†Arizona, Washington, and Guam have adopted regulations, with the effect of law, establishing school entry immunication requirements.
‡Vermont has local option regulations at the school district level, establishing school entry immunization requirements.
§State law was signed in July 1977 and is effective 1 January 1978.
Source: Information received from immunization projects.

by the time they enter school may result in small epidemics even when they are in high school.

2. Doctors have tended to become lax, too, because they no longer have to deal with large outbreaks of infectious diseases, even though many children have not been properly immunized.

3. Parents in lower socioeconomic groups do not think about having their preschoolers immunized, although vaccines are readily available at no cost in public clinics. In many of these homes preventive medicine gives way to more immediate needs.

Concerned school personnel should occupy the forefront in promoting community action to require the immunization of preschool children. Where preschool immunization laws do not exist, the schools should attempt to fill the gap by offering and encouraging immunization of the school population. The general belief among experts is that an 80 percent immunization level among schoolchildren will suffice to prevent outbreaks of the specific diseases. Where preschool immunization clinics are scarce, a considerable need exists for education of adult PTA groups, public health officials, school nurses, and others to convince the population of the indispensability of good immunization levels in the school.

Most states with preschool immunization laws exempt or make allowances for persons who do not want to have their children immunized. Religious grounds, personal reasons, and medical problems are usually the bases of exception. Where such exemptions exist, a well-planned and consistently promoted immunization program will usually help to maintain a sufficiently high level of immunity in the school to ward off outbreaks of disease (see Table 16-3).

A final point: Although immunization is most effective when ad-

TABLE 16-3. Childhood Immunization Schedule Proposed by American Academy of Pediatrics

Age	Vaccine
2 months	DTP,* polio
4 months	DTP, polio
6 months	DTP
1 year	TB test
15 months	Measles, rubella, mumps
18 months	DTP, polio
4–6 years	DTP, polio
14–16 years	TD†

*Diphtheria, tetanus, pertussis.
†Tetanus, diphtheria.

ministered several months or more before exposure to a communicable disease, additional circumstances may warrant its use. Children who have been exposed to an infective disease can be given a "booster" injection if they have previously been immunized or a passive immunization if they have never been immunized. And in addition to immunization, the consistent application of good health habits will render children more resistant to infection.

Minimizing Effects of Infectious Diseases

Community participation in laboratory services, community diagnostic surveys, and community clinics is essential for prompt and early diagnosis of cases of a disease. Early diagnosis helps minimize the risk of spread and initiates effective treatment to reduce morbidity and mortality. Provisions for adequate community-treatment facilities and appropriate follow-up by school nurses and family physicians will help to alleviate the distress of the disease and to avoid complications.

DISEASES OF SPECIAL CONCERN

Table 16–4 lists communicable diseases about which teachers should have a general knowledge. But two types of diseases deserve special attention here because they do affect schoolchildren, they are difficult to control, and their occurrence is widespread. They are skin diseases and venereal diseases.

Skin Diseases

Perhaps the most obvious diseases to the teacher are those that cause skin lesions or rashes. To the medical profession skin diseases offer a peculiar diagnostic challenge, and certainly they should arouse prompt concern in the school for some are contagious (see Table 16–5). Lesions require school personnel to determine whether to remove a child from the classroom. Therefore, where possible, teachers should consult the school nurse whenever lesions cannot be explained on the basis of trauma.

Venereal Diseases

It is difficult to determine the actual incidence of venereal disease in the elementary school population. Certainly, a virtual epidemic exists among teenagers and young adults in certain areas of the United

TABLE 16-4. Major Infectious Diseases

Disease	Pathogen	How Transmitted	Incubation Period	Characteristics of Occurrence	Signs and Symptoms	Prevention
Ascariasis	Nematode	Food contaminated with eggs of the nematode. Raw foods (salads) are usually implicated.	Worms mature in about two months.	Common and world-wide. In U.S. the disease is most prevalent in the South. Preschool and elementary school age children are more frequently and heavily infected than older children and adults. In tropical climate, infection may exceed 50 percent of the population. Eggs are shed in feces.	Vague or absent, ordinarily mild. Heavy infections may cause digestive disturbances, abdominal pain, vomiting, restlessness.	Proper disposal of feces. Education regarding toilet habits and hand-washing before eating.
Chicken pox (varicella)	Virus	Spreads by air, through inhalation. Droplets are directly or indirectly spread.	14–16 days.	Occurs epidemically, mainly in winter and spring. Before age 20, affects both sexes equally. Virus reaches skin from respiratory system via the blood. Virus can affect nerve pathways, causing the disease "shingles" years after the infection.	Mild disease with fever and itching vesicular eruption. Papules make appearance about 24 hours after onset of fever. Lesions are most abundant over the trunk, but also on the face, and spread to mouth, throat, and extremities. Successive crops of lesions may be seen, with general involvement of lymph glands.	Immunizations (somewhat ineffective); gamma globulin prevents some cases.
Cholera	Bacteria	By direct contact with patients in incubation stage; food, utensils, and water contaminated by fecal materials; flies.	1–3 days.	Endemic in certain Asian countries. Few cases occur in U.S. Travelers to countries where cholera is endemic or epidemic should be immunized before departure.	Sudden onset. Copious and frequent watery stools and prostration. Vomiting. Severe dehydration. Loss of as much as 15 percent of body weight in a few hours. Thirst, but patient cannot retain fluids or food. Features become pinched, eyes sunken. Painful cramps. Enfeebled voice. Rapid and weak pulse, low blood pressure. Uremia. Death may sometimes occur in a few hours.	Cholera vaccine is effective for a few months.
Diphtheria	Bacteria	Directly by droplet infection from respiratory discharges, and through contamination of hands, objects and, occasionally, milk.	2–5 days.	Endemic and epidemic where immunization measures neglected.	Abrupt fever, chilliness, malaise, sore throat. Whitish-grey membrane forms on tonsils and then thickens to form yellowish diphtheric membrane. Other areas may also be invaded. Cervical lymph nodes are swollen. Bacteria do not invade the tissues, but produce toxins that cause heart and kidney damage.	Diphtheria-pertussis-tetanus toxoids (DPT) and diphtheria-tetanus toxoids (DT) for pediatric use; special tetanus and diphtheria toxoids (TD) for adult use.

(continued)

283

TABLE 16-4 (Continued)

Disease	Pathogen	How Transmitted	Incubation Period	Characteristics of Occurrence	Signs and Symptoms	Prevention
Encephalitis, viral (arthropod-borne)	Virus	By mosquitoes that feed on birds harboring the virus (without suffering any ill effects).	5–15 days.	Three types of encephalitis viruses cause bulk of infections in U.S.: Eastern equine, St. Louis, and Western. Types of birds that harbor the disease vary, as do types of mosquitoes, but the latter's bite is the source of the virus for man, as well as for horses, mules, and other mammals.	Severity of symptoms varies. In the St. Louis type, high fever, vomiting, headache, vertigo, nuchal rigidity, ataxia, and confusion are among serious symptoms. Western equine type may involve repeated convulsions and deep coma.	
Hepatitis, infectious	Virus	Fecal or oral discharges contaminating food, water, or milk.	15–35 days.	Occurs sporadically and in small local epidemics, which have been traced to sewage-contaminated water or consumption of contaminated food, especially shellfish. Believed that, like serum hepatitis, infectious hepatitis, may also be transmitted by injection equipment.	Headache, fever, and anorexia (in most cases); shaking chills (in half). Nausea and vomiting. Malaise, myalgia (sore muscles); joint stiffness, sore throat, dull upper abdominal pain. Urine darkens. Jaundice. Most cases recover fully within four months. Disease tends to be mild in children and young adults, more serious in older adults.	Gamma globulin after known exposure is helpful, but does not prevent the disease.
Hepatitis, serum	Virus	Inadequately sterilized needles and syringes; blood or blood products.	2–6 mo.; 12–14 weeks average.	Virus may circulate in the blood for eight years or more after patient has recovered. Tests can now detect the virus in the blood and are means of preventing spread of disease by transfusion.	Symptoms resemble those of infectious hepatitis, but are more severe.	Proper blood storage and sterilization techniques; gamma globulin for all persons over age 40 receiving blood transfusions is recommended by some.
Herpes simplex	Virus	Presumably by direct or droplet contact and maybe by indirect association.	Unknown.	Primary herpes simplex is mainly a disease of childhood. In adults, herpes-like episodes may occur during attacks of pneumonia, meningitis, malaria, and other diseases. Virus lives in balance with most tissues and does not reveal its presence until some stress shifts the balance in its favor.	Commonest form of the disease is characterized by painful blisters on lips and gums sometimes associated with fever, irritability, malaise, and swelling of glands. Symptoms may persist for 7 to 10 days. Other sites sometimes affected are the genitalia and the conjunctivae and eye. Most herpes-simplex-like attacks in adults probably caused by other, ill-defined viruses.	
Herpes zoster (shingles)	Virus	Perhaps by air or contact from children with chicken pox. Sometimes accompanies pneumonia and tuberculosis.	7–14 days.	Sporadic occurrence, especially in winter and spring. Rarely seen before age 20. Occurs more often in males than in females.	Onset often marked by severe pain, fever, malaise, and tenderness. Affected area develops small blisters that are often moist and weeping.	

284

Disease	Cause	Mode of transmission	Incubation period	Occurrence	Characteristic symptoms	Prevention/control
Infectious mononucleosis	Virus	Direct contact, secretions.	4–14 days.	Outbreaks in colleges, camps, and institutions, but generally appears sporadically. Typically affects young adults. Very little known about the disease.	Malaise, fever, lymphatic enlargement (neck). Some have jaundice due to hepatitis (difficult to distinguish from infectious hepatitis).	
Influenza	Virus	Droplet infection, soiled articles, direct contact.	24–72 hours.	Sporadic cases, local epidemics, pandemics. May affect up to 50 percent of population within period of 4–6 weeks. Each year the National Institutes of Health, after a careful survey of viruses recovered from recent influenza cases, decides what the exact composition and strength of influenza vaccine should be for the new season, and that becomes the new standard for all U.S. manufacturers.	Sudden onset. Fever of 1–7 days, chills, listlessness, nausea, vomiting, prostration, aches and pains in back and limbs, coryza, sore throat, bronchitis.	Immunization for high-risk individuals, i.e., those with diabetes, chronic respiratory diseases, heart ailments, advanced age.
Measles (rubeola)	Virus	Respiratory discharges (direct or indirect).	9–11 days.	Most outbreaks in late winter and early spring. Epidemics run in 2- to 3-year cycles. Mainly a disease of children; mortality is highest in those under 5 years old and in the aged.	Rhinitis, cough, mild fever, headache, malaise, fatigue, anorexia, conjunctivitis, eye sensitivity to light, and lacrimation. Rash usually appears the second to the fourth day.	Immunization.
German measles (rubella)	Virus	Respiratory discharges (direct or indirect).	9–11 days.	Usually a childhood disease, but fairly common in adults. One attack may confer lifelong immunity. The age group usually affected is from 2 to 15 years. Permanent effects are rare except for damage to the unborn child when the mother is infected in the first 6 months of pregnancy.	Mild rash, slight fever, and swelling of lymph nodes. These symptoms usually appear from 14 to 21 days after exposure and last for only 1 to 4 days.	Immunization; gamma globulin may curtail symptoms; vaccine should not be given to pregnant women.
Mumps	Virus	Infected droplets or direct contact with salivary droplets from infected person.	17–21 days.	Occur most often in 5–15 age group, but disease may attack adults. Because of the low degree of infectivity, many adults have not been exposed to the disease and are susceptible. Many cases are asymptomatic.	Prodromal symptoms (fever, chilliness, malaise, loss of appetite, and headache) may or may not precede swelling of parotid gland. Swelling may affect one or two glands, with tenderness and difficulty in moving jaw. Testes, ovaries, pancreas or thyroid gland can also be involved.	Immunization available, but does not offer full immunity.
Pertussis (whooping cough)	Bacteria	Inhalation of droplets or dusts from infected person.	7–14 days.	Epidemic at 2- to 4-year intervals. Endemic in winter and spring. Mainly disease of infants and very young children; high mortality under 6 months of age. Highly contagious.	Mild cough becomes violent and spasmodic. Coughing followed by loud whooping sounds as the individual attempts to breathe. Disease usually of 6 weeks duration in 3 stages of approximately 2 weeks each: (1) *catarrhal stage*: upper respiratory infection with increasingly intense	Immunization.

(continued)

285

TABLE 16-4 (Continued)

Disease	Pathogen	How Transmitted	Incubation Period	Characteristics of Occurrence	Signs and Symptoms	Prevention
Pertussis					nonproductive; (2) cough and rhinorrhea, sometimes low-grade fever, *spasmodic stage:* in 10 to 14 days cough becomes strangling and explosive, ending with characteristic whoop; thick, ropy mucus; vomiting, exhaustion, mental confusion; (3) *convalescent stage:* gradual decrease in severity of symptoms.	Immunization should only accompany exposure to endemic areas.
Plague	Bacteria	Fleas (from wild rodents), not directly communicable.	2–10 days.	Endemic in Asia; sometimes appears in parts of Africa and South America. Infected ground squirrels and prairie dogs in the western states of the U.S. have been found; these animals can transmit plague to "domestic" rats and thence to man. Disease is spread principally by migration in rat-infested ships.	Plague appears in 3 forms: bubonic, septicemic; and pneumonic. Headache, dizziness, and thirst are early symptoms. High fever, restlessness, rapid breathing, fast pulse. Enlarged lymph nodes or buboes appear on second day. Pneumonic plague is marked by cyanosis, followed by convulsions and coma.	
Poliomyelitis	Virus	Nose and mouth droplets, as well as fecal contamination.	7–14 days.	Children most susceptible; pregnant women vulnerable. Mild infections confer full immunity. There are 3 strains of virus.	Fever, headache, vomiting, malaise, sore throat, stiffness and pain in back, weakness, flaccid paralysis (in spinal type of disease). In bulbar type, respiratory paralysis, inability to swallow or talk clearly.	Immunization with all 3 types of vaccine.
Rabies	Virus	Bites of rabid animals, mainly dogs; sometimes by licks on open sore.	2–6 weeks (10 days in head bites); may be as long as one year.	Sporadic. Epizootics of rabies in wild animals such as wolves, bats, foxes, coyotes, and skunks are potential reservoirs for rabies virus. Disease may spread to a number of domestic animals, including cats and cows, but canine rabies is mainly responsible for urban outbreaks. Head and neck bites cause more infections in man than bites on other parts of the human body.	Sense of apprehension, headache, vague sensory changes. Paralytic manifestations, in 2 or 3 days, first cause spasm on drinking. Delirium, convulsions, respiratory paralysis, death. Once symptoms appear, disease is usually fatal.	Immunization in the event of a bite by rabid animal or to persons in high-risk occupations.
Rocky Mountain spotted fever	Rickettsiae	Tick-borne.	3–10 days.	Majority of cases occur in April and May, when the wood tick is prevalent. People in outdoor occupations are in greatest danger of being bitten by	Disease resembles typhus, including the prodromal symptoms and sudden onset with headache, chills, prostration, and quickly rising fever. Marked muscle and	Immunization.

286

Disease	Causative agent	Mode of transmission	Incubation period	Epidemiology	Symptoms	Prevention and control
					joint pains and often bleeding from the nose. In untreated, severe cases, fever ends late in the third week. Rash resembles that seen in early measles, which fades and is followed by lesions on ankles, wrists, legs, chest.	infected ticks has been disappointing; personal care and immunization are best insurance.
Dysentery (shigellosis)	Bacteria	Fecal-oral, contaminated food, milk, water, carriers.	1–7 days.	Endemic only in areas where poor sanitary practices prevail; may cause epidemics or sporadic outbreaks in the presence of local breakdown of sanitation. Most common in summer and in prisons, camps, and institutions; and in children. Reservoir is usually infected humans.	Acute onset with frequent stools, diarrhea (frequently bloody and mucoid). Cramping in severe cases with fever. The disease is more severe in children because convulsions may occur. Bacteria invade mucus tissues and create abscesses.	Control depends almost entirely on sanitary measures, including surveillance of food handlers and water supplies.
Smallpox	Virus	Contact-inhalation. Virus-laden droplets or dusts are inhaled.	10–12 days.	Formerly endemic and recurrent in some areas of Asia, Africa, South America, and the Middle East. Now considered to be a nonexisting disease.	Sudden onset with backache, headache, and vomiting, followed by eruption of pocks, which start as macules, become papules, then vesicles and finally pustules. Disease varies from mild to severe. Nine different grades of severity have been described with mortality ranging from 0 to 100 percent.	Immunization is usually recommended only for those in high-risk areas or those traveling into endemic areas. Routine immunization no longer recommended.
Tetanus	Bacteria	Usually, contamination of puncture or deep wounds.	4–12 days.	Bacteria found in the soil, but boiling is usually not sufficient to destroy. Disease is painful and fatality approaches 20 percent.	Tightness in neck, general irritability, stiffness of muscles, inability to open mouth. Convulsions and cyanosis. Extensor spasms in which the head and heels are bent backward and the body forward.	Immunization.
Tuberculosis	Bacteria	Contact-inhalation of droplets from infected person; milk from tuberculous cows.	2–10 weeks.	Susceptibility is general; high in children under 3, lowest 3–12 years, relatively high remainder of life; overcrowding and malnutrition contribute to spread.	Malaise, lassitude, fatigue, fever, weight loss, hoarseness, cough, expectoration, and hemorrhage from lungs. In some cases, the infection may spread to bones and kidneys.	Immunization for high-risk persons and pasteurization of milk.
Typhoid/paratyphoid	Bacteria	Contaminated food and water spread through fecal or oral contamination.	10–21 days.	Large epidemics of typhoid fever, once common, have been ended by modern water supply and sewage disposal and milk pasteurization. Remaining cases can be traced to contaminated food and to rare typhoid carriers. Man is the only reservoir. Paratyphoid fever is a closely related disease caused by certain other species of Salmonnellae. It is spread in the same manner as typhoid.	Typhoid fever ranges in severity from a mild disease of 1–2 weeks duration to a "fulminating," rapidly fatal illness. Usually malaise, headache, and fever develop gradually. Anorexia, nausea, vomiting, constipation. Nosebleeds common. Fever in untreated cases gradually rises to 102–104°F (delirium), with sweats and chills. Diarrhea. Paratyphoid has similar symptoms.	Immunization for those traveling into endemic areas. However, vaccine does not offer full protection.

(continued)

TABLE 16-4 (Continued)

Disease	Pathogen	How Transmitted	Incubation Period	Characteristics of Occurrence	Signs and Symptoms	Prevention
Typhus fever (epidemic)	Rickettsiae	Louse-borne.	6–15 days.	Epidemic disease in many African, Asian, and Eastern European countries. Related to, but not identical to, endemic or murine typhus, a mild disease maintained in certain parts of the U.S. Vaccine protects only against louse-borne typhus.	After mild prodromal symptoms, such as fatigue and headache, the disease suddenly manifests itself with severe headache and bodywide pains; fever rises to 104°F and stays there until recovery. A rash usually appears on the fifth day on the back and chest, spreading to the abdomen and extremities, but usually not extending to the face, palms, and soles. Small hemorrhages in these lesions cause them to turn purplish in the second week. Stupor and coma foreshadow a fatal outcome. When contracted by immunized persons, disease symptoms and duration are greatly reduced.	Immunization for those traveling into endemic areas.

TABLE 16-5. Common Skin Disorders and Their Management

Disease	Cause	Symptoms	Treatment
Acne	Emotional stress, hormonal change incident to pubescence, unknown factors; not contagious.	Increased oiliness of skin, blackheads, papules and pustules, cysts on the face, back, and chest.	Proper management of stress, twice daily cleansing with soap, and 8 to 9 hours of sleep nightly. Irritants, such as resorcinol, acetone salicylic acid, and the irritant vitamin A acid are particularly effective treatments. Benzoyl peroxide is useful for closed pustular forms. Antibiotic therapy (tetracycline, clindamycin) is sometimes effective. Of questionable value are radiation treatments, diet and estrogen therapy.
Impetigo	Streptoccus bacterium; contagious.	Formation of crested sore with oozing. Itching leads to scratching, which abrades surrounding skin and infects adjacent areas and other objects or persons. Inadequate treatment may lead to serious renal (kidney) infections.	Oral or injected antibiotics are superior to topical applications. Patient should be excluded from school and readmitted on physician's approval.

(*continued*)

TABLE 16–5 (Continued)

Disease	Cause	Symptoms	Treatment
Pediculosis	Lice; contagious by contact with person or personal articles.	Itching, prescence of lice or nits (eggs) on the hair or clothing. Nits appear as white specks attached to the hair.	Cleanliness, use of antiseptic solutions and medications.
Ringworm	Fungus; contagious by contact with person or contaminated articles.	Hair loss in patches, whitish, greyish, or yellowish scales on scalp.	Treatment is slow. Child remains in school. Screening of class with ultraviolet lamp (Wood's light) is desirable to find and treat new cases and prevent spread.
Scabies	Itch; contagious by direct contact.	Itching with scratching between fingers, in armpits, on genitalia.	Similar to pediculosis.
Warts	Virus, mildly contagious.	Raised, rounded, grayish protrusions on the skin; called "plantar warts" when on soles of feet.	Cauthoridin or liquid nitrogen will not leave scars. Immunity will usually develop followed by spontaneous disappearance.

Source: Communicable Disease Control Center, U.S. Department of Health, Education and Welfare, Atlanta, Ga.

States. In younger age groups, the rate is generally low but may be increasing. *Gonorrhea* is most widespread, to judge from the number of reported cases in this country; syphilis is number three. The high rates of both diseases are rather paradoxical in view of the relative ease of treating them—although a penicillin-resistant strain of gonorrhea has appeared in several states. Part of the control problem is attributable to the fact that female victims do not manifest symptoms until the infection is well advanced and therefore constitute a vast reservoir for the diseases.[17] It is also paradoxical that instead of stressing avoidance of contact with the source of contagion as a preventive measure, education programs emphasize detection, a control procedure that has proven woefully ineffective to date. Meanwhile, increased media enhancement of the "recreational virtues" of sexual activity seems to have paralleled an epidemic spiral of venereal infections. We can safely and at least casually associate increased exposure of children to sex in the media with an increased incidence of venereal diseases in younger age groups.

Discussion of the venereal diseases as part of the topic of communicable diseases keeps it out of value-laden or anatomical and physiological discussions that comprise sex education. Using the disease orientation allows teachers to focus on avoiding contacts as a control measure without inviting accusations of moral preachment.

A synopsis of the facts about common venereal infections appears in Table 16-6. Teachers and parents should be able to talk knowledgeably about venereal diseases with adolescents and should maintain an open, concerned attitude with youngsters who might thereby feel free to approach them about these and other health concerns.

SCHOOL POLICY AND COMMUNICABLE DISEASE CONTROL

The legal responsibility for communicable disease control is vested in the state board of health. Nevertheless, as a cooperative agency, the school should incorporate certain procedures to control diseases more effectively and prevent outbreaks in the school population. Parents should be aware of the control problems facing the school and should cooperate in all policy efforts to keep communicable diseases out of the classroom.

1. Parents and school personnel must be familiar with the legal limitations on the school regarding communicable disease control. School policies on immunization procedures and classroom exclusion and readmission must be in harmony with existing legislation.
2. Policies regarding school attendance need careful study and understanding. A distinct hazard exists in establishing school budgets on the basis of attendance records. Such a policy favors the spread of communicable diseases because it encourages sick children to attend school to maintain budget allocations. This policy might be less detrimental if school personnel could appreciate the relationship between allowing contagious children into class and further increases in absenteeism. The sick child in the classroom will likely create an attendance drop by spreading infection to several other students. A satisfactory alternative to this policy would be to count sick children present when compiling average daily attendance figures.
3. Parents should keep children out of school when they display pro-

TABLE 16-6. The Venereal Diseases

Type	How Transmitted	Symptoms	Treatment	Diagnosis
Gonorrhea (bacteria)	Direct sexual contact to infant during birth.	Incubation period 2–14 days, average of 3 days. Males: inflammation of urethra with painful urination occasionally accompanied by pus discharge. Asymptomatic cases exist. Complications: (1) stricture—closing off of urethra with subsequent difficult urination; (2) Orchitis—inflammation of testes with subsequent sterility. Females: disease is usually mild with slight vaginal irritation and discharge. Nearly 90 percent of infected females are asymptomatic. Complications: (1) spreading to fallopian tubes (salpingitis with subsequent scarring, narrowing or blockage); (2) infertility and ectopic pregnancies may result; (3) arthritis; (4) eye infection of infants during birth	Antibiotic penicillin: 2.4 million units.	Culture from urethra and vagina.
Genital herpes infection (virus)	Contracted during coitus. May spread through oral-genital contact. Once infection has set in, stress initiates recurrence.	Cold-sorelike vesicles on genitalia. Pain especially during coitus. Occasionally virus infects infant during pregnancy, with serious results. Lesions may become secondarily infected with bacteria.	Slow regression within 2 to 4 weeks without treatment. Medications topically applied or acridine dyes plus light. Relapses are common.	Direct inspection of lesions.

| Syphilis (bacteria) | Kissing, direct sexual contact, contaminated hypodermic needles; through placenta during pregnancy. Infectious any time chancre is present or lesions appear. Disease is not infectious during tertiary stage; involvement may produce: (1) paresis (mental illness) due to brain damage; (2) aortitis (enlargement and possible rupture of aorta. | 3 symptomatic stages: (1) Primary: about 3 weeks after contact, painless, hard sore (chancre) appears at site of infection, usually on or near genitalia; chancre, containing infectious spirochetes, heals in 4 to 6 weeks without treatment. (2) Secondary: appears as a rash after disappearance of chancre (2–10 weeks), spirochetes, having entered the general circulation are found in every rash or mucous lesion. If oral lesions are present, disease may be transmitted by kissing; rash lasts weeks or months; about one-half of cases do not progress beyond this stage. (3) Tertiary: (after 5–20 years latency): hypersensitivity reactions to remaining spirochetes; any part of the body may be involved. | Antibiotic therapy; penicillin dosage depends on stage. Tertiary symptoms may be untreatable particularly when neural damage is present. | Examination of exudate from chancre. Serological test. |

dromal symptoms. Without their cooperation, disease control in the school becomes very difficult. The school must ever operate on the assumption that parental cooperation is a distinct asset to the success of nearly every phase of the school program.

Unfortunately, most classroom teachers will frequently encounter, and must be able to detect, obvious symptoms of a communicable disease. Parents should closely inspect their children before sending them out of the door in the morning and should keep them home if signs of illness are present. Too frequently parents ignore coughing, sneezing, a runny nose, and other suggestive signs (see Table 16-7) and hustle them off to school. Consequently teachers are left with the responsibility of taking measures to protect their students against possible infection.

What steps teachers take in the event of suspected infection varies from one school district to another. The availability of a school nurse would suggest a referral for further evaluation and action. Some schools require that the principal or other administrative personnel make the decision to remove the child from the classroom. Frequently, and in most situations appropriately, teachers themselves have the authority to decide whether a child should remain in school and to contact the parents if exclusion seems warranted. Properly handled, the decision should not pose a problem if the parents are knowledgeable. Unfortunately, homebound children may interfere with the parents' daily schedule, particularly if both parents work. In this case exclusion is a bit more difficult.

Following a decision to keep a child out of class, it is necessary to arrange safe transport home. If walking is feasible, another child, perhaps one that is older and more responsible, may accompany the sick child home. Preferably, a parent or a neighbor would call for the child at school and thereby assume full responsibility. It is not appropriate to send an ill child home alone or to an empty house.

When a child is sent home ill, it is necessary to notify the following individuals:

1. The child's teacher, if the decision was made by someone else
2. Local public health personnel, if the symptoms suggest the presence of a reportable disease
3. Other teachers who have siblings of the sick child in their classes or all teachers if the disease is beginning to affect an increasing number of the school population. The teachers may then be sensitive to the possible appearance of new cases. Occasionally, when siblings attend different schools, it may be necessary to notify other schools.

TABLE 16-7. Symptoms and Percentage of Mothers Keeping Children Home from School

	Percent of Mothers	
Symptoms	Black (N = 208)	White (N = 510)
Fever, sore throat	100.0	99.6
Fever, headache, stomach ache	100.0	99.8
Fever, stomach ache, diarrhea	100.0	100.0
Stomach ache, diarrhea	99.5	99.8
Fever, hurts all over	99.5	99.8
Fever, cough, running nose	99.0	99.6
Fever, earache	99.5	99.4
Fever, running nose	98.5	99.2
Fever, cough, sore throat	98.5	96.8
Fever, cough	97.5	97.4
Fever	96.6	96.2
Diarrhea	95.1	93.5
Hurts all over	92.3	82.1
Dizziness	91.3	89.2
Pain in chest	90.3	77.2
Earache	84.1	87.4
Sore throat	79.8	76.2
Stiff neck or back	79.8	62.1
Stomach ache	75.0	60.1
Rash	73.5	71.3
Constipation	59.1	31.1
Headache	56.2	44.5
Nervousness	54.8	23.9
Overtired	49.5	35.0
Cough	41.8	30.3
Sneezing	35.5	20.7
Running nose	33.1	21.5
Loss of appetite	31.7	17.4

Source: Cecil Slome, Wayne Michael Lednar, Doris E. Roberts, and Delores Basco, "Should James Go To School? Mothers Responses to Symptoms," *Journal of School Health,* February 1977, p. 107.

Readmission of The Recovered Child

When a school excludes a child because of illness, readmission depends on established local health laws and codes. In general, the child should bring professional certification that he or she is no longer an infectious hazard to other students. It is desirable that the family physician provide such certification, but a release signed by county health officers is a satisfactory alternate. Obviously, if the law covering exclusion requires certification by a family physician for readmission, the school must have a careful exclusion procedure, because barring the child from the classroom will automatically force the family to incur an additional financial responsibility (i.e., to pay for a physician's services). If such is the procedure, it may be asking too much of teachers to decide to send children home, for pressures to keep prodromal children in class rather than incur the possibility of an error in judgment might outweigh the obligation to act in the best interest of the children.

Some school districts can leave readmission decisions to almost anyone (the school nurse, principal, teacher, or even the parent) and be in compliance with local regulations. Short of the parental decision, this procedure may be adequate, but it certainly falls far short of the protection afforded the other students by a physician's certification.

Procedures in Epidemics

In an agrarian society, particularly in days of yore when living "down on the farm" meant being practically isolated from the rest of the world, the school was a pathogen's paradise, a primary source of disease infection. Before effective treatment was available, it was natural to close the school to try to isolate, or quarantine, the disease, particularly in the face of an epidemic. Studies have shown, however, that school closure is an ineffective means of controlling communicable diseases in urban or suburban settings and is of dubious value in today's rural school as well.[18] Nevertheless, schools frequently come under considerable lay pressure to close when infectious diseases become epidemic in a community. Without closure of other community meeting places and recreational facilities, it is certain that discontinuing school is a greater boon to public relations than it is to communicable disease control. The eyes of watchful teachers who can exclude individual disease cases from the classroom, however, can provide more effective isolation than simply closing the school and allowing the children to mingle together at various community facilities. In any event, if the school remains open it is important to strengthen observational and exclusion processes to minimize the spread of infection.

Implications for Health Education

A good educational program on communicable diseases enables students to exercise control measures that will reduce communicable disease incidence in their own lives and, therefore, in the lives of their close associates. The principles of good nutrition, personal cleanliness, proper use of handkerchiefs, isolation, and immunization are applicable and are particularly teachable in the home environment. School personnel might consider involving the parents in the educational program by encouraging them to instruct and motivate children to:

During Sickness

1. Use separate washcloths, towels, bedding, and other personal items, such as eating utensils.
2. Sleep in a separate room, if possible.
3. Limit direct and indirect physical contact with other family members.
4. Use medical services properly and follow physicians' instructions regarding use of medications.

At Other Times

5. Maintain immunizations.
6. Properly care for pets (immunizations, purchase from authorized dealers, control).
7. Control flies and mosquitoes (proper garbage disposal, elimination of standing water).
8. Keep hands and other objects away from the mouth.

At All Times

9. Maintain proper nutrition, sleep, and exercise.
10. Properly use handkerchiefs (use of disposal bags, etc.).

Parents who are willing to establish an incentive program and want to impress children with the importance of preventive medicine can encourage use of these techniques in the home. They could set up a mock disease situation in the home in order to practice these principles under simulated circumstances and report the results to the school. To check the success of home instruction educators could test children on the material they should have learned from the parents, material that was not part of the classroom presentation.

NOTES

1. American Public Health Association, *Control of Communicable Diseases in Man.* (New York: American Public Health Association, 1970), p. 288.
2. John J. White, "We're Not Immunizing Enough of Our Children," *Today's Health,* September 1973, p. 4.

3. Franklin Top and Paul Wehrle, *Communicable and Infectious Diseases* (St. Louis: C.V. Mosby Co., 1972), p. 10.

4. Parcal J. Imperato, *Treatment and Control of Infectious Diseases in Man* (Springfield, Ill.: Charles C. Thomas, 1974), p. 46.

5. Gaylord W. Anderson, Margaret Arnstein, and Mary Lester, *Communicable Disease Control* (New York: Macmillan Co., 1962), p. 27.

6. Ibid., p. 28.

7. Imperato, p. 55.

8. Ibid., p. 56.

9. Top and Wehrle, p. 4.

10. Dorothy F. Johnston, *Essentials of Communicable Diseases* (St. Louis: C.V. Mosby Co., 1968), p. 41.

11. Ibid.

12. Margaret B. Tewenkle, "Immunization and Communicable Diseases," *Journal of Practical Nursing,* March 1974, pp. 25-28.

13. Ibid.

14. Anderson et al., p. 47.

15. Ibid., p. 62.

16. Mary Lynn M. Luy, "Vaccines: Why Aren't Today's Children Being Fully Immunized," *Modern Medicine,* 30 May 1977, p. 58.

17. Brent Q. Hafen, Alton L. Thygerson, and Ronald L. Rhodes, *Prescriptions for Health* (Provo, Utah: Brigham Young University Press, 1977), p. 421.

18. C.L. Anderson, *Community Health* (St. Louis: C.V. Mosby Co., 1973), p. 175.

CHAPTER 17
Allergies in Children

The presence of allergies, or more scientifically, hypersensitivities, in the school is generally more bothersome than serious. It is generally estimated that 15 to 20 percent of the population have hypersensitivities. The incidence is somewhat higher among youngsters than among adults.[1] Eighty percent of allergies make their appearance by the time a child has finished high school. Severe reactions are not common, but the hypersensitive person may be quite miserable and it is only considerate to make them as comfortable as possible.

Common allergic reactions include hay fever, asthma, urticaria (hives), eczema, angioedema (a swelling of tissues) and hypersensitivity to certain foods, drugs, and stings. Though generally rather harmless, allergies may pose a significant emotional threat to a child. The periodic drama of an asthmatic attack or persistent eczema may stigmatize a child and lead to rejection and isolation by the other students. As a result, the child may withdraw and become frustrated, hostile, and even aggressive in an effort to cope with the situation. Some allergic children use their hypersensitivities in manipulative ways to gain favors and special dispensations that in no way relate to any of the disabilities that might accompany the allergy. The irritation of an allergy in fact may make certain tasks difficult, however. The constant discomfort caused by an allergy may compromise attempts to concentrate. Respiratory allergies may limit physical performance. Nausea and vomiting may necessitate missing school. Obviously teachers must be informed, patient, and prepared to take whatever action seems appropriate in order to minimize the negative effects of an allergy on a child's education.

THE MECHANISM

The exact process by which an individual becomes allergic is still poorly understood, but the basic mechanism seems to be similar to immunity. The typical immune reaction occurs in three steps:

1. Exposure to an antigen: An antigen may be a part of a bacterium, toxin, or other substance (usually containing protein) that the body recognizes as being foreign.
2. Production of antibody: Certain body cells, particularly small plasma cells, respond to the presence of the antigen by manufacturing antibody, which becomes a part of the blood called the gamma globulin.
3. Antigen-antibody reaction: If the now-immune individual encounters the antigen again, an antigen-antibody interaction will prevent the disease process from proceeding.

In a hypersensitivity reaction, the same general steps occur, but there are certain significant variations. The antigen, which is called an *allergen,* causes the production of an antibody that enters into an allergen-antibody reaction, but in contrast to the typical immune response, an allergic reaction causes cells to release chemical compounds—most notably histamine—that cause a localized inflammation, that is, the allergic response (see Figure 17–1).

The allergic reaction always requires prior exposure to the allergen, but exposure may occur many times without the development of an allergy. Why an individual suddenly responds to the allergen in a hypersensitive way is poorly understood, but the current thesis is that infection, heredity, climatic conditions, fatigue, and even emotional stress may predispose to the development of the reaction. Exposure to the allergen under the predisposing conditions may be the result of eating, injecting, inhaling, or just experiencing a surface contact with the offending agent. Once developed, the allergy may last for many years, but it may disappear just as suddenly and mysteriously as it began. For example, food allergies, which are common among infants, may be totally absent by age five.[2]

FIGURE 17-1. *Respiratory and food allergies. Antibody (IgE) attached to the surface of mast cells near the capillary blood vessels binds allergen as it enters the body. The act of combination leads to release of histamine and other chemical mediators. Common sites of reaction are (a) the gastrointestinal tract (diarrhea and vomiting), (b) the nasal passages (hay fever), and (c) the lungs (asthma).*

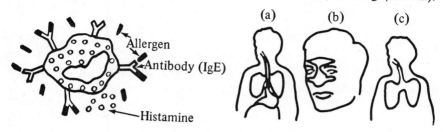

TYPES OF ALLERGIES

Hereditary predisposition to allergies, called *atopy,* may be qualitatively specific; that is, an individual may inherit a tendency toward a specific type of allergy. Upper-respiratory allergies, particularly nasal allergies, are the most common types. The symptoms include wheezing, runny nose, inflamed and reddened eyes, sneezing, and coughing. Sniffling, rubbing and picking the nose, and rubbing the eyes represent the sufferer's attempt to relieve the discomfort of a nasal allergy. The persistent "allergic salute" (pushing upward on the nose) may give rise to a horizontal line across the nose that is a permanent telltale sign of past or present nasal allergies.

Respiratory Allergies

Upper-respiratory allergies may be continuous or seasonal, depending on the offending agent. When pollens from trees, shrubs, flowers, and grasses are to blame, the individual will be most uncomfortable in the spring and early fall. On the other hand, if animal dander (scales from fur), dust-mite residues, or other continuously present substances excite the reaction, symptoms will be evident year-round.

Asthma

A particularly troublesome condition is asthma, which afflicts three out of fifty elementary-school students. It is not a specific disorder, but rather a response to various stimuli. It involves a drastic narrowing of the air passages in the upper-respiratory tract. In the majority of cases, it is a hypersensitivity state, but occasionally other environmental factors such as physical exertion, irritants, emotional stress or infection will precipitate an attack.[3] Frequently, the exciting factor is unknown. An asthma attack starts with a tightening sensation in the chest with wheezing and coughing, which become increasingly severe. Difficulty in breathing to the point of *cyanosis* (bluish color) may occur, and the individual may become disoriented and confused. Generally, sitting up and leaning forward on one's arms is more comfortable than lying down. If the episodes occur frequently, the asthmatic child may carry medication, which the teacher may help administer to abort or ease the attack.

Asthmatic attacks are usually more frightening to the onlooker than to the victim, who has been through it all before. Ordinarily, a child may remain in class until the paroxysms subside, without risk to anyone present. In cases in which attacks are frequent, teachers should consult the school nurse who will investigate the possibility of improving medical control of the condition or in some other way reducing the disruptive influence of frequent episodes in the classroom.

Since, as stated above, various stimuli may precipitate attacks, teachers may effectively modify the environment to decrease the likelihood of an incident by doing the following:

1. Determine what agents are most likely to precipitate an attack, and if possible, eliminate them. (Pollens, animal dander, and foods are sometimes causes.)
2. Avoid excessive excitement in the classroom.
3. Allow asthmatic children to pace themselves in physical activities. They usually know their limitations and will act accordingly, although malingering is possible.
4. Reduce exposure to cold air. Walking on cold days may precipitate an attack by the time the child has reached school.
5. Control communicable disease in the classroom. Viral infections are particularly likely to induce asthmatic attacks.

Skin Allergies

Allergies are not contagious. The problem in skin allergies is determining whether a group of symptoms are allergic or attributable to infection. The following factors may point to an allergy:

1. No history of infection-related symptoms (fever, malaise)
2. Patterning of lesions localized to an area of exposure or contact.
3. Raised whitish areas with red borders
4. Areas of itching and redness followed by scaling and evidence of dry or oozing lesions

Gastrointestinal Allergies

Food allergies may manifest respiratory, skin, or gastrointestinal symptoms. Allergies involving the digestive tract cause nausea, vomiting, or pain and possibly diarrhea. The symptoms usually cause sufficient distress to justify keeping a child at home. Gastrointestinal complaints may be a sign of serious problems and, allergy or not, the parents should be called upon to remove their child from the classroom.

Anaphylactic Reactions

Some hypersensitivities, such as asthma not only can cause great distress but also can be life threatening. Upon exposure to the allergen, an individual may go into shock and collapse. This reaction is called *anaphylaxis* and it usually occurs when the blood stream absorbs a significant quantity of the allergen. Hence, anaphylaxis most often results from injection of the allergen, as in penicillin shots and bee stings or from the absorption of large amounts via the digestive tract. Anaphylaxis constitutes an emergency situation and prompt medical attention is necessary to save the victim's life.

DIAGNOSIS

Teachers should know certain facts to be able to determine whether or not a child is hypersensitive. First of all, determining the cause of an allergy may be very difficult because the number of potential allergens is almost infinite. Inhaled substances such as pollens from weeds and grasses, dust in the home and factory, mold spores, and

TABLE 17-1.   Diagnosis for Hypersensitivities

Scratch test	An area of cleansed skin is lightly scratched and minute amounts of numerous potential allergens are applied. A large wheal, similar to an insect bite, at the site of application of an allergen indicates hypersensitivity.
Patch test	The allergen is applied to cleansed, unbroken skin on a patch that remains on the skin for 24 hours. A reaction resembling the lesions of the original allergy confirms the diagnosis.
Mucus membrane test	The allergen is placed on the conjunctiva of the eye, sprayed in one nostril, or inhaled into the bronchi. The typical allergic response confirms the diagnosis.

animal danders (skin or hair shed by domestic or laboratory animals) are a few common allergens. Drugs, taken by mouth or injected, and foods—eggs, milk, wheat, fish, nuts, chocolate, and many fruits, for example—also cause allergic reactions in sensitized individuals.

The family history that a physician compiles usually notes any inherited allergic tendencies. The environmental circumstances and activity of the patient just before symptoms also may provide clues to causal factors. Then, although a careful history and clinical examination generally identify the allergens, the doctor may make skin tests to confirm the diagnosis (see Table 17–1).

TREATMENT

There are basically three ways in which to control allergies: avoidance of the allergen, desensitization, and drug therapy. Avoiding the allergen implies that the allergen is known and is of such a nature that it can be excluded from the victim's immediate environment. Pollens and dusts in the ambient air will obviously not yield to this approach, although the victim will usually be much more comfortable in an air-conditioned, air-filtered environment than in a non-air-conditioned one. But when it is possible to keep allergen out of the allergic child's surroundings, teachers may be able to make the child comfortable by taking reasonable precautions to control the environment. Such a simple adjustment as removing geranium plants may be sufficient.

Desensitization consists of injecting the allergen in small, increasing amounts at frequent intervals. This approach causes the body to produce blocking antibodies that will prevent the reaction from taking place. Not all conditions are amenable to desensitization, however, and it is necessary to evaluate the potential for success for each case.

Drug therapy may be in the form of bronchodilators, antihistamines, or corticosteroids. These drugs relieve symptoms, but they have no lasting effect on the allergy and they carry certain disadvantages. Long-term use is generally undesirable because the drugs may become less effective with time, and, in some instances, create hypersensitivities of their own.[4] The side effects of corticosteroids are unpleasant, and antihistamines tend to cause attention problems and drowsiness.

Many parents fail to recognize or seek adequate treatment for hypersensitivity reactions. Teachers and other school personnel can encourage them to find a satisfactory management program. Because learning to care adequately for an allergy is an important educational goal for hypersensitive children, parents may cooperate in a home-based incentive program aimed at establishing good control habits. These children should learn to stay away from avoidable allergens and take medication as prescribed. Parents, teachers, and allergic children cooperate in eliminating unnecessary stress and thereby reduce the severity of hypersensitivity reactions when they occur. Parents can play a particularly important role in helping children learn that using allergies as excuse for poor performance in non-allergy-related dimensions of their lives is inappropriate. They can join the teacher in watching for signs of emotional problems stemming from impaired interpersonal relationships or self-demeaning thoughts. Good home-school cooperation should allow allergic children to handle their allergies in such a way that they will be a minimal influence or perhaps even a growth factor in their lives.

NOTES

1. Public Health Service, National Institutes of Health, *Allergy Research: An Introduction* (Washington, D.C.: U.S. Department of Health, Education, and Welfare, 1972).
2. Ibid.
3. John P. McGovern, "Chronic Respiratory Diseases of School-age Children," *Journal of School Health* 46 (June 1976): 347.
4. Public Health Service, *Allergy Research.*

CHAPTER **18**
Chronic
Health Problems
in Children*

At some time every teacher will come in contact either directly or indirectly with students who have health problems. Some problems will be minor and will have little effect upon classroom procedure. No matter how serious the problem, however, it is imperative that the affected student have a sense of belonging and acceptance by the teacher and the other students.[1]

Teachers have the same responsibilities toward chronically ill children that they have toward other students, but the challenge of helping the former is greater. It is easy enough to send home children who are acutely ill and to welcome them back when they are well, but when a child has a chronic illness, an incurable one, or a progressively fatal one, we can not remain detached and merely sympathetic. Sympathy will not do such a child as much good as understanding and help. No one expects teachers to be experts on health problems, but a basic understanding of the problems discussed in this chapter will enable you to support and aid chronically ill students in some circumstances and to refer them to specialists when appropriate.

Perhaps you have never considered the possibility that you—the teacher of a regular class—might have a student with a significant

---

*This chapter is based on U.S. Department of Health, Education, and Welfare, *Responding to Individual Needs in Head Start—Working with the Individual Child* (Washington, D.C.: U.S. Government Printing Office, 1975).

health problem in your classroom. You may feel, to put it in mild terms, less than adequately prepared to cope with the unknown elements of the situation. You do not know exactly how the child will act with you, how the other children will react, or how you will react to the child. You probably underestimate enormously the help you can actually give the child. And you may be worried about whether you will do any harm. These are natural and understandable concerns, but the fact is that the child will probably benefit greatly from being in your classroom.

Remember as you read that we are discussing many different types of problems—they will not all appear in your room at once. Remember, too, that you have an invaluable source of information in the parent as well as the child, for they have been managing the problem as long as it has existed. And, finally, remember that what you have already learned about children in general is much more important than what you do not know about health impairments.

For most people, knowing more about the difficulties with which they are trying to cope makes the task somewhat easier. Teachers will want to know the particular needs generated by the health problems of children in their charge. They should also be well aware of the strengths and special abilities of these children in order to avoid treating them as more handicapped than they actually are. The goal is to develop expectations for the affected child that are neither too high nor too low.

Not all physical (or emotional) problems are equally handicapping. Some, like asthma, involve periodic attacks of shortness of breath, but between attacks the child may seem perfectly normal. Other problems, such as clubfoot or partial-sightedness, are apparent in the physical appearance and behavior of the child at all times. Casts, braces, crutches, wheelchairs, special glasses, and even hearing apparatuses are very visible and both the handicapped child and non-handicapped peers may react negatively to them. On the other hand, physical aids sometimes fascinate nonhandicapped children; they may beg to try them out and even envy rather than fear the wearer.

An important factor in the reactions of health-impaired children to their problems is how others react to them. Their early experiences in the home and in the neighborhood can affect their self-image either positively or negatively. And they bring this self-image into the classroom. Children with a positive self-image can be a real asset to the group. Given normal support and protection against the usual classroom hazards, these children can do very well in school. Children who have a negative self-image, of course, need more help.

What follows in this chapter is background information about some of the physical health problems teachers encounter along with suggestions about how to manage medical aspects of the problem in the classroom. This chapter does not include all of the health impairments you may encounter; it covers problems that may require some teacher understanding and/or assistance and problems that are most common in a classroom situation (hearing, dental, eye, and allergy problems are discussed in other chapters of this book). Of course, all teachers will not encounter most of the conditions this chapter describes. Some of them, for example, hemophilia, are relatively rare.

Some children may have more than one health problem. A child with cerebral palsy may have a severe vision problem or may be slow in mental development. A mentally slow child may be overaggressive in the classroom or quite passive and lacking in initiative. Understandably, children who are subject to seizures or who have chronic asthma may be frightened of separating from their mothers and remaining in the classroom. It is a good idea to keep in mind that children with physical handicaps may develop emotional reactions to their handicap: some may be frightened at separating from their home and parents, some may be ashamed of being different from other children, some may feel more helpless and impaired than they actually are, and some may not recognize the limitations their handicap imposes and thus may get into dangerous situations.

Most students with chronic health problems require neither a modification in the curriculum nor unusual methods of instruction. They do require special management that takes into consideration reduced energy, strength, motivation, and personality variables. In addition, they require help from the teacher in developing positive self-concepts. Frequent negative reactions to a handicap usually result in low self-esteem, fear of school failure, and hostility toward others. Regardless of the severity of their illness, these children need to succeed, to win recognition from peers and teachers by earning at least average grades and excelling in something. If they are intelligent enough to "win" in spite of school absences, they can overcome, at least in part, the handicap of illness.

A teacher's attitude often determines an ailing child's school adjustment. Parents frequently complain that teachers seem to have no understanding of their children's chronic disorders. Some teachers panic and are unnecessarily protective. The American Academy of Pediatrics recommends against unduly protecting chronically ill children and advocates a cooperative effort by physicians, parents, children, and the school to devise individualized plans for minimizing handicaps.[2]

BLEEDING DISORDERS

As medical problems go, bleeding disorders are not very common, but now and then a child with one of the three major types will appear in a classroom.

Prolonged, excessive, or unexpected bleeding out of proportion to the severity of an injury is the common characteristic of bleeding disorders. After a minor fall, a joint swells with blood. Brushing the teeth causes the gums to bleed, and the socket of a pulled tooth oozes blood hours after the procedure ended. Large bruises discolor the skin after even a mild bump. The three major groups of blood disorders are:

1. The *hemophilias*, characterized by abnormalities of the amounts or kinds of blood proteins responsible for blood clotting
2. A reduction in the number of blood cells (platelets) that help to stop bleeding when a blood vessel is injured
3. *Von Willebrand's disease*, which involves abnormalities of both platelets and clotting proteins

The hemophilias are the bleeding disorders that teachers are most likely to see. Some types of hemophilia are passed by the mother to her male offspring only. The world knows this type as the "royal disease" transmitted by Queen Victoria of England to a number of the crown heads of Europe. Other hemophilias develop spontaneously.

Platelets, the blood cells that help to stop bleeding, may decline in number in reaction to medication or as the result of an infection. Most often, however, the cause is unknown, and in this case, the condition is called *idiopathic thrombocytopenic prupura.* The chief characteristic of this disorder is the abnormal susceptibility to bruising due to a deficiency of platelets.

Recent years have seen major progress in the treatment of all the bleeding disorders. Transfusions, protein injections, use of cortisone and other methods have eliminated the need for excessive precautions with affected children. Overprotection may spare a child some bleeding episodes and a few trips to the doctor, but the psychological price to the child may outweigh the benefits. Teachers who have hemophiliac children in their classrooms need not fear that they will bleed to death at the slightest injury.

The principles of first aid for a bleeder are simple. Treat any cut or skin scrape as you would for a normal child. The best way to stop bleeding is to apply pressure directly to the wound with clean gauze or other dressing. Call the doctor only if you cannot stop the bleeding in what seems to be a reasonable length of time.

In the event of injury to an ankle, elbow, knee, or other joint, have the hemophiliac child assume a comfortable position. Wrap the joint to immobilize it; use a sling to immobilize an albow. Fill a plastic bag with ice cubes, wrap it in a towel and apply it to the injured joint. Then call the child's parents or physician.

One word of caution: the one location where bleeding can be immediately dangerous is the neck or throat. A large collection of blood there can obstruct breathing. In this rare event, the child will complain of pain or swelling and show obvious signs of difficulty in breathing. This is an emergency, and a doctor should see the child at once.

After receiving medical treatment for an injured joint, a hemophiliac child may be on crutches or have an arm in a sling for a few days. At these times teacher support and frequent reminders not to try running without crutches are necessary.

Certain common drugs such as aspirin, phenergan (an antihistamine contained in many cough medicines), glyceral guaiacolate (a common expectorant in cough medicines), and tranquilizers can aggravate bleeding tendencies. Accordingly, it is unwise to give a child with a bleeding disorder any medication without a doctor's prescription. In general, it is unwise for anyone other than knowledgeable school personnel to administer even aspirin to *any* child. No one should give medicine to a child with a specific medical condition without a written order from a physician or parent.

Personality development can take several courses in hemophiliac children. Some may be able to accept the disease and cope with the limitations. Others may become so fearful of injury that they sink into a passive existence. Still others may turn into hemophiliac daredevils who seem to go out of their way to expose themselves to danger. Whatever course the personality is taking, a pattern will already be apparent by the time the child reaches school. Teachers will not find it easy to keep a balance between overprotection and permissiveness with these children, but consultation with the parents will help. As in the case of other kinds of handicaps, teachers will find that the parents have had to develop sound ideas about the child's condition and the requirements for safety.

Fear of hemophilia is an all-too-common manifestation of misunderstanding about external bleeding or fatal accident, and the concern that many overburdened teachers feel about one more problem is not unusual. Misapprehension, however, is not sufficient to justify denying hemophiliac children the opportunity for regular school attendance.

CEREBRAL PALSY

Cerebral palsy is a disorder of movement (muscle action) or posture caused by brain damage. The muscle deficiency is a permanent disability, but it can change over time in quality and intensity. Although cerebral palsy may affect intelligence, often it is normal. Until a thorough assessment has been made, teachers should never assume that the intelligence of cerebral palsy victims is defective or that they will have learning problems. Between 50 and 60 percent of these children are retarded, so the other 40 to 50 percent have a global intelligence score of 70 or above, which usually indicates the possibility of successful school achievement within regular school programs.[3]

The kind of brain damage that leads to cerebral palsy has many causes, among them excessive jaundice in the newborn, deprivation of oxygen at birth, head injury, infections of the brain and spinal cord, and lead poisoning. Although brain damage is irreparable improvement in spastic muscle control is possible.

Cerebral palsy ranges in severity from barely noticeable clumsiness (ataxia) to obvious crippling that requires braces and wheelchair. At birth a baby with cerebral palsy may have a weak or paralyzed arm or leg. Later on, the muscles of the affected limb may become tense (spastic), bending the arm at the elbow or pulling the thigh up toward the abdomen while the lower leg remains flexed and the foot extended downward. Some children with cerebral palsy cannot totally control their movements (athetosis). Grimacing and a peculiar posture are common. The muscles used in talking may be impaired, and consequently the victim's speech may be indistinct and halting.[4]

A physical complication of constant muscle spasm is shortening (contracture) of the *tendons,* which are the sinewy bands that attach muscles to bones near a joint. For example, the heel cord, or Achilles tendon, may shorten due to constant spasm of the calf muscles and downward positioning of the foot. Consequently, the foot may not be able to move into any other position. Contractures of tendons seriously interfere with function. Even with braces, a child with a foot locked in a downward position will not be able to walk.

Minimizing contractures is a major objective of medical treatment, which entails moving the joints through the full range of motion to stretch the tendons and keep them supple. Physical therapists teach these exercises to the parents, who perform them each day. Other exercises actively involve the child to strengthen weakened muscles. Surgery may be necessary to lengthen contracted tendons and to shift spastic muscles to new locations. Braces give support to weakened legs and thereby permit walking.[5]

Teachers of cerebral palsy children may need to know how to remove and put on braces and how to adjust them. The child's parents can provide this instruction, as well as information about the child's abilities and special problems. The effort required to help children with severe cerebral palsy use their bodies at maximum effectiveness often aids their developmental progress.

Educators must be aware of other abnormalities that commonly accompany cerebral palsy, including mental retardation, seizures, visual impairment, and auditory and speech abnormalities. Teachers can provide considerable emotional support to pupils with cerebral palsy.[6]

CLEFT PALATE

Children with cleft lip (harelip) and cleft palate will arrive in school with a long history of disability and traumatic experiences that will have influenced their personalities in different ways. Cleft lip is a general anomaly that develops prior to birth. It may be a small indentation of the lip or a more serious defect in which a fissure extends to the nostril, giving to the face a characteristic appearance. A cleft palate also can range from mild to severe. It can occur with or without cleft lip. Usually surgical repair is possible when a child is about eighteen months old, but very often several operations will be necessary in order to fully correct the condition. Imagine how traumatic it could be for children so young to go through all those procedures. Certainly the experience has an impact on future behavior. Babies with cleft palates tend to accumulate fluid in the ear and to develop repeated ear infections. Not only is this a very painful condition, but it also can cause impaired hearing, an additional factor that contributes to communication difficulties. Speech development is usually delayed. A child with cleft palate will often make articulation errors and will have a nasal voice that is difficult to understand. The hurt and the relative social isolation of a child who talks but is often not understood and who not only looks but also sounds different from other children is tremendous.

Children with cleft lips and palates usually are self-conscious about their appearance. If they are fortunate enough to have an accepting family, they may be able to relate readily to their peers. Others may need considerable assistance in learning to interact comfortably with peers and the public. Teachers can try to include them in the group and should also be alert for hearing problems, which may be the source of inattentiveness, poor school performance, or social withdrawal.[7]

CYSTIC FIBROSIS

Cystic fibrosis is one of the most common of the serious chronic diseases of childhood. For some unknown reason, it occurs less frequently in black children than in Caucasian children. The cause of the disease also is unknown, although it is believed that children who have it lack some substance or substances that are essential to the normal functioning of a number of organs.

The main feature of cystic fibrosis is the production of abnormally thick and viscous gluelike mucus by the membranes that line several organs. This abnormally thick mucus clogs the bronchial passages, impeding breathing and predisposing the child to pneumonia. It also blocks ducts that deliver enzymes from the pancreas and thus interferes with normal processes in the small intestine. Consequently digestion also is difficult. Cystic fibrosis is not contagious.

Cystic fibrosis affects the functioning of the lungs, sweat glands, and digestive system. Whereas normal mucus lubricates the lungs and enables us to clear the lungs by coughing up accumulations of mucus, the thick mucus of cystic fibrosis clings and clogs, becoming a fertile medium for the growth of bacteria.

Children with cystic fibrosis are likely to do a great deal of coughing in the classroom. Teachers should make a point of accepting the cough in a matter-of-fact way, and the other children will follow their lead. Taking part in physical games is good for these children because the exertion will tend to make them bring up mucus. Many of these children lack the stamina to compete on equal terms and thus need encouragement as well as a watchful eye to detect when they are pushing themselves toward exhaustion.[8]

The involvement of the lungs in cystic fibrosis sometimes arouses fear of contagion. On the contrary, children with cystic fibrosis are not spreaders of contagion but are easy victims. To them any pulmonary contagion is a very real menace, and the appearance of flu in the school is a signal to keep them at home. Nevertheless, many of these children have better-than-average attendance records.

Obstruction of the pancreatic ducts in cystic fibrosis causes victims to have trouble digesting fats, carbohydrates, and proteins, because digestive juices secreted by the pancreas do not reach the small intestine. As a result, children with cystic fibrosis may eat more—a great deal more—than normal children. They may take capsules of pancreatic enzymes to aid digestion. With or without these capsules, these children may have increased bowel movements. Teachers who are aware of this possibility can treat the occurrence as natural and avoid problems.

A problem unique to cystic fibrosis is the feeling of shame common to the school-age child. Although feelings of being different are common among children with major chronic illnesses, no other group known has the peculiar difficulty that arises from the pervasive odor of foul stools and flatulence, or gas. The bad odor of undigested fat in the stools is difficult for others to tolerate and embarrassing for the child.

Excessive sweating is another characteristic of cystic fibrosis. From infancy the skin of cystic fibrosis victims has a salty taste. To compensate for salt losses in sweating, these children may layer their food with salt, and in hot weather they may need to take supplementary salt tablets—but only on a doctor's prescription, of course.[9]

Children with cystic fibrosis need peer acceptance. Because their lack of stamina restricts their playground activities, they sometimes feel left out. At home their condition has gained them special attention since babyhood, and they may have difficulty adjusting to group situations in which they must share the spotlight. The teacher's assistance in making the adjustment is most important.

DIABETES

Diabetes occurs at all ages and affects some 10 million people in the United States. Of these, about 10 percent have onset in childhood. Juvenile-onset diabetes is a more severe form of diabetes than the type that strikes mature individuals. It usually appears abruptly in childhood or young adulthood and can progress rapidly. Complications may develop and life expectancy may decrease.[10] Its exact cause and means of prevention are not yet known. Many diabetic children have a family history of diabetes. Sometimes diabetes develops in an older family member after onset in a child. The general consensus among doctors and researchers is that a hereditary contribution from both parents is necessary to cause a child to manifest the disease.

Normally, sugar moves smoothly from the blood into fat and muscle cells as needed for energy and the level of sugar in the blood remains fairly constant. As the cells need more sugar, the pancreas releases *insulin,* a hormone that facilitates the passage of sugar from the bloodstream into the cells. As the cells' fuel needs are met, insulin output encourages conversion of blood sugar to fat.

The problem in diabetes is insufficient useable insulin. In juvenile diabetes, the pancreas usually does not produce any insulin at all. If sugar cannot get into the cells the bloodstream absorbs more in an effort to overcome the blockage. The blood sugar level rises and eventually the kidneys pass the excess sugar into the urine (see Figure 18-1). The sugar spilled in the urine takes with it a great deal of water. The result is frequent urination and excessive thirst. (One common symptom of diabetes is bedwetting in an otherwise dry child.) Deprived of sugar, starving body cells stimulate the breakdown of body fat into fatty acids, which, in the absence of sugar, cells use for energy. The mobilization of fat leads to weight loss and increased appetite, both of which are characteristic signs of diabetes. Burning fatty acids for energy causes the blood to become acidic, and this condition, in turn, leads to quickened, deep breathing. The fatty acids are processed into acetone, which appears in the urine along with the sugar. Without treatment, the course of childhood diabetes is progressive deterioration, including weight loss, dehydration, coma, and death. This group of symptoms and signs of untreated diabetes is known as *diabetic keto-acidosis.* It is usually the presenting picture in new diabetics, but diabetics who are under treatment can experience it when their diabetes is out of control.

FIGURE 18-1. *Insulin and utilization of food.*

Normal Person

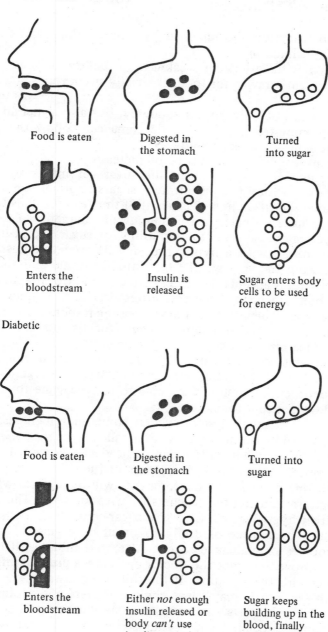

Food is eaten

Digested in
the stomach

Turned
into sugar

Enters the
bloodstream

Insulin is
released

Sugar enters body
cells to be used
for energy

Diabetic

Food is eaten

Digested in
the stomach

Turned into
sugar

Enters the
bloodstream

Either *not* enough
insulin released or
body *can't* use
insulin properly

Sugar keeps
building up in the
blood, finally
spills over into the
urine and leaves
the body

Many newly detected cases of juvenile diabetes undergo hospital treatment for their first episode of keto-acidosis.

In summary, the sudden appearance of the following behaviors are characteristic of juvenile-onset diabetes:[11]

1. Frequent urination accompanied by unusual thirst and excessive drinking of fluids
2. Weight loss with easy tiring, weakness, irritability, or nausea
3. Uncontrollable craving for food, especially sweet foods and candy

The symptoms not only appear suddenly, but also signal an urgent need for prompt treatment. Diabetic coma can follow the appearance of the symptoms very rapidly.

Treatment of diabetes consists of increasing blood insulin with daily injections in order to help the sugar get into cells, a well-balanced diet without concentrated sugars, normal amounts of exercise, and education in management of the disorder. Pills to lower blood sugar have no place in treating juvenile diabetics. The family and the patient must learn to test urine for sugar and acetone, to administer insulin with a hypodermic needle, and to adjust insulin dosage to keep the spillage of sugar into the urine and the blood sugar level within acceptable ranges. They learn how infection, exercise, and diet can change the insulin requirement. As diabetic children grow older, they must assume increasing responsibility for their own care. Attendance at a summer camp for diabetic children may aid them in learning to accept this responsibility.

Diabetic children can do everything that normal children do. There should be no restrictions on their activity. With regard to food, most diabetic children should be able to eat the same foods as the other children, except for sweets.

Intake of too much insulin, which sometimes happens, lowers blood sugar below normal, a condition called *hypoglycemia*. Symptoms of hypoglycemia include fussiness, headache, hunger, drowsiness and inattention, sweating, and coolness of the skin. The symptoms vary from one child to the next. Parents will be familiar with their child's pattern and can tell teachers what to look for. The quickest way to treat hypoglycemia is to give sugar-containing foods such as orange juice or a piece of candy followed by a glass of milk and several cookies or graham crackers. After five minutes, if the child has not improved contact the doctor or follow a predetermined plan for dealing with the situation. If the child is not awake, give nothing by mouth because it may cause choking. Severe and prolonged depression of the blood sugar causes unconsciousness and coma. The hypoglycemia associated with administered insulin is known as an *insulin reaction* or *insulin shock*.

Thus, the two most serious emergencies for diabetic children are

TABLE 18-1.   Diabetic Crises

Hypoglycemia (Rapid Onset)	Diabetic Coma (Slow Onset)

Causes
    Too much insulin
    Not eating enough food
    An unusual amount of exercise
    Delayed meal
	Causes
	    Too little insulin
	    Failure to follow diet
	    Infection, fever, emotional stress

Signs
    Excessive sweating, faintness
    Headache
    Hunger
    Pounding of heart, trembling,
      impaired vision
    Not able to awaken
    Irritability
    Personality change
	Signs
	    Increased thirst and urination
	    Large amounts of sugar and
	      ketones in urine
	    Weakness, abdominal pains,
	      generalized aches
	    Loss of appetite, nausea, and
	      vomiting

What to do
    Give the child sugar or any food
      containing sugar (fruit juice, candy)
    Call the doctor
    Do not give the child insulin
	What to do
	    Call the doctor at once
	    Put the child to bed and keep
	      warm
	    Give the child fluids without
	      sugar

Source: National Institutes of Health, Washington, D.C., *Diabetes,* PHS Publication No. 870, 1976, p. 4.

hypoglycemia (low blood sugar), which manifests usually in minutes or a few hours, and *acidosis,* or diabetic coma, which develops gradually over a few hours or days.[12] It is important to distinguish between the two because each condition requires completely different but immediate treatments. Table 18-1 summarizes the causes and symptoms of both conditions and indicates what immediate action to take while waiting for more specific instructions from the doctor.

The possibility of hypoglycemic reaction exists even when diabetic children receive the best care. They should always carry some form of sugar to take at the first sign of a hypoglycemic reaction. Packaged sugar lumps or a small candy bar should never be far away, particularly during exercise.

The reason for avoiding hypoglycemic reactions in the well-controlled child is that the brain must have an adequate supply of sugar as an energy source in order to function properly. When the sugar content of the blood falls to a low level, the brain does not operate at full efficiency. The blood sugar level must be restored to normal so that the brain can function normally.

If a diabetic coma occurs, medical attention is vital. In fact, if unconsciousness occurs, it is important to get the child to a doctor or a hospital as quickly as possible for diagnosis and treatment.

With rare exceptions, when children develop diabetes they have it permanently. The overall outlook for survival and for a comfortable life is problematic. The first generation of treated childhood diabetics is only now in the adult age group. Many adults who have had this type of diabetes for as long as fifteen to twenty years have developed complications such as kidney disease, high blood pressure, arteriosclerosis, changes in the blood vessels of the retina, and cataracts in the lenses of the eyes (both eye complications interfere with vision).[13]

In school, teachers should treat diabetic children like other children although recognizing that sometimes they may require special attention. All teachers should know the symptoms of both low and high blood sugar.

Children who look "normal" and attend regular schools do not have the advantage that some handicapped children have, namely, a teacher who has had special training in work with exceptional children. Teachers, who represent adult authority, are potential friends or enemies in the child's emotional adjustment and should help to plan a program to aid the diabetic child who is having difficulty maintaining control. Psychological stress raises blood sugar levels and teachers can try to minimize it in the classroom.[14]

EPILEPSY

An estimated 3 million Americans have epilepsy. This figure indicates a high probability of encountering an epileptic child in the classroom sometime. It also suggests that teachers should know how to deal with an epileptic seizure.

The first important fact to know about epilepsy is that it has nothing whatever to do with insanity. Most epileptics are normal and healthy in other respects and have average or better-than-average intelligence. Many great musicians, writers, and thinkers have had epilepsy, and the handicap did not prevent them from leading richly productive lives. Persons with epilepsy differ from the rest of us mainly in their tendency to have seizures, which range in severity from momentary conditions of clouded consciousness to the startling convulsive episodes known as *grand mal*. It is grand mal, which may cause the person to lose consciousness, froth at the mouth, and turn blue, that aroused superstitious dread in ancient times and even today may frighten onlookers quite unnecessarily.

In most cases of epilepsy the cause is never known, except in a general way. It is assumed usually that a brain injury is to blame. The injury may occur before or during birth. It may come from a bad fall or severe blow. Or it may be the result of an infectious disease, such as meningitis. In any event, seizures are believed to occur when a group of brain cells becomes overactive. It may involve only a small area of the brain, or the overactivity may spread from one region to others and over the entire brain. The severity of the seizure possibly depends on the location or on the extent of the regions affected.

It is not likely that a teacher will be the one to discover that a child has grand mal, but a teacher conceivably might be the first to notice something amiss in a child whose epilepsy previously manifested only petit mal or psychomotor seizures. *Petit mal* is a simple "absence" without any of the frightening convulsions characteristic of grand mal. Although a petit mal seizure does suspend consciousness for a few seconds, the victim does not fall to the ground or thrash about. The only visible sign of a petit mal attack may be a rhythmic fluttering of the eyelids. On regaining full consciousness, the person usually resumes normal activity as though nothing has happened. The episode is so fleeting and so unnoticeable that unaware or unobservant bystanders could mistake it for daydreaming. In *psychomotor epilepsy,* during a seizure the victim tends to repeat over and over some complex movement—chewing or swallowing or fingering some object—or to wander aimlessly about the room. These physical actions are performed in a vacant manner suggestive of sleepwalking. The attack lasts a minute or so and is followed by a period of confusion lasting another minute or so. The person hears no call or command during the attack and has no memory of the episode. Again, the circumstances are such that an unbriefed or unobservant teacher could mistake the attack for classroom misbehavior. Teachers who observe symptoms suggesting petit mal or psychomotor seizure but have no information to link the child with epilepsy should report the incident to the child's parents and to the appropriate school specialist.

If a child goes into grand mal in the classroom, there will be no mistaking the attack for daydreaming or misbehavior. The child may or may not have a brief warning of the impending seizure. The seizure will begin with loss of consciousness and the child will fall, toppling off a chair if seated. All the muscles will contract violently and this muscular rigidity usually gives way to convulsive jerking of the arms and legs. The eyes will roll up and froth may appear around the mouth. The victim may turn very pale, even blue, and may lose control of bladder and intestinal control. Possibly the child will bite his or her tongue or the inside of the cheek.

A grand mal seizure usually lasts only a few minutes. Afterward the child will appear to be confused and may complain of headache. Exhaustion and deep sleep may ensue. Although victims of grand mal have no memory of an attack, in a general way they may give the appearance of being embarrassed and deeply disturbed.

Although educated persons long ago discarded superstitions about "fits" and "spells" (see Table 18-2), the first encounter with epileptic seizure does seem to leave most lay persons feeling helpless, at least. Knowledge of several simple facts will ease that feeling and enable the onlooker to be useful:

1. The seizure will not last long.
2. The victim is not suffering any pain.
3. The victim is not going to die and is unlikely to suffer serious injury.
4. Onlookers are not in danger unless, in a mistaken notion of how to be helpful, someone puts a finger in the victim's mouth and is bitten.

Many epileptics experience a warning, called an *aura,* prior to an attack. A child may not be able to finds words to describe the sensations, but the aura apparently includes peculiar feelings in the stomach region, spots before the eyes, odd sensations of taste or smell, flashing memories of old events, and unusual tensions and anxiety. In the classroom the aura may give the teacher time to help the child to a safe place to lie down during the attack.

Since the epileptic in grand mal is almost sure to fall, the first step is to try to prevent him or her from hitting a sharp edge or corner and thereby suffering injury. The safest place for an epileptic in grand mal is on a mattress, a soft rug, or a pile of blankets or clothing on the floor.

Loosen tight clothing, especially at the neck. Wipe away any froth or saliva around the mouth and nose to aid breathing. At one time inserting a hard object or finger between the teeth was recommended to keep epileptics from biting their tongues, but don't do it. The violent muscle contractions could cause damage to the victim's teeth from a hard object, or to your own finger if you were to use it. Do not try to hold the person down. Restraint will only cause a more violent reaction and may cause wrenched or strained muscles. It is helpful to cradle the head in your arm to prevent injury. It is best to leave the child alone in a safe place, preferably on a soft surface, to recover from the attack. A face-down position, head turned toward the side also might be helpful.

Teachers should try to observe closely and to remember what happens in the early stages of the attack. This information will be useful to the specialist in charge of the case.

As the foregoing descriptions suggest, epileptic seizures ordinarily do not constitute medical emergencies. A rare exception to this rule of thumb is *status epilepticus,* a series of convulsions, each of

TABLE 18–2. Myths about Epilepsy

Myth	Fact
Epilepsy is passed on from father to son.	Most epilepsy is caused by brain injury.
All epileptics foam at the mouth and have convulsions.	Only those suffering from grand mal have this type of seizure.
An epileptic attack is easy to spot.	Not always. Victims of some psychomotor attacks have symptoms quite similar to drunkenness (slurred speech, unsteady gait, irrational behavior, etc.). Some victims of cerebrovascular disease exhibit symptoms similar to the epileptic's.
Epileptics can't drive cars.	Thirty-five states have no prohibitions against epileptics driving; others (with 2 exceptions) allow epileptics to drive if their seizures are fully controlled.
In most epileptics, seizures can be completely controlled.	If the ability to go 2 years without any seizure is taken as a criterion for "complete control," only 30 percent of epileptics fall in this group. However, 80 percent can have their seizures under control most of the time.
Most epileptics have only one form of epilepsy.	Two-thirds have 2 or more forms of seizure.
The type of seizure doesn't change.	It can change with age or with changes in body condition because the brain damage that causes it may improve or grow worse.
There is no surgical procedure for epilepsy.	Anterior temporal lobectomy can completely free certain types of epileptics from seizures. The operation takes from 5 to 12 hours and may cost $12,000.

Source: Helen K. Branion, "The Epileptic—How You Can Help," *RN*, June 1972, p. 51. Reprinted with permission of *RN* magazine.

which occurs before the victim has fully recovered from the previous convulsion. The duration and severity of the symptoms will be unmistakable. This type of attack calls for immediate hospitalization.

In dealing with a child who has had a seizure, teachers must control their attitude and manner. The child is likely to be confused and embarrassed, and the best comfort is quiet assurance that all is well. Calm and the appearance of confidence will benefit the other children as well as the one who has had the seizure. When there is an epileptic child in the class, it may be wise to discuss the condition (not the child), along with other kinds of chronic problems, with the entire class to dispel fears and promote healthy attitudes.

The main goal should be to avoid alarming the children during or after an attack. Assure them that the episode was not serious and that the epileptic child will soon be all right. If the child has never had an attack in your classroom, you should notify the parents as quickly as possible. They may wish to call a doctor.

Control of epilepsy requires anticonvulsant drugs, which the epileptic must take on a fairly rigorous schedule.[15] Teachers who have epileptic children in their care should make doubly sure what medication they must take during school hours and what the correct dosage is. Because the doctor may vary prescriptions with changes in a child's condition, it would be wise to double-check medication requirements from time to time.

Children who have epilepsy should take part in normal classroom activities. The possibility that seizures may occur should not occasion changes in the curriculum to accommodate them, nor it is a sufficient reason to keep them from participating in group activities. Subject to contrary instructions from a physician, epileptic children need not refrain from engaging in most playground sports and games. For children who experience seizures, crossing busy streets and such activities as bicycle riding and swimming perhaps pose special risks, but common sense will prevent careless accidents. Teachers should make an effort to find out from parents or doctors how often seizures are likely to occur.

How seizures affect an epileptic child's classmates depends on the attitude and influence of the teacher. As with other handicaps, the way a teacher cares for a convulsing child can provide a practical and vivid lesson in first aid and human relations from which the other children may benefit.

Children with seizure disorders are prone to certain behavior problems. Their attention spans may be short, and they may be given to some destructiveness. This sort of behavior will be more noticeable in younger children. The anticonvulsant medicines prescribed for children with seizure disorders may depress the mental function, especially if the dosage is heavy, and teachers should be aware of this condition. The children may develop severe anxieties about their condition, which parents may accentuate if they make an elaborate show of concealing the facts. For this reason, the companionship and respect of peers are important to children with epilepsy.

Teachers have a unique opportunity to normalize the life of epileptic children. By teaching the facts about epilepsy to the entire class, they can lessen the social stigma attached to it, and through this effort they will make it easier for epileptic children to function as truly normal individuals.[16] As in the case of any other handicapping condition, it is also important to direct the attention of the class to the needs of the handicapped student.[17]

Sometimes teachers allow parents of handicapped children to persuade them to give their child special privileges, such as frequent rest periods and less homework, and to refrain from reprimanding or scolding the child. Coddling an epileptic student in this way may cause more emotional harm to the child than normal management. Epileptic students should receive the same treatment as all of their classmates unless their personal physician has given other instructions.

HEART DISEASE

Another handicapping condition that teachers are likely to see in children is heart disease. Approximately 1,700,000 school-age children have congenital heart disease and 150,000 have rheumatic heart disease. Describing each one of the conditions that can produce cardiac disability is beyond the scope of this book, but a few general words are in order.

The heart is a four-chambered pump with valves that control entry into and exit from each chamber. Its function is to pump blood through the body. The heart can sustain damage in various stages of development. Before birth, during pregnancy, the heart may develop abnormally in ways that will affect its function. For instance, communication between the chambers may be faulty, or the valves may develop in such a way that complete closing or opening cannot occur. After birth other kinds of problems may develop. The most common cause is *rheumatic fever,* a disease that leaves valves impaired after a specific microorganism (streptococcus) has infected a distant part of the body (for instance, the throat). Permanent scarring of one or more valves can result from this condition. Modern surgical advances have made it possible to correct many of these defects.

Rheumatic fever—usually thought of as a childhood disease—most frequently strikes between ages five and fifteen. It always follows streptococcal infection, usually a throat infection. Not all "strep" infections lead to rheumatic fever and not all cases of rheumatic fever produce heart complications.

After an initial attack, rheumatic fever is apt to recur. That is why it is important for those who suffered rheumatic fever in childhood to remain on long-term penicillin or other antibiotic therapy, which will prevent recurrence of strep infection, rheumatic fever, and rheumatic heart disease, in which scarring and deformation of the heart valves occurs.

Rheumatic heart disease can not only shorten life but also seriously impair the quality of life. Although rheumatic fever and rheumatic heart disease are preventable, incidence rates remain far too high, particularly among disadvantaged groups.

Prevention of rheumatic heart disease is a two-step process. The first step is identification of streptococcal infection. Often termed *primary prevention,* identification occurs in schools, clinics and private physicians' offices. The second step is effective treatment for streptococcal infection.

Children with heart disease do not all behave the same way. A child with a mild abnormality and almost no disability will be indistinguishable from normal children. Other children may be far less able to tolerate physical exercise than normal children due to more severe involvement. Another group comprises children with mild cases who are so anxiety-ridden that they behave as if their disability were great. More often than not this type of reaction directly reflects the way the parents have adapted to the situation.

Children with *congenital heart disease* (present at birth) may complain of shortness of breath, limited exercise tolerance, and a few may have *cyanosis* (blue appearance of the skin due to poor oxygenation of the blood). Children with congenital heart defects who have reached school age generally are not likely to have a life-threatening problem. Many will have undergone complete surgical correction of the defect in early childhood.[18] Children who have heart disease generally know their limits. It is not necessary to restrain them from everyday exercise. Those children whose tolerance is markedly diminished will need help adjusting to the fact that they are different from other children and cannot participate in all the classroom activities. With help, they will be able to recognize their limitations and at the same time acquire confidence by developing other skills. By achieving their full potential children with heart disease, like other handicapped children, will have a better adjustment to life.[19]

Some school-age children who have heart conditions have strong feelings of being different from others and express their anxiety about it either through excitation or through withdrawal. A body image of disjointedness and incapacity may also be evident. Teachers can help these children adjust by avoiding undue restrictions and providing optimistic and positive feedback.

SICKLE-CELL ANEMIA

Generally sickle-cell anemia is not considered a handicapping condition. Sickle-cell anemia is always severe, however. In a sickle-cell crisis, afflicted children may require hospitalization. They may tire easily, and they tend to get infections frequently. These problems do affect a child's adaptation to the school program, so it is helpful for teachers to know something about the disease.

Sickle-cell anemia is an inherited disease, primarily among blacks, that causes the red blood cells to flatten out into the shape of a half-moon or sickle. These cells do not survive as long as normal cells (120 days). They form small clots, which cause attacks of pain and impair function in some parts of the body. In general, the production of new red cells cannot keep pace with the constant removal of the sickled cells, and this imbalance produces anemia, an inadequate supply of red blood cells. Sometimes the rate of red blood cell destruction increases markedly. At other times the production of new red cells temporarily stalls. Both problems increase the severity of the anemia.

Children with sickle-cell anemia are chronically ill, but as in all diseases, the intensity of symptoms varies from one child to another and in the same child from one time to another. Often the child will look normal except for gangly arms and legs and eyes that have a yellow cast (jaundice). During a crisis, the child may show fatigue, paleness (seen best in black children in the nail beds and inner parts of the eyelid), susceptibility to infection, and attacks of pain (commonly in the abdomen and extremities). Fatigue varies in degrees and over time, but a general lassitude seems to be a constant characteristic. Some children periodically have trouble sitting through a class. Getting to school or walking from one class to another can be tiring. Especially when loss of sleep from pain as well as joint tenderness and swelling add to the general fatigue, the child cannot attend school. There is no cure yet for the disease itself, although treatment exists for severe anemia and painful attacks.

When anemia is not severe, children with sickle-cell anemia require no special classroom precautions. They can be fully active, and teachers should treat them like normal children.

To have sickle-cell anemia, a child must inherit the tendency from both parents, who are said to be *carriers* of the tendency, or trait. If one parent is a carrier, the offspring will not manifest the disease, but they may be carriers. Only under extraordinary circumstances does a carrier develop sickel-cell symptoms but a carrier's red blood cells can be made to sickle under proper laboratory conditions. Knowledge of being a carrier is important information for a person who is considering having children. By not marrying another carrier it is possible to avoid having affected children. When two carriers marry, there is a 25 percent chance that they will produce a child with sickle-cell anemia and a fifty percent chance of having a child who is neither a carrier nor a victim of the disease.

There is little practical point in knowing whether a child is a carrier before the reproductive years, except perhaps to encourage the parents to take the test themselves. A good time to check children is when they are in high school. Carriers are generally not ill or at risk for developing any complications. The information about the carrier state is useful primarily to guide decisions about reproduction. Dangerously, people may think that if they do not manifest the disease, they have no problem because they do not understand the difference between being a carrier and having the disease.

Education is especially important for children with sickle-cell anemia because they lack the stamina to undertake unskilled labor or outdoor jobs that involve significant exertion.

EMOTIONAL AND BEHAVIOR IMPACTS
OF PHYSICAL ILLNESS[20]

Like other health problems, chronic illness can significantly influence emotional and mental health, thereby influencing an individual's behavior and general response to the educational experience. Almost everyone knows about *psychosomatic illness,* in which the symptoms are physical and the cause is at least partly mental or emotional. The great majority of the people who go to doctors have a psychosomatic disorder. But many people, including some doctors, are only dimly aware of illness whose nature is the reverse of psychosomatic. This type has been called *somatopsychic,* because the symptoms are mental or emotional although the cause is somatic, or physical. Like its opposite, somatopsychic illness is widespread. Moreover, children who have psychological problems are sometimes in treatment by psychiatrists or psychologists for months and even years without effect, simply because their trouble lies not in the mind but in the body. For example, hypoglycemia commonly produces abnormal behavior because very low blood-sugar levels affect the brain's functioning. Young children become irritable and fretful; older children become confused, negativistic, and possibly violent. Another sign of hypoglycemia is violent excitability in a usually quiet and withdrawn child. Involuntary twitching, impaired ability to execute coordinated movements, restlessness, insomnia, daytime drowsiness, inability to concentrate, weakness, and depression are other symptoms. Prolonged hypoglycemia can cause brain damage.

Another "hypo-" disorder that has serious implications is *hypothyroidism,* or an abnormally low level of thyroid hormone. This condition may exist at birth and it may develop in children and adults. Without adequate treatment, in the form of hormone therapy, children born with hypothyroidism become mentally retarded.

When children have congenital hypothyroidism, research indicates, the earlier treatment begins, the less brain damage they suffer. The IQs of three-year-old congenitally hypothyroid children who began therapy prior to three months of age range from 64 to 107.

For those who started receiving treatment at age seven months the range was 25-80.[23]

Among the signs of untreated hypothyroidism are feeding problems, unwanted gains in weight, lethargy, and evidence of mental dysfunction. The last symptom includes *perseveration,* or giving the same response to a variety of questions; *periphrasis,* using unnecessarily long forms of expression; and *aphasia,* in which the ability to use language diminishes or disappears. After treatment has started, other problems may arise. Rebelliousness, extreme assertiveness, and obstinacy are common side effects, but they disappear once the body has become accustomed to the hormone.

When the body's level of thyroid activity is too high, *hyperthyroidism,* or *thyrotoxicosis,* exists. More often than hypothyroidism this physical state gives rise to symptoms that are easily confused with those of psychiatric disorder, such as nervousness, irritability, crying spells, temper tantrums, difficulties with school work, lack of concentration, and hyperactivity. Investigators have found also that anxiety and emotional instability are common. Hyperthyroid children are easily excitable, quarrelsome, and hostile. They may have fainting spells, and suicidal tendencies, poor coordination of the fine muscles, a tendency toward enuresis, or bedwetting, and morbid concern about their health. The common assumption that hyperthyroidism is rare sometimes prevents correct diagnosis and forces worried parents and upset youngsters to seek help from mental health practitioners.

Attempts to explain children's behavioral problems often fail to include tests for still another physical disorder: *iron-deficiency anemia,* which results from the depletion of the body's iron. Iron-deficient persons lose their appetite, become irritable, and suffer from fatigue, weakness, and inability to concentrate. Many children who are iron deficient become breath holders. Anemic children misbehave in school more often than other children and may also show disturbances in attention and perception. They throw more tantrums than other children, fight more, cry more often, have more sleep disturbances, are more likely to be finger suckers and nail biters, and more often are enuretic. A poor home environment may compound these effects.

Recognition that emotional problems can have significant effects on the body (psychosomatic) is ages old, but the influence of illness on the mind (somatopsychic) is no less noteworthy. Physical illness and injuries and the life changes they bring about affect psychological health regardless of whether the patient is an adult or a child. But pain, weakness, fatigue, and alterations in daily routine and emotional climate are particularly troubling for children, who have not yet learned that they are bearable and will most likely pass. Children react to their own physical disabilities in one of two principal ways: they seek extra love and attention or they withdraw from their immediate world and concentrate on their bodily needs.[21]

Even minor sickness may have a disturbing emotional impact on a child. Physical illness of whatever severity often leads to a regression to earlier developmental behaviors such as bedwetting and school phobias. New symptoms may develop, too. For example, the relationship with parents and siblings may change, self-confidence may disintegrate, and mood swings may occur.

The psychological problems that may follow physical illness fall into five major categories:[22]

1. Behavior disorders, including night terrors, sleep walking, fear of the dark or of hidden dangers, hypochondria, and excessive irritability
2. Disturbances in interpersonal relationships, such as withdrawal from social contacts, shyness and timidity, outbursts of temper, and an increase in demands on the mother
3. Habit disorders such as nail biting, rejection of food, bedwetting
4. Conduct disorders—for example, stealing—to draw attention and concern
5. Learning problems

Among both children and adults, the most common reaction to illness, in general, combines regression and anxiety. But there are others. For instance, many youngsters believe that illness is punishment for misbehavior. Some of them fear that the outcome will be death, which they regard also as punishment. Feelings of helplessness and low self-esteem are common, as are anger and resentment. Physical restrictions on movement may lead to increased irritability and aggressiveness.

Physical handicaps, whatever their nature, also may prove psychologically damaging, and a child with a mild handicap may well develop more psychiatric problems than a child who has been stricken more severely. Severely handicapped children are more ready to accept their limitations. For the child with a mild handicap, however, such acceptance comes hard. The ability to participate in many but not all activities can be highly frustrating.

Crippled children generally appear to be cheerful, optimistic, cooperative, and nonaggressive. This posture, however, often gives way to crying spells, displays of stubbornness and temper, and a desire to make normal people realize what it means to be crippled. Because of their handicap, these children have an inner world filled with fears of death, fragmentation, loss of love, and punishment. This world also contains the fear of their own aggressiveness. Commonly, they carry a burden of guilt, both because they consider the handicap to be a punishment and because they wish it had been visited upon somebody else.

NOTES

1. Brent Hafen, *Health for the Secondary Teacher* (Dubuque, Iowa: Wm. C. Brown Co., 1972), p. 188.
2. Georgia Travis, *Chronic Illness in Children* (Palo Alto, Calif.: Stanford University Press, 1976), p. 45.
3. Donald B. Tower, "Cerebral Palsy," *Pharmacy Times*, February 1977, pp. 48-53.
4. Ibid.
5. Ibid.
6. Robert H.A. Haslam and Peter J. Vallentutti, *Medical Problems in the Classroom* (Baltimore, Md.: University Park Press, 1975), p. 155.
7. Brent Hafen, Alton L. Thygerson, and Ronald L. Rhodes, *Prescriptions for Health* (Provo, Utah: Brigham Young University Press, 1977), p. 193.
8. Ibid., p. 195.
9. Travis, p. 271.
10. Judith M. McFarlane, "The Child with Diabetes Mellitus," *Pediatric Nursing*, September/October 1975, pp. 6-9.
11. Judith M. McFarlane, *Care of the Child With Diabetes*, (Baltimore, Md.: Ames Company, 1975).
12. Judith M. McFarlane, *What You Need to Know About Diabetes*, (New York: American Diabetes Association, 1976).
13. Travis, p. 345.
14. Haslam and Vallentutti, *Medical Problems*, p. 78.
15. Robert H.A. Haslam and Peter J. Vallentutti, "On Growing Up Epileptic," *Emergency Medicine*, March 1977, pp. 195-205.
16. Ibid., p. 198.
17. Haslam and Vallentutti, *Medical Problems*, p. 61.
18. Dan G. MacNamara, "Management of Congenital Heart Disease," *Pediatric Clinics of North America*, November 1971, p. 1197.
19. Haslam and Vallentutti, *Medical Problems*.
20. Adapted from J.R. Wasseritein and H. Yahoraes, *The Child's Emotions: How Physical Illness Can Affect Them* (Bethesda, Md.: *National Institute of Mental Health*, 1977).
21. Paul D. Steinhauser et al., "Psychological Aspects of Chronic Illness," *Pediatric Clinics of North America*, November 1974, pp. 825-40.
22. Ibid., p. 826.
23. Ibid., p. 833.

RESOURCES

American Cancer Society, Pennsylvania Division, Inc. (or local division), 3309 Spring Street, Harrisburg, Pa. 17111. (Materials: television materials, posters, films, radio transcriptions.)

American Diabetes Association, 18 East 48th Street, New York, N.Y. 10017.

American Heart Association, Inquiries Section (or local Heart Association), 44 East 23rd Street, New York, N.Y. 10010.

American Medical Association, Bureau of Health Education, 535 N. Dearborn Street, Chicago, Ill. 60610 (Materials: pamphlets, posters, films, radio scripts. Request publications list.)

National Epilepsy League, 203 N. Wabash Avenue, Chicago, Ill. 60610. (Materials: films, pamphlets, quarterly newspaper *Horizons*).

National Foundation, division of Scientific and Health Information, 800 Second Avenue, New York, N.Y. 10017. (Materials: publications on birth defects, arthritis, polio, genetics. Request publications list.)

National Multiple Sclerosis Society (or local chapter), 257 Fourth Avenue, New York, 10010. (Request publications list.)

National Tuberculosis and Respiratory Disease Society, 1790 Broadway, New York, N.Y. 10019.

United Cerebral Palsy Association, Inc., 369 Lexington Avenue, New York, N.Y. 10017.

John Hancock Mutual Life Insurance Company, Health Education Service, 200 Berkeley Street, Boston, Mass. 02116 (Materials: publications on mental health, accidents, disease.)

Heart Disease Control Program, Division of Special Health Services, U.S. Public Health Service, U.S. Department of Human Resources, Washington, D.C. 20025.

Heart Information Center, National Heart Institute, U.S. Public Health Service, Bethesda, Md. 20014.

National Center for Chronic Disease Control, Office of Information, 4040 N. Fairfax Drive, Arlington, Va.

National Institutes of Health, U.S. Department of Health, Education and Welfare, U.S. Department of Human Resources, Bethesda, Md. 20014 (Currently undergoing complete reorganization. There will be new department titles and addresses. (Materials: publications on allergy and infectious disease, arthritis and metabolic diseases, cancer, child health and human development, dental research, general medical services, heart, mental health, neurological diseases and blindness.))

State and county health departments usually have free literature on the following subjects:

Aging	Amebiasis
Adolescent health	Arthritis
Alcoholism	Asthma
Allergy in children	Mumps
Cancer	Nutrition
Child health	Overweight
Chronic disease (general)	Poliomyelitis
Cleft lip and cleft palate	Rheumatic fever
Colds	Safety
Communicable disease and	Sight conservation
immunization	Sleep
Community health	Smallpox

Dental health
Diabetes
Diphtheria
Drugs
First aid
Fluoridation
Food
Hay fever
Heart disease
Hepatitis
Immunization and travel
Influenza
Louse infestation
Maternal and child health
Meningitis

Snakebite
Social hygiene
Stroke
Sunstroke
Swimming
Syphilis
Teeth
Tetanus
Tuberculosis
Typhoid fever
Venereal disease
Whooping cough
Malaria
Measles

U.S. Public Health Service, Public Inquiries Branch, Washington, D.C. 20201. (Materials: list of health information pamphlets of the Public Health Service and list of government films on medicine and allied sciences).

Superintendent of Documents, U.S. Government Printing Office, Washington, D.C. 20205. (Materials: biweekly list of publications for Education [PL 31], health [PL 51], children's bureau and civil defense [PL 71])

U.S. Department of Human Resources, Washington, D.C. 20201. (Materials: child health and safety [Children's Bureau], food and drugs [Food and Drug Administration], health [Office of Education], rehabilitation [Office of Vocational Rehabilitation].)

CHAPTER 19
Safety Programs and Policies

One of the major health problems of elementary schoolchildren is accidental injury. In the age group five to fourteen, accidents account for more deaths than all diseases combined! Another tragedy is that for every accidental death five or six children suffer some degree of permanent disability as the result of accidents. Table 19–1 indicates accidental death rates among elementary schoolchildren:

These statistics point to a great need for careful planning for a safe school environment and a program of emergency control. Schools and classroom teachers need to assume direct responsibility for the provision of a safe environment, for the development of positive safety attitudes through safety instruction, and the nurture of positive emotional well-being.

SAFETY EDUCATION IN THE ELEMENTARY SCHOOL

In the past few years concern for safety has grown dramatically. Today an increased emphasis on the value of human life and on the protection of the earth's resources is causing people to ask why accidents claim thousands of lives, cause millions of injuries, and cost billions of dollars every year. What began at the turn of the century as a plea for safer working conditions has blossomed into a national

TABLE 19-1. Accidental Deaths of School-Age Children Five to Fourteen Years (1977) per 100,000 Population*

	Deaths	*Rate*
TOTAL	6,305	17
Motor vehicle	3,142	9
Drowning	1,110	3
Fires, burns	550	1
Other	1,159	3

*National Safety Council, *Accident Facts,* 1979 edition, p. 8.

effort to provide safer surroundings for everyone all the time. Safer autos, better packaging of potentially hazardous products, flame-retardant sleep wear, and safer toys are representative of the fruits of this movement.

In order to survive, people have always sought safety from the elements. Today we have even more to fear from our own inventions. The fast pace of the mechanized world requires that we adapt to new situations almost daily. So far, our record in meeting these challenges has not been very good. Not only are accidents the leading cause of death for American children aged one to fourteen, but they also are the leading cause of permanent and temporary disabilities among those over the age of one year. Furthermore, accident costs in the United States amount to more than $500,000 every ten minutes.

With the desire for an accident-free environment has come recognition that all the new devices in the world offer no protection from a person's own unsafe behavior. The need for sound safety education—with emphasis on positive attitudes and values—is urgent. But where do we start? Most people agree that to be effective, safety education must begin with children, and the younger the better. Early instruction in the home can be invaluable, but parents, educators, and lawmakers alike feel that safety education is so crucial that the schools must provide it.

Will safety education for children really help reduce this toll? Yes, if the safety program focuses not only on helping children confront specific safety problems in everyday life, but also on developing a "safety consciousness" or "safe attitude" as a frame of reference for safe behavior in any situation. Such a program can have widespread ramifications. People who live safely increase the safety and the safety-mindedness of the people around them. By preventing accidents, they safeguard the lives of their families and others in the community. And by exercising a respect for safe behavior, they encourage others—particularly their children—to confront safety problems reasonably and to develop a safety consciousness of their own. If the school can provide the initial spark in this self-perpetuating system, it will indeed brighten the future of accident prevention.

Obviously, accident prevention is the chief aim of safety education, but good safety education, by its very nature, does more. Not a restrictive set of "don'ts," good safety education can actually give children more freedom in everyday activities. By helping them to improve their judgment, skills, knowledge and ability to estimate hazards, it affords them more opportunities for worthwhile pursuits— even adventurous ones that entail calculated risk—with fewer mishaps likely to sideline them along the way.

A good safety education program can also move children toward the general goal of self-realization. Through a good program, they come to understand how the environment works and how their activities affect it. They learn to assess their own mental, physical, and emotional capacities and to explore their own values, attitudes, and beliefs. Their experiences in the program teach them to make sound, independent decisions. As they grow older, they begin to accept responsibility for themselves and others and for the community and to initiate beneficial projects. And perhaps most important, through a good safety education program, children acquire a sense of their own worth and respect for life, health, and property.

Broadly conceived, *safety education* is the process of coordinating administrative procedures, protection measures, and planned instruction in a comprehensive school program designed to conserve human and material resources. In a living environment that daily confronts every individual with hazards, the school must meet its obligation to the community by equipping students with the know-how to stay alive and to live efficiently in a technological world. Obviously, a school program is not complete if it concentrates on developing the minds and bodies of young people without instilling in them those traits that will enable them to protect themselves and others from injury and even death.

The central purpose of safety education is to conserve life, limb, and property through the reduction of both the frequency and the severity of accidents. It is essential, therefore, to understand the true nature of accidents. A popular notion is that an accident is some sort of unexpected incident that unavoidably results in property damage, bodily injury, or death. The implication is that such chance occurrences are unpredictable and thus no one can control the accident-producing circumstances. Carried to the extreme, this attitude would make meaningless all engineering endeavors designed to create environments as free as possible from hazards as well as the application of common-sense rules for human behavior within faulty environments and efforts to educate people for safe living. Accumulated research contradicts this point of view. Indeed, authorities tell us that the word "accident" itself may be a misnomer. Careful analysis has demonstrated that an accident consists of a complex series of events rather than a singular incident. Moreover, factors contributing to the injury-producing incident do not necessarily cause an immediate accident. We can describe any accident, then, as a series of identifiable events moving toward predictable consequences. By changing one or more events in the series it is possible to change the outcome.

Research in safety is by no means definitive, but authorities generally agree that engineering, enforcement, and education can effectively (1) alter human behavior in a manner that will lower the likelihood of injury-producing acts or conditions and (2) reduce the severity of damage when such events take place or such conditions exist. The challenge to educators, therefore, is to utilize the principles of education as well as principles from the social, psychological, and physical sciences to make safety education an integral part of the school curriculum. Safety education experiences designed to enhance knowledge, develop skills, and improve behavioral traits are essential for modern life and must be a fundamental objective of education. Safety instruction, therefore, should be part of every curricular offering to which it is appropriate.

Learning to live safely in an increasingly unsafe environment is vital for children. To develop this capacity, our youth not only need to know how to identify unsafe situations in their environment, but must also learn when and how to modify their environment to eliminate or minimize as many unsafe situations as possible. They must also learn to recognize their own handicaps and limitations and to compensate for them.

Safe living has become an important and complicated problem in the modern world. The home has failed to tackle this problem adequately, and as a result, the school must assume responsibility for preparing young people to live reasonably safely. Society's recognition of the school's responsibility for safety shows in legislative enactments requiring the teaching of safety in grades 1–12 and requiring teacher-training institutions to offer safety courses. The quality of a safety education program depends primarily on effective instruction by qualified personnel.

Although classroom instruction is the most vital element, a good children's safety program includes all community activities directed toward safer living. It provides for the elimination or control of hazardous conditions in the environment. It means safe school buildings and school grounds. It includes protection by the police, fire department, and other protective agencies. It presupposes safe pupil transportation. It depends on safe conditions in homes and in public places. A good children's safety program involves the cooperation of many community agencies.

School administrators and teachers hold key positions in the development of a children's safety program. A properly organized and

supervised school program will elicit the cooperation of community
agencies.

WHY CHILDREN HAVE ACCIDENTS

The very nature of growing children invites danger! Who are the really
curious creatures? Who are the adventurous ones? Whose imagina-
tions are most fertile? Who are flexing their muscles and trying out
their developing bodies? Whose wholeheartedness throws them head
over heels into much trouble? Surely the people who have all these
characteristics are children and young people—and who would want
them any other way?

Elementary schoolchildren are particularly vulnerable to traffic
hazards. They walk a great deal—more than the average adult. They
walk to and from school and recreation areas. They run errands and
attend community gatherings. They roller-skate, and ride wagons,
bicycles, school, and commercial buses. They also are frequent pas-
sengers in the family automobile. In general, children in this age
group engage in an increasing number of activities that place their
lives in jeopardy.

During the first few years of school, children assume greater and
greater degrees of personal responsibility and independence. At times
they eagerly plunge impulsively into new adventures, without sufficient knowledge about or concern for potential hazards. At other
times, they crave guidance and protection from parents, teachers,
adults, and other children.

Although the muscular coordination of young children is not yet
well developed, this age group possesses boundless energy, ready for
any release—running, jumping, climbing, wrestling. In every group
there are a few "show-offs" who either feel insecure or aspire to leadership. Others tend to follow such "leaders," regardless of danger. No
child wants to be branded a coward. A significant characteristic of
young children is that they tend to value approval by classmates as
much as approval by parents or teachers. Restlessness, experimentation, and competition may produce a serious lack of concern for
others.

As a child's physical growth rate increases, coordination fails to
keep pace. Yet the tendency is for parents and teachers to grant more
and more independence with less and less supervision when children
enter the intermediate grades. At this age, children have a wide range
of interests, and they are prone to overconfidence and misjudgment.
The general feeling appears to be that, if an older youth or adult can
perform a given activity with apparent ease, then there is no good
reason why they cannot acquire the observed skills immediately. The

following points about children and safety make very good reasons, however:[1]

1. Young children depend very much on adults for safety and protection.
2. Children under emotional stress or strain are not alert in their thinking.
3. Children from homes in which there is emotional stress need more learning experiences to develop understanding and knowledge.
4. Knowing what is right gives assurance. Practicing "the right way" makes it an automatic response.
5. Children are not always capable of recognizing potential dangers.
6. Fears are learned from experience or teaching.
7. Physical defects such as poor vision or slow coordination can be safety hazards.
8. Large muscle coordination and hand-eye coordination lag in some children.
9. Young children who overextend themselves and become fatigued are accident-prone.
10. Pre-adolescents have periods of rapid muscular growth, which lead to awkwardness and restlessness. These conditions may encourage poor safety habits.
11. Children like rough-and-tumble play.
12. Pre-adolescents are often argumentative, outspoken, and critical of adults.
13. Children often become rebellious and uncooperative as they approach adolescence.
14. Teasing between boys and girls of the pre-adolescent period creates safety hazards.

Typical primary and intermediate schoolchildren need firm and consistent training in all of the best safety rules that parents, teachers, and society can devise. To expect them to know how to ride a bus or bicycle safely without specific instruction is to deny them an opportunity for constructive and satisfying learning. Failure to demand that children consistently observe reasonable rules of safety robs them of the sense of security that they can gain only through effective interaction with their environment. Educators tend to blame parents for poor behavior in children, but who is really to blame if they do not know how to conduct themselves safely to and from school? Is it realistic to think that young children can effectively transfer safety practices from their homes to the school situation? The answer is yes.

Elementary school teachers know that all children have certain

basic physical, mental, social, and emotional needs: the need for frequent physical activity in guided work and play and in unsupervised
"free play"; the need for a feeling of security within their families
and within the classroom; the need for challenge to their growing
mental capacities, provided by a well-planned succession of learning
experiences. Good planning and direction will insure that the school
safety program serves all of these needs and at the same time protects
children from actual physical harm.

In order to benefit from the safety program, children must first
understand its purposes. They need help to become aware, but not
unduly fearful, of the hazards to which daily living exposes them—at
home, at school, at play, on the farm, on the road, and in the streets.
They need guidance to recognize and analyze these hazards for themselves and to work out safety precautions. They must have constant
practice in self-protection, until their eyes, ears, and muscles respond
automatically to safeguard them against danger.

During regular class periods safety instruction can provide experience in recognizing and analyzing hazards and can help children
devise safety precautions to avoid them. Class instruction alone, however, will not develop automatic responses. Safety must be part of
every activity of every school day. Teachers, administrators, and children all have a responsibility to develop automatic safety habits.

The best way to teach safety in primary and intermediate grades is
by integrating appropriate learning experiences into subject areas
such as social science, natural science, health, language arts, physical
education, and arithmetic, as well as by presenting special units designed to place timely emphasis on specific needs of particular
student groups.

Teachers should make certain that all of the younger students are
aware of their physical and social environment. For instance, they
should know:

1. Name, address, telephone number, parents' names, parents' place
   of employment, and family doctor's name
2. Why avoidance of injury-producing incidents is important to themselves, their families, and society
3. The school's attitude toward safety
4. What safety programs exist in the local and wider community

The overall safety program should successfully convince children to
consistently exercise *safe behavior*, defined as the optimum performance of the seven dynamic processes described in the following
list.[2] A child exercises safe behavior when he or she:

1. *Identifies* hazards to her- or himself, to others and/or to the environment.

2. *Assesses* risks in terms of his own mental, emotional, and physical capabilities and the capabilities of others and of the environment.
3. *Decides* what to do by selecting those actions that allow maximum fulfillment of life goals and mental, physical, and emotional needs, while assuming only a reasonable amount of risk.
4. *Performs* the selected tasks by correctly using the skills necessary to complete the tasks as desired.
5. *Evaluates* the results by weighing the advantages and disadvantages of the outcome.
6. *Modifies,* if necessary, the concept of the hazards, the perception of the risks, and the correctness of the decision or the way it was carried out.
7. *Applies* the experience gained to new situations when it is appropriate.

TEACHERS AND ACCIDENTS

So far we have talked only about pupils and accidents. What about the teachers in elementary schools? Do they have accidents, and if so, why? The National Safety Council, in a report on a very informative study completed in New York City, stated that hundreds of teachers had accidents in New York City Schools each year.[3] In seventeen years the teacher accident rate had multiplied by a shocking 600 percent. An extensive survey of teacher accidents uncovered some surprising facts. Women teachers had a far higher number of accidents than their male colleagues. Among women between the ages of 25 and 39 the incidence of accidents was relatively low, but among older women the rate was higher. The great majority of female accident victims were over 45, and approximately one-third of them were 55 or older. For men teachers the greatest accident "zone" was the 25–34 age group. Further, almost half the men's accidents occurred in specially equipped areas, such as shops, gymnasiums, and playgrounds. Men were much more likely to have accidents while supervising physical activities, lifting heavy objects, and using machinery and tools.

The incidence of cuts, overexertion and strain was three times as high for men as for women in the New York Study. The causes of accidents involving women were more subtle and correlate to physical and emotional difficulties of the middle and advanced years of life. The report stated that the female susceptibility to accidents may be a symptom of personal stress due to emotional and other health problems.

In addition, the study revealed that school physical plants were not unsafe places so much as people were. More than a quarter of all teacher accidents involved children. Mechanical causes stemmed usually from poor housekeeping. Falls over books, clothing, and so on comprised 43 percent of all women's accidents. The most dangerous place in the school building is the stairway; the classroom is the safest. Of all levels, the elementary schools had the highest accident rates.

Based on the statistics, the New York study suggested the following precautionary measures:

1. To prevent falls, make corridors and stairs physically safe.
2. Give older women teachers with health or known emotional problems first-floor rooms so that they will not have to climb stairs.
3. Because many accidents are caused by pupils in motion, institute procedures for orderly passage through the halls.
4. Young and inexperienced teachers certainly would benefit from training in classroom management. Male teachers especially should learn how to use supplies and equipment properly and how to perform activities that require physical exertion safely. In fact, teacher preparatory institutions might do well to instruct students in these methods before they begin their careers.
5. In the final analysis, the best way to decrease teacher accidents in the school is to *study the accident record first.* General warnings like "let's all be more careful" do very little good, but specific action to counter specifically known hazards is bound to bring results.

ADMINISTRATIVE CONSIDERATIONS

A good safety-education program is a continuous program that coincides with the purposes of the school and is well integrated in the total program. Also, it is a cooperative that involves not only all school personnel but also the community and all community agencies.

The most effective learning in the elementary school takes place only when everyone concerned shows interest in the process. Therefore the habits and attitudes necessary for safe living will take root only when real interest in this phase of learning permeates the community, school administration, instructional staff, and individual classroom. The program should reflect truly cooperative thoughts and action. Only when it does will sound, gradual growth in safety habits and attitudes take place rather than spasmodic progress. In order to achieve unity of effort in the school program, responsible individuals, including parents, need to define areas of responsibility and action.

District school boards, superintendents, and principals have direct responsibility for planning and implementing school safety-education programs. Each school district should establish a definite procedure for meeting the needs of the students and the community. Although active participation of all persons in the school system characterizes the better safety-education programs, dedicated commitment on the part of the school leadership is of primary importance. To demonstrate concern, school administrators can adopt a formal school safety policy and designate a specialist to coordinate the safety education program. Planning and implementing such a program requires mobilization of a broad base of experience, including community resources. Implementation entails administrative action, maintenance of a school environment that is free from unnecessary hazards, and timely instruction by every teacher at every grade level.

A good safety education program requires careful planning and execution. The planning process should involve representatives of the student body, teachers, and administrative and classified personnel. Community resources include safety councils, automobile clubs, civil defense officials, health organizations, police departments, and fire agencies. A prudent first step is to designate a qualified person to serve as safety education coordinator. With the advice of a representative safety education planning committee, the coordinator should examine records of (1) accidents in the school itself, (2) accidents to school-age youths outside the school, and (3) statistical trends in other sections of the county, state, and nation. In the absence of complete local reports and records, planners should analyze statistical information gathered from similar communities.

A major function of leadership responsibility at the district level is to develop and implement a policy statement or "set of principles" governing the administration of the safety program. Examples of the goals that this statement might include are:

1. The protection of child health is a *major* educational objective that requires careful planning.
2. A continuous appraisal of a safe physical plant and effective safety instruction is imperative.
3. Safety education should be positive and should not dwell on the morbid consequences of unsafe behavior. The program should avoid developing unnecessary inhibitions and needless fears in children.
4. Participation in the safety program should include every child and member of the school staff. To achieve this goal the coordinator can organize in-service workshops for teachers and staff, direct and participate in student patrol activity, direct and participate in emergency drills, and coordinate and participate in school safety procedures, to name but a few.
5. A system for recording school accidents is a necessary part of planning for safety.
6. Dramatic appeal will make many phases of safety instruction more effective.

7. The safety instruction program should have a seasonal orientation to meet changing needs and lend variety to the program.
8. Many activities can increase the popularity of safety considerations and safety education. Examples are poster contests, radio and TV programs, safety plays, and puppet shows, invited guests, special excursions, and a school "safety week."
9. The foremost goal of the school and community safety programs should be to develop proper safety attitudes, for therein lies the key to safe behavior.
10. The school and community safety programs should dovetail and their personnel should cooperate in planning, eliminating safety hazards, and utilizing the total resources of the community.
11. Program evaluation for the school and community program should note:
    a. Amount and quality of participation in safety programs
    b. Community and school attitudes concerning safety
    c. Any change in the number and seriousness of accidents

School administrators hold the greatest responsibility for safety in the schools. The safety of pupils in the school building, on the playground, and in all areas surrounding the school come under their jurisdiction. According to the Pennsylvania Department of Public Instruction, the duties of administrators are the following:

In the Building and Building Areas

1. Enforcement of established safety rules and regulations
2. Elimination of projecting hazards
3. Investigation of the hazards of screened windows and doors
4. Provision for:
    a. Proper and safe equipment
    b. Proper maintenance of the building and the equipment
    c. Careful storage of inflammable materials
    d. Emergency lighting in buildings which are used at night
    e. A high-grade, non-slip treatment for floors
5. Periodical inspection of:
    a. The fire alarm system
    b. The fire escapes and exits
    c. All fire extinguishers
    d. All corridors, stairs, and handrails
    e. The cleanliness of lavatories
    f. The storage areas
    g. The cafeteria and its equipment

On the Playground

1. Adequate drainage
2. Proper surfacing of play areas—rubber-base asphalt, hard-surface asphalt, sand, etc.
3. Proper zoning of areas adjacent to apparatus

4. Elimination of overlapping play areas
5. Scheduling a daily inspection of playground equipment
6. Scheduling daily supervision for the playground
7. Proper housekeeping for the playground—keep free of broken glass, fruit peels, stones, etc.
8. An annual budget for additions to and the replacement of playground equipment
9. Protective fence or hedge as needed
10. Control of operation of bicycles on or near the playground

Traffic Within School Areas

1. Marking of all walk and crossing areas and loading/unloading zones. Safety devices where feasible.
2. Establishment of loading/unloading zones for school buses within the school grounds
3. Placement of bicycle racks apart from play spaces and areas where other vehicles operate
4. Establishment of motor vehicle parking areas involving permanent and clear signs and pavement markings. Where possible, these parking areas should not be adjacent to play areas.
5. Removing all possible risks from coal chutes, areaways, fire escapes and/or other prevalent hazard areas[4]

Intercommunication and Signal Systems

Communication and signal systems should suit the size and plan of the building. Their design and location should provide ready internal and external communication in the event of safety and health emergencies.

The fire alarm system should meet all legal standards and requirements. Inside bells and other signals should have as soft a tone as possible.

Telephone service should be available wherever practicable, including one-room schools, for use in cases of illness or accident and as a means of enhancing the home-school relationship. Children and teachers should formulate sensible regulations about the use of the telephone, with which parents also should comply in order to avoid "nuisance" situations.

The School Administrator's Disaster Checklist

It is the responsibility of school administrators to:

1. Inform themselves about local disaster threats and the means to meet them. Acquaint themselves with local agencies and local plans to survive disaster.

2. Call the school board's attention to the need for a disaster survival program and a disaster curriculum. Secure board authorization to initiate such programs.
3. Become part of local government's civil defense program. Set up working arrangements for emergency operations between their schools and local government.
4. Organize a committee to plan a disaster protection program.
5. Secure board approval of the disaster protection program and make it official.
6. Make the program operational:
   a. Fill all positions in the chain of command. Take measures that all participants in this program understand their assignments and are competent to carry them out.
   b. Set up and periodically test the alert chain.
   c. Provide shelter areas for protection from fallout and severe storms (e.g., tornadoes), either by designating them in existing buildings or by converting existing facilities or by building them. Equip these areas for shelter use.
   d. Drill pupils and staff in the proper use of these shelter areas or in building evacuation.
   e. Set up, in conformity with the community evacuation plan, an overall school evacuation plan.
   f. Insure that individual schools tailor this overall evacuation plan to their needs.
   g. Authorize drills to test this plan and to develop its skillful execution.
   h. Intensify the "safe person" aspects of the pupil safety program.
   i. Build community understanding and support of the school's disaster survival program.
   j. Take measures to protect school buildings, equipment, and grounds, and to remove records beyond the area where heavy damage is likely to occur.
   k. Recommend that the board allocate funds to provide training and materials for the program and to cover related costs.
   l. Develop working arrangements with neighboring school systems for mutual support in the event disaster strikes.
7. Take the usual steps to develop a curriculum guide in disaster protection.
8. Secure the authorization of the board to make this guide official for use in the schools.
9. Set up a program to interpret this guide to the staffs. Check on its use. Revise it as facts and needs involved in disaster protection change.
10. Give staff members an opportunity to gain such immunities for disaster operation as the law provides (e.g., proper training in emergency care).

In the event of imminent disaster, responsibilities of administrators are likewise consistent with their leadership role:

In the Face of Disaster

1. Take their place in the chain of command and give the orders that will set the plan in motion.
2. Carry out any personal assignments that the plan dictates.
3. Keep calm.

Immediately After Disaster

1. Give the orders necessary to put postdisaster plans into operation.
2. Give priority to plans to save lives over plans to save property.
3. Work to reestablish communications within the schools and with civil defense and other local protection agencies.
4. Assess and report damage.
5. Assume leadership in rescue and other operations affecting schools.
6. Assume leadership by making school facilities available for non-school disaster relief and recovery purposes.

During the Prolonged Postdisaster Period

1. Continue to take inventory of damage. Assess inventory and re-sources necessary for reopening schools.
2. Represent the community, the schools, and displaced staff, and pupils. Assist in making arrangements for their temporary school-ing in evacuation areas.
3. Serve as contact agent in the chain of command.
4. Assist recovery by organizing and making available school records.
5. Serve as the school's representative in contacts with other govern-mental agencies and with the chief state school officer.
6. Take leadership in reopening schools in the stricken community and in restoring school operations.

ACCIDENT REPORTING AND RECORDING

Accident records can serve a real purpose. Recording and reporting accidents for statistical purposes only are a waste of valuable time An adequate accident reporting system can provide:

1. Materials for continuous and intelligent curriculum planning. Rec-ords help answer the question of what safety practices and atti-tudes to teach and when.
2. Problems for student organizations to study when developing safety programs. The traffic squad, for example, can learn where

the traffic accidents occur, and the playground supervisor can discover what equipment needs special supervision.

3. Information to help the supervisor decide on a course of study and practices in safety instruction; information for assigning responsibility for safety teaching or supervision.

4. Data that principals can use to plan their programs, to solicit the aid and cooperation of other community agencies, and to publicize the seriousness of the local accident situation, by means of graphs, spot maps, and so on.

5. Assistance for individual student guidance. What special personal characteristics contributed to the accident? What hazards face the child outside the school?

6. Identification of hazards in order to modify and improve the structure and use of school buildings or playgrounds and equipment.

7. Questions to raise in parent conferences.

8. Legal data for school personnel and the school board in case of accident litigation.

9. Accident facts that suggest special drives and campaigns to convince board members and parents of the necessity to remove hazards and to stimulate greater community interest.

Location, age, grade level, activity, and season of year all have a bearing on accident statistics. Each of these factors deserves note in the school's accident records. The student accident report prepared by the National Safety Council suggests the format for a monthly report. Although individual schools should adopt a report plan that meets community needs and that school personnel can easily follow, the reporting system should be coordinated with the reports of the National Safety Council whenever possible.

EVALUATION OF THE SAFETY PROGRAM

Many schools have been content to have only a safety patrol, the organization, stimulation, operation, and support of which are incidental. Without discounting the importance and dramatic appeal of the patrol, it is appropriate to point out that efficient safety programs are far less complacent.

A rapidly increasing number of schools encourage students to produce assembly programs on safety and include a variety of classroom safety activities in the curriculum. In a full-scale safety program these activities are not haphazard. Planned to convey specific informational content, these programs aim to incorporate safety instruction in classroom activities in an interesting way. In a cooperative effort, staff and students analyze objectives and carefully build the program around them.

The next development in establishing a comprehensive safety program usually is the organization of safety groups to insure a higher degree of participation by the staff and students, both on a school-wide basis and within individual classrooms. At this stage safety councils, safety clubs, courts, safety research, and reports appear.

The ultimate safety program requires a coordinated school-community approach. The adults in the neighborhood, the community council, the police, and local welfare agencies all take active parts in planning the program and they all participate to some degree in executing it. The participants share responsibility. The community cooperates and coordinates, and the students come to regard safety as a civic enterprise.

The foregoing is an attempt to simplify the typical process of developing a comprehensive safety program for children. It represents an expansion that is taking place in many localities. You should ask yourself the question "At what level is my school?"

OTHER ROLES IN SAFETY EDUCATION PROGRAMS

A survey of professional personnel, safety agencies, and lay persons in Pennsylvania revealed many activities that are representative of different kinds of school-community cooperation. The following list divides these activities into three groups: (1) a group of activities for which the principal usually, but by no means always, assumes initiatory responsibility; (2) activities usually initiated by the classroom teacher; and (3) activities for which a variety of people are essential in a well-balanced program of safety education. An asterisk (*) indicates high frequency of mention by survey participants.

The Principal

The principal usually assumes these responsibilities:

* 1. Organizes safety patrol
* 2. Provides for organization of safety committees throughout the school
* 3. Plans the program, the cooperative assistance
* 4. Sets up safety clubs
* 5. Gives special safety talks in assemblies
* 6. Sets up safety committees among staff
* 7. Conducts safety demonstrations
* 8. Arranges for state or local police to address pupils
* 9. Participates in safety drives
*10. Organizes patrol for in-school service

*11. Organizes fire drills
*12. Organizes first aid classes
*13. Stimulates use of visual aids and other materials
*14. Arranges for PTA activities by students
*15. Evaluates safety procedures with appropriate cooperation
*16. Prepares and distributes safety checklists
*17. Develops community activities
*18. Organizes junior safety council
*19. Organizes poster displays
*20. Commissions survey of school-related motor vehicle traffic
*21. Organizes school bus safety procedures
*22. Makes effective use of school newspaper
 23. Organizes Junior Firefighters
 24. Considers school membership in national and local safety councils
 25. Organizes bicycle clubs and inspections
 26. Prepares and distributes safety letters to parents
 27. Organizes safety clipping service for school
 28. Encourages dramatization and improved teaching techniques
 29. Commissions neighborhood safety-hazard survey
 30. Encourages "hazard" reporting
 31. Organizes model traffic setup
 32. Assists in the elimination of community hazards
 33. Organizes accident reporting system; evaluates findings for instructional use
 34. Assists in surveying causes of fire in the community

In addition to the foregoing list of activities, the principal has a major role in determining:

 1. Safety needs of pupils and community
 2. Amount of safety education in the curriculum
 3. Status and efficiency of the accident reporting system
 4. Degree of safety consciousness in the organization
 5. Adequacy and use of instructional materials
 6. Problems involving pupil transportation
 7. Activities of pupil safety organizations
 8. Need for in-service education of teachers
 9. Relation to local police authorities
10. Compliance with safety laws, such as fire-drill regulations
11. Hazards in or near the school
12. All other decisions affecting current safety and the role of education in insuring pupils' future safety

The principal's function goes even further to include the initiation of appropriate measures to satisfy all other responsibilities.

The Classroom Teacher

In general, teachers set the specific objectives for teaching safety within their own classrooms. They determine individual, class, and community needs and fit their instruction into the classroom program. Although principals may offer suggestions and provide materials of instruction, it is the teachers' responsibility to become acquainted with successful instructional practices, available material, and sources of assistance on the subject of safety.

Teacher contributions to faculty planning in safety are an important part of the school safety program. Special committees on playground safety, courses of study, safety habits, and coordination of school and community efforts are appropriate activities for teacher participation. In addition, the classroom teacher usually assumes these responsibilities:

* 1. Includes safety instruction wherever and whenever appropriate
* 2. Sponsors safety patrol
* 3. Sponsors safety clubs
* 4. Uses assemblies for safety presentations, including dramatization, citations for safety, and so on
* 5. Provides pupil leaders in gymnasium, play, classrooms
* 6. Prepares for and properly conducts fire drills
* 7. Stimulates preparation of safety posters and safety demonstrations
* 8. Provides opportunity for preparation of classroom safety codes
* 9. Encourages safety talks by pupils
*10. Conducts safety inspections
 11. Uses safety clippings from newspapers
 12. Conducts tours and excursions
 13. Develops radio scripts on safety
 14. Provides opportunities for tours that focus on safety
 15. Stimulates safety stories in class news sheet
 16. Provides opportunities for constructive activities
 17. Plans safe routes to school, especially for beginners
 18. Suggests safety letters
 19. Organizes "brother and sister" or "buddy" safety system for special events
 20. Aids in study of plant (e.g., poison ivy) recognition
 21. Conducts "hazard hunt"
 22. Makes own safety pictures (photographs, slides, and movies)
 23. Develops safety songs, slogans, and poems as class projects

The medical inspector and the school nurse are assets to the safety program. A medical examination is a good way to begin safety planning, particularly at the kindergarten or first-grade level. Good health is essential to safety. Those children who appear prone to accidents should receive vision examinations. Many accidents that do not appear to be serious may justify consultation with the nurse or doctor. Notations of accidents and treatments should appear on the cumulative school record of each student. Follow-up procedures will confirm treatment and corrections.

School custodians also should participate in the safety program. They should be familiar with the aims and objectives of the program. All causes of potential accidents relating to the structure and condition of the building need their attention. Participation in safety council conferences and planning sessions will increase their interest in school safety.

School bus drivers play an important role in the school safety program, too. They need the support of the school to make bus transportation safe. Their problems may make a good assembly program. For example, they may want to discuss:

1. Discipline on the bus
2. Safety monitors
*3. Getting on and off the bus
4. Protection for children while they wait for the bus
5. Bus safety inspection reports
6. Bus schedule and pupil load
7. Bus accident reports

Still another key role in the safety program is the one played by teachers in charge of physical education and health. Because many school accidents occur in the gymnasium and on the playground, their special knowledge of the proper play equipment, organization of the program, and the types of games that fit special needs is a valuable asset. They are probably specially qualified in the techniques of first aid, too. In addition, physical fitness augments the effectiveness of accident prevention programs.

Teachers of art and music need to understand fully the goals of the school safety program. They can help design safety posters, advise on safety activities, and inspire children through creative work.

SAFETY LIABILITY

The last point to consider in the administration of a school safety program is the ever-present liability for injuries and the threat of court suits. School administrators and teachers assigned to supervise school grounds and free play, as well as those who teach physical activities, are legally responsible for any accidents that occur, if it can be proven that they were negligent in their duty—for example, if they were not with the children under their direct supervision. Recess activities need to be well planned and play equipment must be safe. Proper supervision and adequate space is essential. The following teacher obligations, if acted upon, will combat liability suits:

1. Check and keep all equipment in good repair at all times.
2. Find all hazards with pupils and mark them in bright yellow paints.
3. Direct all pupils in safety measures to be taken.
4. Teach all children how to use all apparatus and equipment correctly.
5. Discuss with the class why they should not do anything on the playground which might interfere with the safety of anyone else.
6. Use activities which minimize accident possibilities.
7. Insist that all children wear suitable apparel for all activities.
8. Do not permit pupils to try new, more dangerous activities until they become skilled enough to do so.
9. Insist that all game rules be obeyed at all times.
10. Never leave an assigned group.[5]

In 1971, McGhehey, a noted authority on the legal problems of education, gave a speech in which he discussed governmental immunity.[6] In his words, "a school district could not be sued in damages for injuries to pupils, patrols or employees arising out of the exercise of the governmental function of maintaining school district operations." Lately many states have abolished the concept of governmental immunity. Now approximately half of the states permit liability suits against school districts. Citizens also are increasingly willing to sue school employees, school-board members and school districts for "negligence." By maintaining a safe physical plant, an effective safety-education program, and continuous safety in-service by school personnel, school districts can minimize the likelihood of a successful negligence lawsuit against them and their personnel.

THE SCHOOL SAFETY HANDBOOK

Each school or school district will find it immensely useful to prepare a school safety handbook and to insure that administrators and teachers become familiar with it. It may keep the school personnel out of court and other unpleasant situations.

A safety handbook serves several needs:[7]

1. A ready reference in cases of emergency
2. An administrative guide defining areas of responsibility and authority
3. A source of technical, how-to information
4. A compilation and codification of school, municipal, county, state, and federal safety rules and regulations
5. Safety information that applies specifically to the school or district

The following outline for a school safety handbook is the work of a committee of safety-education supervisors.

Due to geographic location and immediate environment every school is unique. Therefore, it is impossible to describe a set pattern of events for every school's safety program. It is suggested that each school administrator or supervisor follow the outline step by step and formulate his program in view of needs, policies, procedures, and evaluation.

A. Procedures in school accidents and unexpected illness
    1. Pupil illness or accident
        a. First aid in accidents
        b. Emergency care
        c. Responsibility of administrators and employees
        d. Procedures for handling athletic injuries
        e. Emergency telephone calls
        f. Procedure for reporting accidents and utilization of report forms
    2. Policy on release of information and records
    3. Annual accident report
B. Disaster preparedness and survival procedures
    1. Organization
        a. Liaison with state and local civil defense organizations
        b. Responsibilities of administrators and employees
        c. Identification for pupils
    2. Designation of shelter areas
    3. Essential equipment
        a. First aid kits, location and utilization
        b. Transistor radios—purpose and location
        c. Radiological instruments for intensity of fallout
        d. Emergency lighting and power
        e. Water and food supply
        f. Sanitation equipment and supplies
    4. Emergency procedures
        a. Alerting system(s)
        b. Types, practices and frequency of drills
        c. Instruction in survival techniques
        d. Recovery plans
C. Fire prevention and drill technique
    1. Organization
        a. Responsibilities of administrators and employees
    2. Essential equipment
        a. Alarm system
        b. Fire extinguisher—location and operation
        c. Location of blankets
        d. Building code for sprinkler system
        e. Exit lights and signs
    3. Prevention techniques
        a. Inspections of school building
        b. Housekeeping regulations
        c. Emergency devices
        d. Controls for false alarms

    4. Drills
        a. Signals and instructional procedures
        b. Procedures for evacuation
        c. Requirements of fire department
D. Traffic regulations and safety education
    1. Traffic code
        a. Pedestrians
        b. Motor vehicle
        c. Bicycle
        d. School bus
    2. Safety patrol
        a. Authorization and permission
        b. Responsibilities of principals and employees
        c. Rules for operation
    3. Safety engineering school area
        a. Responsibilities of administrators and employees
        b. Procedures to follow
        c. Off-street parking
        d. Loading zone
        e. Control signs and traffic signs
E. Safety policies within the school
    1. General safety policies and responsibilities
        a. Authorized activities
        b. Approval of materials and supplies
        c. Health practices
        d. Community use of facilities
    2. Instruction program
        a. Gymnasium area
        b. Swimming pool area
        c. Science area
        d. Industrial arts area
        e. Lunchroom and cafeteria area
        f. Music area
        g. Art area
        h. Business education area
        i. General classroom
        j. Audio-visual aid area
        k. R.O.T.C. and rifle range
        l. Stage and auditorium
        m. Stairs and corridors
        n. Elevators
    3. Student safety organization(s)
F. Procedures for safety on the school grounds
    1. General safety policies and responsibilities
        a. Authorized activities
        b. Approval of materials and supplies
        c. Approval of playground equipment
        d. Health practices
    2. Specific safety policies and responsibilities
        a. School grounds and athletic fields

   b. Summer recreation
   c. After-school recreation
   d. Evening recreation
   e. Off-street parking
   f. Authorized activities
   g. Community use of facilities
G. Safe school operation and maintenance
   1. State and city building safety codes
      a. Responsibilities for compliance of code
      b. Safety inspections
      c. Repairs or replacements of machines and equipment
      d. Approval of building materials and authorized repairs
H. Administrative safety regulations for employees
   1. Reporting illness or accidents of employees
   2. Safety training programs
   3. Procedures to follow for Workman's Compensation Law
   4. In-service training program for preparation in emergencies, disasters, civil defense and security procedures.[8]

NOTES

1. Adapted from *Safety Action* (Dover, Del.: State Department of Public Instruction, 1968), p. 5.
2. *Safety Education in the Elementary Schools* (Harrisburg, Pa.: Pennsylvania Department of Public Instruction, 1968), pp. 12-14. Reprinted with permission.
3. Frederick Shaw, *How Teachers Get Hurt* (Washington, D.C.: National Safety Council, 1963). p. 3.
4. *Safety Education in the Elementary Schools* (Harrisburg, Pa.: Pennsylvania Department of Public Instruction, 1968) (pamphlet). Reprinted with permission.
5. Maryhelen Vannier, *Teaching Health in Elementary Schools* (New York: Harper and Row, 1963), p. 56.
6. Marion A. McGhehey, "Is Liability a Factor Affecting School Safety Patrol Programs Today?" AAA, 1971, pp. 1-5.
7. National Safety Council, "Help," *Safety Education* March 1965, pp. 6-9.
8. Shaw, p. 5.

RESOURCES

Books for Elementary Children

Joan Barry. *Fireman Fred.* Chicago: Whitman.
J. Beim. *Anoy and the School Bus.* New York: Morrow.
J. Beim. *Country Fireman.* New York: Morrow.
Margaret W. Brown. *Dr. Squash, the Doll Doctor.* New York: Simon and Schuster.

Rosalie and Bill Brown. *Forest Fireman.* New York: Coward-McCann-Geoghegan.
Mary Elting. *First Book of Fireman.* New York: Watts.
F. Freidman. *Pat and Lee Policeman.* New York: Morrow.
Hardie Gramatsky. *Hercules: Story of an Old Fashioned Fire Engine.* New York: Putnam.
James Joseph. *Better Water Skiing for Boys.* New York: Dodd, Mead, 1964.
Murro Leaf. *Safety Can Be Fun.* Philadelphia: Lippincott, 1964.
Tina Lee. *Manners to Grow On.* New York: Doubleday, 1955.
H.B. Lent. *The Firefighters.* New York: Macmillan.
Golden MacDonald. *Red Light, Green Light.* New York: Doubleday, 1944.
Tom McNally. *Hunting for Boys.* Chicago: Follett, 1962.
National Safety Council. *Rhyme and Reason for Safety.* 1963.
National Safety Council. Showmanship in Safety. 1963.
Martha Sharp. *Let's Find Out About Safety.* New York: Watt, 1964.
Noah Smaridge. *Watch Out.* Tennessee: Abingdon, 1965.
Ruth Tooze. *Policeman Mike's Brass Buttons.* Chicago: Melmont, 1951.

Books for Teacher Reference

A.E. Florio and B.T. Stafford. *Safety Education,* New York: McGraw-Hill Book Co., 1962.
Education for Safety. Sacramento, Calif.: State Department of Education, 1963.
John T. Foror and Gust Dalis. *Health Instruction: Theory and Application.* Philadelphia: Lea and Febiger, 1966.
Ruth E. Grout. *Health Teaching in School.* Philadelphia: W.B. Saunders, 1963.
William Haddon, Jr. et al. *Accident Research.* New York: Harper and Row, 1964.
Maxwell N. Halsey, ed. *Accident Prevention.* New York: McGraw-Hill Book Co., 1961.
Irwin, Cornacchia and Staton. *Health in Elementary Schools.* St. Louis: C.V. Mosby Co., 1966.
Gladys Gardner Jenkins. *Health and Safety for Teenagers.* 1962.
Gary D. Lawson. *Safe and Sound.* 1965.
Marland K. Strasser, ed. *21 Fundamentals of Safety Education.* New York: Macmillan, 1964.

Transparencies

Social Science Packet No. 4: *The ABC's of Safety,* 3M Company, Visual Products Division, St. Paul, Minn., 1964.

Periodicals

Family Safety (National Safety Council, 425 N. Michigan Avenue, Chicago, Ill.)
Journal of Health, Physical Education and Recreation
Parent's Magazine,
Safe Driver (National Safety Council)

Safety Education (National Safety Council)
Safety: Journal of Administration, Instruction and Protection (Safety Education
    Commission, NEA)
School Safety (National Safety Council)
Today's Health
Traffic Safety (National Safety Council)

Resource Booklets

A Directory of National Organizations with Interest in School Health (February
    1977 or current edition), U.S. Department of Health and Human Resources,
    Division of Community Health Services.
Free and Inexpensive Learning Materials (Fourteenth Biennial Edition or current
    edition), Division of Surveys and Field Services, George Peabody College for
    Teachers, Nashville, Tenn. 37203.
Publication Catalog (1977–78 or current edition), Publication Division, National
    Education Association, 1201 16th Street, N.W., Washington, D.C. 20036.

Records

Mickey Mouse Record Club (Walt Disney)
Golden Record Library (Affiliated Publishers, Rockefeller Center, New York,
    N.Y.)
Decca Distributing Company (Camden, N.J.)
Educational Record Sales (New York, N.Y.)
Keystone Enterprises (Hershey, Pa.)

Sources of Free and Inexpensive Materials

Contact the following local resources:

Community safety council	Insurance companies
Police and fire departments	Civil defense office
Health agencies	Recreation department

Contact specific organizations listed in the following sections.

Organizations with Interest in School Safety

American Red Cross, National Headquarters, Washington, D.C. 20006 (or local
    office). (Publications: *Primary Study Guide* (Arc 1446), *Programs for Elemen-
    tary Schools, Be a Hazard Hunter* (Arc 1447–revised, 1968).)
National Commission on Safety Education, NEA, 1201 16th Street, N.W., Wash-
    ington, D.C. 20036. (Publications: *Safety Guides for You–In the Intermedi-
    ate Grade* (No. 461-13912), *Safety Guides for You–In the Primary Grades*

(No. 461–13856), *Teaching Safety in the Elementary School, Suggested School Safety Policies: Accident Prevention in Physical Education, Athletics and Recreation, Annual Safety Education Review, 1965, Accident Research for Better Safety Teaching, Checklist of Safety and Safety Education in Your School, Our Schools Plan Safe Living, Classroom Poster Series.)*
National Safety Council, 444 N. Michigan Ave., Chicago, Ill. 60611. (Materials: posters, films, slides, stickers, table teasers, "pop" posters, booklets, leaflets.)

Areas of Special Interest

Bicycle safety
Civil defense and disaster
Fire safety
First Aid

Home and school safety
Poison precautions
Recreation safety
Traffic and pedestrian safety

Bicycle Safety

American Automobile Association, 1712 F. Street, N.W., Washington, D.C., Publication: *Bicycling Is Great Fun.*
Bicycle Institute of America, Inc., 122 E. 42nd Street, New York, N.Y. 10017. Materials: *Bicycle Safety Tests, Bike Fun . . . , How to Plan Successful Bike Safety Programs,* posters, and pamphlets.
Goodyear Tire and Rubber Company, Public Relations Department, 1144 E. Market Street, Akron, Ohio 44316. Publication: *Bicycle Blue Book.*
Kemper Insurance Company, Chicago, Ill.
National Commission on Safety Education, NEA, 1201 16th Street, N.W., Washington, D.C. 20036. Publication: *Bicycle Safety in Action* and posters.
National Education Association.

Civil Defense and Disaster (Local and State Offices)

American Journal of Public Health, American Public Health Association, 1790 Broadway, New York, N.Y. 10019.
American Red Cross, 17th and D Streets, N.W., Washington, D.C. 20000.
Civil Defense Adult Education, Room 318, Towne House, Harrisburg, Pa. 17101.
Disaster Readiness in Undergraduate Education, Office of Civil Defense Mobilization, Battle Creek, Mich. (or through local, state, and regional offices).
Medical Self Help Section, Department of Health, P. O. Box 90, Harrisburg, Pa.
National Education Association, Safety Education Commission, 1201 16th Street, N.W., Washington, D.C. 20036. (Ask for *Schools and Civil Defense.*)
Office of Civil Defense, Department of Defense, The Pentagon, Washington, D.C. 20310. (State type of material desired.)
Public Health Reports, U.S. Public Health Service, U.S. Department of Human Resources, Washington, D.C.

Fire Safety

American Insurance Association, Engineering and Safety Department, 85 John Street, New York, N.Y. 10038. Materials: *The Careless Family, The Do-little's House,* and other pamphlets on fire prevention in farms and homes.

Paul W. Kearney. *How to Make Your Home Firesafe*. New York: William Frederick Press, 1968.

Kemper Insurance Company. Chicago, Ill.

National Fire Protection Association, Public Relations Department, Boston, Mass. 02100 Materials: *Early Man and Fire* and other pamphlets on fire safety.

First Aid

American Insurance Association, Engineering and Safety Department, 85 John Street, New York, N.Y. 10038. (Publication: *An Emergency First Aid Guide*.)

American Red Cross, National Headquarters, Washington, D.C. 20006 (or local chapter). (Materials: *American Red Cross Standard* (or *Advanced*) *First Aid Textbook*, instructional charts, films (*Checking for Injuries, Disaster and You, First Aid: Parts* I and II), and other, free and inexpensive materials.)

Arthur D. Belilios et al. *Handbook of First Aid and Bandaging*. Baltimore, Md.: Williams and Wilkins, 1963.

Brent Q. Hafen and Keith J. Karren. *First Aid and Emergency Care Workbook*. Denver, Colo.: Morton Publishing, 1980.

Johnson and Johnson, c/o Director, Consumer Relations, New Brunswick, N.J. 08900. (Materials: first aid information.)

New York State Department of Health (Materials: films (*First Aid, Rescue Breathing*).)

Young American Films, McGraw-Hill, Inc., 1221 Avenue of the Americas, New York, N.Y. 10019. (Materials: films (*First Aid Services*).)

Home and School Safety

Aetna Life Affiliated Companies, Information and Education Department, Hartford, Conn. Materials: packet of free booklets on home safety.

American Automobile Association, 1712 G. Street, N.W., Washington, D.C. 20006.

American Red Cross, National Headquarters, Washington, D.C. 20006 (or local chapter).

Educators Mutual Life Insurance Company, Lancaster, Pa. 17600.

Equitable Life Assurance Society of the United States, Office of Community Services and Health Education, 1285 Avenue of the Americas, New York, N.Y. 10019.

Institute of Makers of Explosives, 420 Lexington Avenue, New York, N.Y. 10017.

Metropolitan Life Insurance Company, 1 Madison Avenue, New York, N.Y. 10016.

National Board of Fire Underwriters, American Insurance Association, 85 John Street, New York, N.Y. 10038.

National Education Association, Safety Education Commission, 1201 16th Street, N.W., Washington, D.C. 20036. Materials: posters.

National Safety Council, Chicago, Ill. 60600

Prudential Insurance Company of America, Newark, N.J. 07100

Travelers Insurance Company, Hartford, Conn. 06100

U.S. Department of Health and Human Resources, Washington, D.C. 20000

Poison Precautions

American Medical Association, Department of Community Health and Health Education, 535 N. Dearborn Street, Chicago, Ill. 60610. Publication: *Dennis the Menace Takes a Poke at Poison.*

Food and Drug Administration, U.S. Department of Health and Human Resources, Washington, D.C.

Public Health Service, U.S. Department of Health, Education and Welfare, Division of Accident Prevention, Washington, D.C. 20201. Publication: *Teaching Poison Prevention in Kindergarten and Primary Grades.*

Recreation Safety

American Recreation Journal (American Recreation Society, Washington, D.C. 20000).

American Rifleman (National Rifle Association of America, Washington, D.C. 20000).

Journal of Health, Physical Education and Recreation (AAHPER, Washington, D.C. 20000).

Junior Red Cross Journal (American Red Cross, National Headquarters, Washington, D.C. 20006).

National Rifle Association Hunter Safety Handbook, NRA of America, Washington, D.C. 20000.

Free and Inexpensive Materials: National Recreation Association, National Safety Council, National Rifle Association.

Traffic and Pedestrian Safety

Aetna Life Affiliated Companies, Information and Education Department, 151 Farmington Avenue, Hartford, Conn. 06115. Materials: packet of free booklets on highway safety and films.

Allstate Insurance Company, Publication: *A Teenage Pattern.*

American Association for Health, Physical Education, and Recreation, 1201 16th Street, N.W., Washington, D.C. 20036. Publication: *Suggested School Safety Policies.*

American Association of Motor Vehicle Administrators, Washington, D.C.

American Automobile Association, 1712 G Street, Washington, D.C. 20006. Materials: "Driver Education Materials Kit."

American Medical Association, Department of Commercial Health and Health Education, Chicago, Ill. 60600.

American Red Cross, National Headquarters, Washington, D.C. 20006 (or local chapter).

American Trucking Associates, Inc., Public Relations Department, Washington, D.C. Materials: pamphlets.

Automotive Industries Highway Safety Committee, 2000 K Street, N.W., Washington, D.C. Materials: films and other resources.

Bicycle Institute of America

Center for Safety Education

DCA Educational Products Materials: transparencies. Defensive Driving Course, National Safety Council.

Ford Motor Company, Educational Affairs Department, The American Road,

Dearborn, Mich. 48121. Materials: automotive booklets, wall charts, and films.

General Motors Educational Aids (Driver Training Aids), General Motors Building, Detroit, Mich.

B.F. Goodrich Company, Akron, Ohio Publication: *Tommy Gets the Keys.*

Goodyear Tire and Rubber Company

Insurance Institute for Highway Safety, Washington, D.C. 20000.

Kemper Insurance Company, Chicago, Ill. 60600.

Keystone Automobile Club, Traffic Safety Department, 220 South Broad Street, Philadelphia, Pa. 19102.

Metropolitan Life Insurance Company, School Health Bureau, Health and Welfare Division, 1 Madison Avenue, New York, N.Y. 10016.

National Commission on Safety Education, NEA, 1201 16th Street, N.W., Washington, D.C. 20036.

Motor Cycle Scooter and Allied Trades Association.

National Safety Council, 444 N. Michigan Ave., Chicago, Ill. 60611.

Pennsylvania Department of Motor Vehicles, Traffic Safety Division, Harrisburg, Pa. 17101.

Pennsylvania Drivers Manual, Pennsylvania Department of Motor Vehicles, President's Committee on Traffic Safety, Washington, D.C.

Safety Education and Traffic Safety. Chicago, Ill.: National Safety Council.

Sports Illustrated Book of Safe Driving. Philadelphia: Lippincott, 1962.

Traveler's Insurance Company, Hartford, Conn. Publication: *A Tragedy of Errors.*

What Makes a Safe Driver. New York: William Frederick Press, 1971.

Preferred Resources Used in the Development of This Unit

Oliver E. Byrd. Health. Philadelphia: W.B. Saunders, 1961.

Harold Cornacchia, and Wesley Staton. *Health in Elementary Schools.* St. Louis: C.V. Mosby, 1974.

Course of Study in Health Education, K-3, 4-6, 7-9. Philadelphia: Division of Physical and Health Education, Philadelphia Public Schools, 1963.

Ruth Engs, and Molly Wantz. *Teaching Health Education in the Elementary School.* Houghton-Mifflin Co., 1978.

Fire Safety: A Resource Unit for Elementary Secondary Schools (curriculum guide). Milwaukee, Wis.: Milwaukee Public Schools, 1962.

Walter H. Greene, Frank H. Jenne, and Patricia M. Legas. *Health Education in the Elementary School.* New York: Macmillan Publishing Co., 1978.

Health Education Guide to Better Health. Olympia, Wash.: State Office of Public Instruction, 1976.

Health Education in Oregon Elementary Schools. Salem, Ore.: State Department of Education, 1975.

Health, Physical Education and Recreation: A Guide to Teaching. Minneapolis, Minn.: Minneapolis Public Schools, 1960.

Fred V. Hein and Dana L. Farnsworth. *Living,* Chicago: Scott, Foresman, 1965.

Bernice R. Moss, Southworth, and Reichert, eds. *Health Education.* Washington, D.C.: National Education Association, 1961.

Safety Education in the Elementary School. Harrisburg, Pa.: Commonwealth of Pennsylvania, 1960.

Safety Education in the Elementary Schools (curriculum guide). Philadelphia: Philadelphia Public Schools, 1972.

Justus J. Schifferes. *Healthier Living.* New York: John Wiley and Sons, 1970.

Walter D. Sorochan and Stephen J. Bender. *Teaching Elementary Health Science.* Reading, Mass.: Addison-Wesley Publishing Co., 1979.

Teaching Safety in the Elementary School. Washington, D.C.: American Association for Health, Physical Education, and Recreation, 1962.

Pedestrian Safety: A Resource Unit. Harrisburg, Pa.: Commonwealth of Pennsylvania, 1967.

Carl E. Willgoose. *Health Education in the Elementary Schools.* Philadelphia: W.B. Saunders, 1969.

CHAPTER **20**

Developing
a School
Emergency Program

As our society and environment become more complex, the chances of natural and man-made disasters increase. A necessary part of the school safety program is disaster preparedness.

EMERGENCY PLANNING

An emergency plan must be unique to each school system. The type of training necessary depends on the geographical location of the school and the likelihood of floods, blizzards, hurricanes, seismic sea waves, nuclear fallout, and so on in the area. Consequently, the school should develop the program in conjunction with local and state emergency services personnel, perhaps with the help of the following checklist.*

---

*Reprinted from *Emergency Planning for Oregon Schools* (Salem, Ore.: Oregon Board of Education, 1970). Authors recommend this publication as an excellent guideline.

Yes

1. Obtain a resolution from the local board of education. —
2. Appoint a school district disaster coordinator. —
3. Contact advisory personnel regarding development of plan. —
4. Correlate plan progress with local emergency operations plan. —
5. Compile information for plan into a written document. —
6. Review plan with local officials (civil defense, police and others). —
7. Obtain legal advice for school property in the event of disaster. —
8. Present plan to board of education for approval. —
9. Notify parents of plan. —
10. Have drill which is outlined in school disaster plan. —
    a. Evacuation of all persons according to plan. —
    b. Drill to occupy shelter area. —
    c. Evaluate drills for efficiency. —
11. Evaluate warning system when used in drills. —
12. Train teachers in disaster preparedness classes. —
13. Integrate training into curriculum. —

The first consideration in the development of a school emergency plan is its organization. To begin, the board of education should prepare a resolution giving the authority and support necessary to develop a school-disaster–readiness program. The next steps are the appointment of a coordinator and assignment of responsibilities to school personnel (the board of education, superintendent of schools, principals, teachers, nurses, nonteaching personnel, cafeteria managers and cooks, custodians and maintenance personnel, bussing personnel, and students). Appropriate personnel should draw up an inventory for the disaster plan (supplies, safety, protection, etc.) and establish objectives and classroom activities for the classroom instructional program.

Disaster plans should include the following possibilities:

1. Floods
2. Snow and blizzards
3. Earthquakes
4. Windstorms
5. Nuclear disasters
6. Civil disturbances
7. Bomb threats
8. Fires and explosions
9. School-sponsored field trips and outings

Following testing and approval by the board of education, the final plan should be publicized throughout the school system and in the community for best results. Periodic review of the disaster plan is necessary to insure continued effectiveness.

Regular evaluation of school safety conditions should be part of the emergency plan.

The following checklist outlines the direction this procedure should take.

Fire Precautions

1. Are fire drills held at scheduled irregular intervals?
2. Are records kept of all fire drills?
3. Is there a definite evacuation plan showing which exits and alternate routes of escape are to be used?

Fire Alarms

1. Is there a special fire alarm gong which can be heard in all parts of the school?
2. Is someone assigned to give the alarm immediately when a fire is discovered?
3. Is the school equipped with an automatic alarm system?
4. Do teachers and children know the signal?
5. Is there either an alarm box outside the school or is the school alarm connected to the fire department?
6. If not, is there a definite plan to call the fire department?

Exits

1. Do all doors open outward?
2. Are there two methods of escape from each floor?
3. Are doors to the exterior marked with EXIT lights?
4. Are doors that need to be locked equipped with emergency exit hardware?
5. Is there a sufficient number of exits (1 door 22 inches wide per each 100 pupils or 60 pupils if a stair exit)?

Waste Disposal

1. Is there a rubbish room with self-closing fire doors and automatic sprinklers?
2. Is waste collected daily?
3. Are old records and papers stored in steel cabinets?
4. Are shavings and sawdust from manual training rooms removed to rubbish room daily?

5. Are waste materials removed from school premises at least twice a week?
6. Are oily rags kept in an approved container?

Interior Finish

1. Is wood trim painted with a flame retardant paint?
2. If floors are of wood, has the use of sweeping compounds containing oils or oiled sawdust been discontinued?
3. Are corridor walls and ceiling of fire retardant construction?
4. Are lockers of steel construction?

Fire Holding Devices

1. If school is old or of a temporary nature, has a sprinkler system been installed?
2. Are there adequate fire extinguishers and are they inspected and recharged periodically?
3. Do the staff, teachers and older children know where they are and how to use extinguishers? (Remember—call the fire department before attempting to fight the fire.)
4. Are there fire hydrants just outside the school premises?
5. Is the stage equipped with a fire curtain and flameproofed drapery?

Stairways

1. Are the stairways enclosed to prevent upward spread of fire and smoke?
2. Are stairway doors self-closing and kept closed at all times?
3. Are doors that must be kept open held with automatic fire releasing devices and not wedges?
4. Are any stairway doors missing?

Heating Devices

1. Are benches on which devices are used covered with an incombustible surface?
2. Are heating devices using electricity (soldering irons, kilns, glue pots, etc.) outlets equipped with a pilot light to show when devices are in use?
3. Are extinguishers in vicinity of electrical heating devices (and electrical equipment) of a type approved for electrical fires?
4. Are boiler rooms kept free from rubbish and with no burnable materials near the boiler?

Safety Precautions

1. Does the school have a student safety committee with shop representatives serving on the committee?
2. Are medical records kept of each accident, no matter how trivial, so that corrective measures may be studied and taught?
3. Are safety precautions taught as an integral part of each vocational course?

Shops

1. Are students properly indoctrinated in the use of power equipment?
2. Do all power tools have a properly installed three-wire ground electrical system?
3. Are belts, blades, etc. of saws, drill presses, printing presses, planers, etc. provided with proper guards?
4. Are hand tools kept in sharp condition to avoid injury from unnecessary pressures?
5. Are solvents and toxic materials suitably labeled and kept in proper containers?
6. Are safety goggles provided for use at grinding wheels and re-melt pots?
7. Are aisles and floors kept clear and clean to avoid tripping hazards?
8. Are machines shut off when unattended?
9. Are high-voltage electrical control cabinets kept locked?

Home Economics

1. Are electrical machines (washers, etc.) properly grounded?
2. Are fire extinguishers in vicinity of cooking stoves of a type to fight grease fires?
3. Are exhaust hoods and fans cleaned at regular intervals?
4. Are pilot lights provided for electric irons?

Physical Education

1. Are safety rules enforced in the gymnasium and swimming pool to prevent injury from youthful exuberance?
2. Are vapor proof lights installed and maintained in locker and shower rooms?
3. Are safety walks installed leading to locker rooms from pool and showers?
4. Is damaged equipment removed promptly until repairs can be made?

5. Are lockers of steel construction rather than wood?
6. Is first-aid equipment kept by pool or in gymnasium?

FIRE SAFETY

In 1974, a total of 35,500 fires in schools and colleges cost Americans $124.8 million. Obviously the need for fire protection and organization is tremendous. Designated school personnel, in cooperation with the local fire department, should organize a fire protection program that takes into account building construction and materials storage.

Buildings design should provide for maximum traffic flow. Panic hardware belongs on all exits and exit signs should be illuminated and easily visible. Fire doors, extinguishers, and alarms should be in good working order and strategically located. A workable fire-evacuation program with which all school personnel are familiar is essential.

Stone et al. suggest that a fire evacuation plan should include the following provisions:

1. Careful training of all school personnel
2. Posted evacuation routes in all rooms
3. Assigned personnel to check that all school areas are cleared
4. A minimum of five fire drills per year (or satisfaction of state regulations)
5. Emphasis on school fire safety in early fall
6. Established exit rules that include no talking, single file, no pushing, and walking only
7. Fire drills that are announced, unannounced, and obstructed at unusual times
8. Planned analysis and discussion periods following each exit or disaster drill
9. Rooms given designated areas in which to assemble outside of the building where roll call can be taken
10. Coordination with the local fire department
11. No one may reenter the building until an appropriate reentry signal is given
12. Designated first aid and communication stations
13. Designated area for the meeting of fire drill monitors
14. All students and personnel participate in each drill.[1]

FIRST AID

Every school should have careful plans and procedures for the proper care of ill or injured students. It is advisable for all public school teachers to have first aid training that is at least equivalent to the American Red Cross standard first aid and safety course.

First Aid Responsibilities of the School

Planning and preparation for emergency care in case of sudden illness or accidental injury is the responsibility of the school administration. Administrators must establish and assign personnel responsibilities in advance in order for the plan to be effective. In addition, it is their responsibility to see that school personnel receive training in first aid procedures, that first aid equipment and supples are always available in the school, and that first aid policies are acceptable to and understood by school personnel and parents. All first aid policies should have the approval of the local medical society.

The main objective of emergency care in schools, then, is to provide adequate facilities and properly trained personnel to handle emergencies. The American Medical Association points out that schools are not medical resources, so any medical treatment should be temporary and only on an emergency basis. Usually, the administration of medication by school personnel is unwise. School personnel who abide by the approved first aid policies should not have to worry about legal entanglements!

The main responsibilities of school personnel in emergency first-aid situations are:

1. Properly administer urgently necessary first aid.
2. Notify the parents of the victim.
3. Make certain the victim is placed in the care of parents or a physician designated by the parents. (Never send sick children home by themselves.)

A good asset to the emergency care program in a school is a first aid room equipped with functional first-aid supplies. All school personnel should know how to treat the following emergencies:

1. Airway is closed.
2. Breathing ceases or becomes inadequate (includes choking).
3. Circulation of blood stops because of heart failure or an open wound is causing loss of blood.
4. Poisoning occurs from drugs, contaminated food, acid or alkali, petroleum products, or the like.
5. Shock results from a forceful blow, emotional reaction, diabetic reaction, blood loss, or the like.
6. Sudden illness develops.
7. Epileptic seizure occurs.

8. Bone fracture is evident.
9. Burns occur from chemicals, hot flames, boiling water or steam, electricity, or the like.

Remember that first aid is emergency care and does *not* include care for injuries or illnesses after the victim has received medical aid. When administering first aid, keep in mind the following points:

1. The victim may suffer further injury through improper emergency care, so take the time necessary to prepare and plan well.
2. In many cases the failure to receive proper emergency care can result in permanent damage and even death.
3. The first-aider should know what *not* to do, as well as what to do.
4. Any victim of an accident or illness needs a quick but thorough exam, performed as follows:
   a. Start at the head. Make sure the victim is breathing and check the victim's heart pulse by feeling the carotid arteries in the neck with two fingers (not the thumbs). If there is profuse bleeding, use direct pressure to control it. Check the pupils of the eyes for any noticeable abnormality. Run your hands gently around the scalp for any indentations, lumps, or cuts. Any indentation or soft, mushy-feeling lump is dangerous and needs immediate medical attention.
   b. Carefully and gently feel the neck and spinal column to ascertain any fractured vertebrae. If you suspect a fractured or twisted vertebra, *do not move* the victim. Keep the head and neck in alignment and wait for the ambulance or for a physician to take over.
   c. Check the chest and abdomen for any indentations, cuts, or rigid areas in the abdomen, which may signify internal injuries.
   d. Finally, check the arms and legs for any cuts or fractures.

Specific First Aid

Breathing Stoppage

Oxygen is necessary for energy production by the body's cells. Without oxygen, the cells begin to die within four to six minutes.

People stop breathing under any of a number of circumstances. One common cause is the blockage of the trachea (windpipe) entrance by a large piece of food or candy or some other mechanical object, such as a coin. Various methods will dislodge the obstruction from the throat. If the victim is lying down, turn him or her on the side and administer a thump or slap between the shoulder blades.

FIGURE 20-1. *Use of the Heimlich maneuver on a choking victim.*

The victim of food choking:

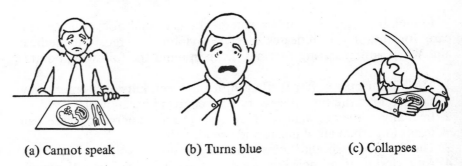

(a) Cannot speak   (b) Turns blue   (c) Collapses

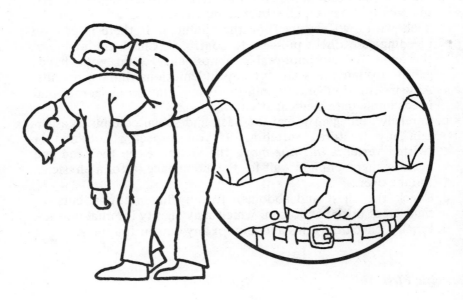

Another very effective method is the *Heimlich maneuver.* Figure 20-1 illustrates choking symptoms and the use of the Heimlich maneuver to force the obstruction from the throat.

Other reasons that people stop breathing include drowning, electrical shock, gas poisoning, strangulation, and drug overdose. If an individual stops breathing, you can artificially ventilate the lungs by artificial respiration. The most efficient and practical method is mouth-to-mouth or mouth-to-nose resuscitation. The following directions will guide you through this procedure.

Objectives

1. To maintain an open airway through the mouth and nose (or through the *stoma,* an opening made through the neck to the windpipe through which a person breathes when normal breathing is not possible).
2. To restore breathing by maintaining an alternating increase and decrease in the expansion of the chest.

General Information

1. The average person may die in six minutes or less without oxygen. It is often impossible to tell exactly when a person has stopped breathing; death may be very near by the time you come upon the scene. Therefore, always start artificial respiration as rapidly as possible.
2. Recovery is usually rapid except in cases of carbon monoxide poisoning, drug overdose, and electrical shock. In these cases it is often necessary to continue artificial respiration for a long time.
3. When a victim revives, administer treatment for shock. A physician's care is necessary during the recovery period.
4. Always continue artificial respiration until:
    a. The victim begins to breathe again.
    b. You become exhausted and cannot continue.
    c. A doctor pronounces the victim dead.

Mouth-to-mouth (Mouth-to-nose) Method

1. Tilt the victim's head backward so that the chin is pointing upward.
    a. In this supine position, an unconscious patient's tongue may drop back and block the throat. To open the air passage, place one hand beneath the victim's neck and lift. Place the heel of the other hand on the victim's forehead and rotate or tilt the head backward into the maximum extension position shown in Figure 20–2.
    b. For mouth-to-mouth ventilation, maintain the head in this position, because it clears the airway by keeping the tongue away from the back of the victim's throat. If a greater opening is necessary, thrust the lower jaw forward into a jutting-out position—the jaw-thrust method.
2. Pinch the victim's nostrils shut with the thumb and index finger of the hand that you are pressing on the victim's forehead. This action prevents air from escaping through the nose while you are

FIGURE 20-2. *Tilt back the head of a nonbreathing, unconscious patient to prevent the tongue from obstructing the throat during mouth-to-mouth resuscitation. (Redrawn from* Standard First Aid and Personal Safety *Copyright © 1973 by the American National Red Cross. Reproduced with permission.)*

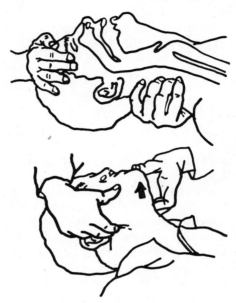

inflating the lungs through the mouth (see Figure 20-3). (Another way is to press your cheek against the victim's nose.)
3. Blow air into the victim's mouth.
   a. Open your mouth widely.
   b. Take a deep breath.
   c. Seal your mouth tightly around the victim's mouth and, with your mouth forming a wide-open circle, exhale into the mouth, as shown in Figure 20-4.
   d. Provide sufficient air. Volume is important. Start at a high rate and then provide at least one breath every five seconds for adults (or twelve per minute).
   e. If the airway is clear, you will feel only moderate resistance to the air pressure.
4. Watch for the victim's chest to rise.
5. Stop respiring when the victim's chest is expanded; raise your mouth; turn your head to the side and listen for the victim to exhale.

FIGURE 20-3. *During mouth-to-mouth resuscitation, keep the patient's nostrils closed. (Redrawn from* Standard First Aid and Personal Safety. *Copyright © 1973 by The American National Red Cross. Reproduced with permission.)*

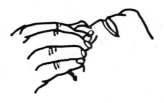

FIGURE 20-4. *Mouth-to-mouth resuscitation. (Redrawn from* Standard First Aid and Personal Safety. *Copyright © 1973 by The American National Red Cross. Reproduced with permission.)*

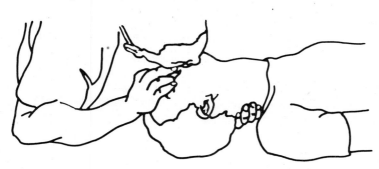

6. Watch the chest to see that it falls (see Figure 20–5).
7. Repeat the resuscitation cycle.
8. For the mouth-to-nose method, maintain the backward head tilt with your hand on the victim's forehead. Use your other hand to close the victim's mouth. Open your mouth widely, take a deep breath, seal your mouth tightly around the victim's nose, and blow into the victim's nose. During the exhalation phase, open the victim's mouth to allow air to escape. *Note:* For small children and infants administer mouth-to-mouth or mouth-to-nose resuscitation as described above, but do not tilt the head as far back as you would for adults or large children. Seal off both the mouth and nose of the infant or small child with your mouth. Blow into the child's mouth and nose every three seconds (about twenty breaths per minute) with less pressure and volume than you would use for an adult, the amount depending on the size of the child. Very small puffs of air will suffice for infants (see Figure 20–6).

FIGURE 20-5. *Listen for the patient to exhale. (Redrawn from* Standard First Aid and Personal Safety. *Copyright © 1973 by The American National Red Cross. Reproduced with permission.)*

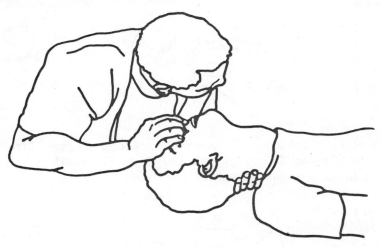

FIGURE 20-6. *Reviving an infant who has stopped breathing. (Redrawn from* Standard First Aid and Personal Safety. *Copyright © 1973 by The American National Red Cross. Reproduced with permission.)*

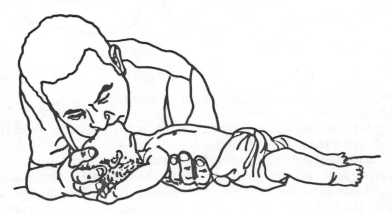

9. If you are not getting air exchange, be certain the position of the head and jaw is correct, and check again for foreign matter in the back of the mouth that may be obstructing the air passage.
10. If foreign matter is preventing ventilation, as a last resort, turn the victim on the side and administer sharp blows between the shoulder blades to jar the material free. You may suspend a child momentarily by the ankles or turn him or her upside down over

one arm and give two or three sharp blows between the shoulder blades. Wipe any obvious foreign matter from the mouth with a "sweeping" motion of the forefinger.

11. Clear the mouth again, reposition, and repeat mouth-to-mouth or mouth-to-nose respiration. If the victim's stomach is bulging, air may have gone into the stomach, particularly if the air passage is obstructed or the pressure of inflation is excessive. Although inflation of the stomach is not dangerous, it may make lung ventilation more difficult and it increases the likelihood of vomiting. If the stomach is bulging, turn the victim's head to one side and be prepared to clear the mouth before pressing your hand briefly and firmly over the upper abdomen, between the rib margin and the navel. This procedure will force air out of the stomach, but it may also cause regurgitation.

Some persons who require artificial respiration never stop breathing completely, but gasp irregularly. Efforts toward breathing assist in recovery, but they should not encourage you to abandon mouth-to-mouth resuscitation until a normal pattern of respiration has returned. Coordinate blowing with the victim's inhalation.

Mouth-to-stoma Method

1. About 25,000 Americans have had their larynxes completely or partially removed by surgery. The operation is called a *laryngectomy*. Those who have had the operation are *laryngectomees*. A laryngectomee breathes through an opening called a *stoma* in the trachea in the front of the neck; neither the nose nor the mouth function for breathing (see Figure 20–7).

2. First aid for laryngectomees:
   a. When examining a victim of an accident or sudden illness, check the front of the neck to determine if the victim is a laryngectomee. (Most laryngectomees carry a card or other identification stating that they cannot breathe through the nose or mouth.)
   b. Do not inadvertently block the stoma when carrying out other first aid. The sound of escaping air, especially in combination with postinjury secretions or blood flow in the neck area, may mislead the first-aider to conclude that the injury constitutes a sucking wound of the chest and may thus attempt to block the stoma with a pressure dressing. Blockage is dangerous because it could cause death from asphyxiation.
   c. Give artificial respiration using the same general procedure as for mouth-to-mouth resuscitation, but place your mouth firmly over the victim's stoma. Exhale at the same rate as you would

FIGURE 20-7. *In a laryngectomee, an artificial opening, or stoma, in the neck permits breathing.* (*Redrawn from* Standard First Aid and Personal Safety. *Copyright © 1973 by The American National Red Cross. Reproduced with permission.*)

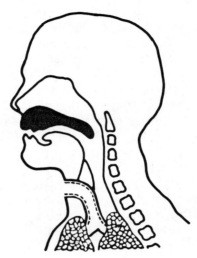

if the victim normally breathed through the nose or mouth and watch the victim's chest for inflow of air.

   d. Keep the victim's head straight. It is not necessary to tilt the head backward and to close off the victim's head and mouth.

   e. Avoid twisting the victim's head. Twisting might change the shape of or close the stoma.

   f. Do not worry about the victim's tongue or dentures blocking the airway.

   g. If the laryngectomy was partial instead of complete, the person breathes both through the stoma and the mouth and nose. If the stoma is clear and the victim's chest does not rise when you blow into the stoma, tilt the victim's head back, close off the mouth and nose, and continue the respiration efforts through the stoma (see Figure 20–8).

3. Advantages of the mouth-to-stoma method:

   a. The mouth-to-stoma approach is more sanitary than mouth-to-mouth resuscitation because air coming from the stoma is cleaner than air coming from the mouth. Also, the contents of the laryngectomee's stomach will not spill into the first-aider's mouth because there is no connection between the stomach and the stoma.

   b. The mouth-to-stoma method is preferable to a manual method because it is much more effective. The use of the Silvester

FIGURE 20-8. *Resuscitation of a laryngectomee. (Redrawn from* Standard First Aid and Personal Safety. *Copyright © 1973 by The American National Red Cross. Reproduced with permission.)*

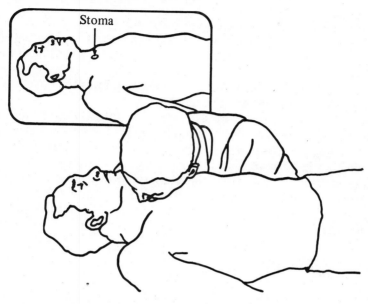

method is justifiable only when the only first-aider available is also a laryngectomee.

Chest Pressure-arm Lift Method (Silvester Method)

The Silvester method is known as a manual method. A manual method of resuscitation is *not recommended* unless mouth-to-mouth resuscitation is impossible because the rescuer is a laryngectomee or the victim has massive facial injuries that make the mouth-to-mouth approach very inefficient.

1. If foreign matter is visible in the victim's mouth, wipe it out quickly with your fingers, preferably with a cloth wrapped around them.
2. Place the victim in a face-up position. Maintain an open airway by placing something under the victim's shoulders to raise them several inches and allowing the head to drop backward. Turn the head to the side. A second helper, if present, should lift the lower jaw or maintain the head in a backward-tilt position.
3. Kneel at the top of the victim's head, grasp the wrists, and cross them over the lower chest.

4. Rock forward until your arms are approximately vertical and allow the weight of the upper part of your body to exert steady, even pressure downward. This action will cause air to flow out of the victim's chest.
5. Immediately release the pressure by rocking back, pulling the victim's arms outward and upward over the head and backward as far as possible (see Figure 20–9). This procedure should cause air to flow in.
6. Repeat this cycle about twelve times per minute, checking the victim's mouth often for obstruction.
7. There is always danger of aspirating vomitus, blood, or blood clots. You can reduce the likelihood of this hazard by keeping the victim's head a little lower than the trunk. A helper should pull the victim's jaw forward and up and be alert to detect the presence of any stomach contents in the victim's mouth. Keep the victim's mouth as clean as possible at all times. Remove any airway obstruction, as described in the technique for mouth-to-mouth breathing.

FIGURE 20-9. *The Silvester method of resuscitation, to be used only when other approaches are impossible. (Redrawn from* Standard First Aid and Personal Safety. *Copyright © 1973 by The American National Red Cross. Reproduced with permission.)*

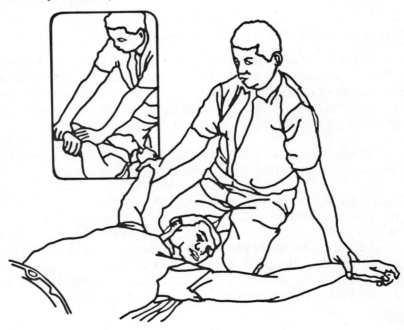

Heart Failure

It is quite unlikely that an elementary student will experience heart failure, but adult school personnel may. Heart failure occurs when the heart does not receive enough blood and consequently lacks sufficient oxygen and nutrients to supply its muscles. In this situation, the heart muscle quits functioning. If much of the heart muscle ceases operation, the whole heart may stop.

The method of artificially circulating oxygenated blood by squeezing and compressing the heart between the sternum (breastbone) and the backbone and giving mouth-to-mouth resuscitation is known as *cardiopulmonary resuscitation*. Unless done properly and practiced often, (on a mannequin), however, this technique can prove more harmful to the victim than it is helpful. Elementary school teachers should contact the local chapter of the American Heart Association for this training.

Bleeding

Serious hemorrhage or bleeding is classed as one of the three kinds of first aid emergency (the other two are absence of breathing and poisoning), because a victim can bleed to death in three minutes or less. Shock and loss of consciousness may result from the rapid loss of even a quart of blood. For this reason, prompt action is essential.

The most efficient way to control bleeding is to elevate the wound and apply direct pressure on the wound with your hand over a dressing. A last resort to stem uncontrolled bleeding is the tourniquet. This technique is potentially dangerous and should be used only in cases of severe, uncontrolled hemorrhage that defy control by the other methods. The American Red Cross warns that "the decision to apply a tourniquet is in reality a decision to risk sacrifice of a limb in order to save life."[2]

A tourniquet should be at least two inches wide. It is placed above the wound, wrapped tightly around the limb twice and tied in a half-knot. Then, after placing a strong, short stick or similar object on the overhand knot, the rescuer ties two additional overhand knots on top of the stick, twists the stick until the bleeding has stopped, and then secures the stick in place. The rescuer writes down the time of tourniquet application where it will not be lost and sees that the tourniquet remains in place until the victim is with a physician.

A thick cloth dressing held between the hand and the wound helps to control bleeding by absorbing the blood and allowing the blood to clot. When the bleeding is under control, the soaked bandage should remain in place and another added if it seems desirable.

FIGURE 20-10. *Pressure point technique for controlling excessive bleeding. (Redrawn from* Standard First Aid and Personal Safety. *Copyright © 1973 by The American National Red Cross. Reproduced with permission.)*

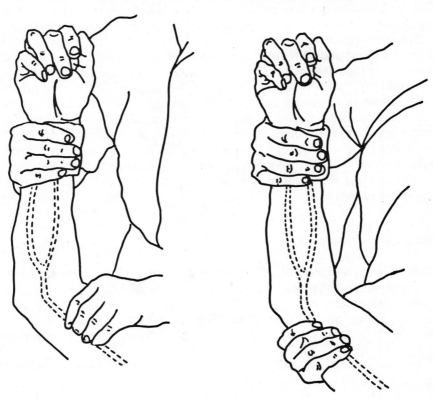

Removing the first dressing may disturb blood clots. The rescuer should hold the dressings in place with a pressure bandage that is firm enough to sustain direct pressure on the wound but not so tight as to cut off circulation. A pulse should be evident below the bandage and skin color will indicate whether the bandage is too tight.

If severe bleeding from an open wound in the arm or leg fails to stop after application of direct pressure and elevation, compression of the supplying artery against underlying bone may be necessary. This method, known as the *pressure point technique* (see Figure 20-10), should be used in conjunction with elevation and direct pressure.

Nosebleed

One of the most common experiences of children is a nosebleed. Nosebleeds call for the following procedures:

1. Place the child in a sitting position with the head slightly tilted forward.
2. Have the child blow all clots and blood from the nose.
3. Into the bleeding nostril place a piece of cotton moistened with cold water or hydrogen peroxide. (Make sure part of the packing remains outside the nostril so the child will not "sniff" the packing into the nostril.
4. Apply firm pressure by pressing the bleeding nostril against the middle partition of the nose for ten minutes.
5. Apply cold packs externally.
6. If the nosebleed persists or if the child has frequent nosebleeds, contact the parents and advise medical care.

Poisoning

Any substance that impairs health or causes death when introduced into or onto the surface of the body is called a *poison*. Poisons can be inhaled, ingested, injected, and absorbed. They may depress, stimulate, irritate, corrode, and otherwise injure body tissues.

The symptoms of poisoning vary greatly. Some of the general symptoms are nausea, stomach cramps, vomiting, burns around the mouth and lips, diarrhea, breath odor, and contraction of eye pupils to the size of a pin point. Table 20–1 explains what to do in the event of poisoning.

Shock

Shock is a condition that results from the depression of certain vital body functions. Causes of shock include trauma to the body and

TABLE 20–1. First Aid for a Poisoning Victim

You Do Not Know What the Poison Is	You Know that the Poison Is Not a Strong Acid, Alkali, or Petroleum Product
Dilute the poison with water or milk.	Dilute the poison with water or milk.
Try to find out from the victim, a container, or some other source, what the poison was.	Induce vomiting (use Ipecac, raw egg, tickle back of throat).
Get medical aid immediately (poison control center, paramedics).	Get medical aid immediately.

In all cases watch respiration and other vital functions closely and take appropriate action should problems arise.

consequent bleeding, severe infection, drug overdose, lack of oxygen, insulin excess, and many other mishaps. Because pain, delay of treatment, and rough handling may increase the severity of shock, it is important for teachers to be able to recognize shock and to know what first aid measures to give.

In the early stages of shock development, the body compensates for poor blood circulation by constricting blood flow to the peripheral areas of the body (skin, skeletal muscles, soft tissues). This action produces the following body signs:

1. The skin may be cool and clammy and may look pale or bluish. If the victim has dark skin, check the color under the eyelids, in nail beds, or in the mucous membranes on the inside of the mouth.
2. The victim will feel weak, faint, and probably nauseated.
3. The heart pulse will probably be weak and rapid. Check it at the carotid artery in the neck.
4. Breathing will be quickened and shallow or possibly deep and irregular.
5. The victim may appear restless and anxious and may complain of severe thirst.
6. In the later stages, the eyes may appear sunken and the expression vacant, and the skin may be blotchy as well.

Shock is a serious condition that may result in death. Proper first aid, as detailed in the following steps, is essential.

1. Take care of any urgently necessary first aid (e.g., restore breathing, stop bleeding, relieve severe pain).
2. Lay the victim in a supine position or, if there is any bleeding or vomiting, on the side. Raise the feet eight to twelve inches. (If this makes the victim uncomfortable, lower them again.)
3. Maintain the victim's body temperature at as normal a level as possible. Give water to drink if you do not suspect internal injuries and if the victim is not nauseated.

Sudden Illness

Sometimes an acute illness or a crisis in a chronic illness will create a sudden need for first aid. When these crises are not serious or long-lasting, teachers can give immediate, effective aid. For example, nosebleeds, fainting, and headache are easy to handle. More serious illnesses, such as heart attack and stroke, require quick and safe transportation of the victim to immediate medical attention. Here we shall discuss only the less serious sudden illnesses.

Fainting

Fainting is the loss of some degree of consciousness because of an acute reduction in the brain's blood supply. The signs and symptoms of a person about to faint include:

1. Extreme paleness and sweaty coolness of the skin
2. Dizziness and accompanying nausea
3. Numbness and tingling of the hands and feet

If a person complains of feeling faint, suggest lying down for a while. The first aid for a simple fainting episode is as follows:

1. Try to catch the victim before he or she collapses so the head will not be injured.
2. Lay the victim in a supine or sideways position and loosen any tight clothing. If vomiting occurs, roll the victim on the side and clean the mouth of vomitus.
3. Make sure the airway remains open and the victim is breathing.
4. Take care of any injuries that may have occurred during a fall.
5. Give the victim ample time to recover normal respiration and heartbeat.
6. If recovery is not prompt or if the fainting attacks continue, seek medical attention for the victim.

Convulsions

Many elementary school teachers know nothing about convulsions and consequently fear them. It is important to understand what a convulsion is and what measures to take when it occurs.

A convulsion is the result of excessive electrochemical activity in the central nervous system. Messages are sent to muscle groups that cause them to contract. The amount of messages sent varies according to the stimuli. Hence, the degree and seriousness of convulsions also varies.

Convulsions may be associated with brain injury, infectious diseases, brain tumors, abscesses, and hemorrhage. A very small child may experience a convulsion during a high fever or gastrointestinal illness. The most common type of convulsion experienced by school-children, however, is an epileptic seizure.

It is important for teachers to read the school records of every child and note medical problems such as epilepsy. A discussion with parents of an epileptic child at the start of the school year is imperative. Find out if the child is on medication and has had recent convulsions. Make sure you know whom to contact if a convulsion does occur.

The signs and symptoms of a convulsion vary from brief twitching of muscles and momentary loss of contact with the environment to rigidity of skeletal muscles followed by jerking movements. The face and lips may turn a bluish or greyish color and the victim may drool from the mouth. The victim may severely bite his tongue, lose control of the bladder and bowel, and possibly stop breathing.

Before administering first aid to a convulsed individual, or any other individual, be sure you know what not to do as well as what to do. First aid for convulsions comprises the following steps:

1. Do *not* restrain or hold the victim down.
2. Do *not* force any object into the victim's mouth. If the victim's mouth is open you may insert something soft (e.g., a handkerchief) between the teeth.
3. Do *not* place the victim in a tub of water.

The following procedures will aid in successful treatment:

1. Try to interrupt the victim's fall to prevent injury.
2. Move objects that the victim might thrash against.
3. Loosen any clothing around the neck.
4. Turn the victim on the side if secretions interfere with breathing.
5. If breathing stops, give mouth-to-mouth resuscitation.
6. Calmly reassure the victim after the convulsion has subsided.
7. If the victim is fatigued after the convulsion, a nap of several hours is advisable.

Preparing the class beforehand, if possible, is almost as important as proper first aid for the victim. Do not allow people to crowd around and stare during the convulsion. Above all, protect the victim from embarrassment.

Sprains and Fractures

Playground and in-school accidents may cause injury to the skeletal system and accompanying tissues. One of the most common injuries of this type is the sprain. A *sprain* is an injury to a joint ligament or a muscle tendon in the region of a joint. In addition, blood vessels and other tissues in the immediate area may stretch or tear. The signs of a sprain include immediate swelling, discoloration, tenderness, and pain upon motion. If you suspect a student has sprained an ankle, do not allow walking. If possible, remove the shoe and sock, cover the ankle with a thin towel to protect the skin, and apply a small bag of crushed ice or cold, wet packs to the sprained joint. Do *not* pack the joint in ice, and *do not* immerse

FIGURE 20-11. *Two types of bone fractures. (Redrawn from* Standard First Aid and Personal Safety. *Copyright © 1973 by The American National Red Cross. Reproduced with permission.)*

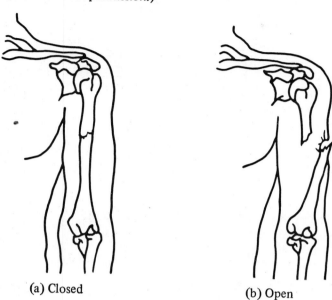

(a) Closed   (b) Open

the injured joint in ice water. After the cold treatment, the child should keep the injured joint raised for at least twenty-four hours. If your responsibility is only to safely transport the victim of a sprained ankle to the school nurse and not to treat the injury, lossen the shoelace, apply a pillow or blanket splint, and elevate the victim's leg to combat swelling. If a sprain victim complains of swelling and pain a few days after the accident, arrange to have the joint x-rayed for a possible closed fracture.

A *fracture* is a bone break. It may be either open or closed (see Figure 20-11). Signs and symptoms of a fracture include the following:

1. The victim heard or felt a bone snap or break.
2. The victim has trouble moving the injured part and complains of pain and tenderness.
3. The victim reports feeling the broken bone ends rubbing together (grating).
4. You may be able to see an obvious deformity or differences in length and shape of corresponding bones.

As soon as you suspect that a fracture has occurred, send someone to call for an ambulance. Do not move the victim unless there is

FIGURE 20-12. *Before moving a person whose leg is broken, tie the broken leg to the other leg. (Redrawn from* Standard First Aid and Personal Safety. *Copyright © 1973 by The American National Red Cross. Reproduced with permission.)*

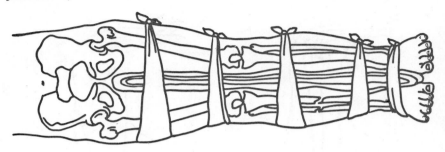

further danger. Keep the injured parts and adjacent joints still. If you have to move the victim, take time to splint the appendage, bind an injured arm to the individual's chest or side, or tie an injured leg to the uninjured one (see Figure 20–12).

It is best to make the victim as comfortable as possible and elevate the involved area, if possible, without disturbing the suspected fracture. If an open fracture has occurred, cover the bone ends and the torn tissue with large sterile dressings and use direct pressure to control the bleeding. Always treat a fracture victim for shock and bring a doctor, nurse, or ambulance to the scene.

If you suspect a fractured neck or back, keep the victim perfectly still. Make sure the victim is breathing and has a heart beat, and keep the head and neck in alignment. Do *not* allow the head to move from side to side. If it is absolutely necessary to move the victim before medical help arrives, use enough helpers (four or five) to lift the victim without any body movement and place the victim on a large, rigid door or stretcher. Keep one person at the victim's head and stabilize the victim on the rigid stretcher. Remember that one wrong move may permanently paralyze or even kill the victim.

Another dangerous injury is skull fracture. Signs and symptoms include a blow to the head, an indentation of the skull, bleeding from the nose and ear, headache with dizziness and vomiting, eye pupils of unequal size, a pale or flushed face, convulsions, and loss of bowel and bladder control.

In the event of a suspected skull fracture, call for an ambulance equipped with oxygen. Keep the victim lying flat and still. Try to maintain normal body temperature. Make sure the victim has an open airway and is breathing. Put a small padding (pillow or coat) under the victim's head and shoulders. Take care of any bleeding, record the extent and duration of unconsciousness, and keep the victim completely still until medical assistance arrives.

FIGURE 20-13. *Treatment for a first-degree burn. (Redrawn from* Standard First Aid and Personal Safety. *Copyright © 1973 by The American National Red Cross. Reproduced with permission.)*

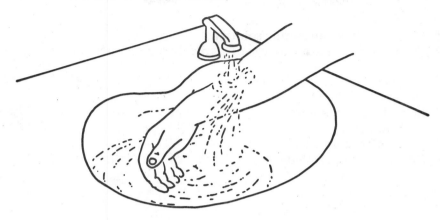

Burns

Chemical agents, radiation, and heat can burn body tissue. Burns are classified according to the severity of injury: reddened skin is a first-degree burn, blistered skin is a second-degree burn, and deeper tissue destruction is a third-degree burn.

The first aid for a burn depends on the degree of damage. For first-degree burns, submerge the burn in cold water and, if necessary, apply a dry dressing (see Figure 20–13). For second-degree burns, submerge the burned area in cold water until the pain subsides, gently blot dry, and cover with a dry, sterile dressing. Do not break any blisters and do not apply *any* medication to the burn. Elevate the area if it is on an appendage and make sure the victim sees a doctor. For a third-degree burn, do not touch the area or remove adhered particles of charred clothing. Cover with thick, sterile dressing or freshly laundered linen. Treat the victim for shock and get medical aid as quickly as possible.

A Brief First Aid Review and Guide

Principals, teachers, nurses, and other school personnel should administer first aid to students or others who need it according to the procedures outlined in this section. Except in cases of very minor injury, notify the family immediately and advise them to secure medical supervision. Teachers and other school personnel should immediately inform the principal of accidents.

The simple first aid procedures that follow correspond to American Red Cross procedures, but before adopting them, have the local county health officer edit and approve them.

Care of Minor Cuts and Scratches

1. Cleanse with an antiseptic solution.
2. Cover with adhesive bandage or sterile dressing, if necessary.

Minor Burns

1. Immediately immerse in cold water and soak for approximately ten minutes.
2. Cover with sterile dressing.
3. *Do not* apply petroleum jelly or grease of any kind.

Wounds

1. Cover with sterile gauze and secure with bandage or adhesive tape.
2. Do not change dressings unless you have written direction to do so from the family physician.

Bites

1. Animal bites:
   a. Wash the wound with soap and clean water. Hold under running water for five minutes.
   b. Apply dressing and call the doctor immediately.
   c. Report to your local county health department (sanitation division) and give description of the animal. If possible, confine the animal but do not kill it.
2. Insect bite:
   a. Remove stinger if it remains in the wound, but do not squeeze the poison sack attached to the end of the stinger.
   b. Apply a compress of aromatic spirits of ammonia, alcohol, or a paste of baking soda.
   c. Watch for generalized allergic reaction, such as hives and swelling of the throat. If severe swelling occurs, urge immediate care. (See pp. 369–375.)

Nosebleed

1. Have the patient sit with head titled slightly *forward.* Avoid exertion such as coughing, talking, or blowing nose.
2. Apply firm pressure to side of nose that is bleeding and maintain for ten minutes.

3. If nosebleed persists, refer to family for medical care.
4. Refer a child who often has nosebleeds to the nurse.

Shock

1. Gently lay patient down so that the *head is level with the rest of the body.*
2. In case of a chest or head injury or difficult breathing, elevate head and shoulders slightly.
3. Keep the person from chilling.
4. *Never attempt to give fluids to an unconscious person.*

Bleeding

1. Cover wound with sterile (if possible) or clean dressing or cloth and apply direct pressure with hand or fingers. Continue pressure until bleeding has stopped. This procedure may take ten to thirty minutes.
2. If blood soaks through dressing, *do not remove it,* but apply more dressing. Bandage firmly to continue pressure.
3. Reassure patient and keep calm.
4. Call doctor, ambulance, or person experienced in first aid.
5. *Do not apply a tourniquet* unless the loss of the limb is inevitable.

Fractures and Dislocations

1. Do not move the patient. Be sure all students and teachers are so advised.
2. Make the patient comfortable. Keep the patient warm and send for doctor, ambulance, or person trained in first aid.

Sprains

1. Elevate the injured area.
2. Apply an ice pack or cold cloth for twenty-five minutes right after injury.
3. If swelling is unusual, do not allow use of injured joint until after a physician has treated it.

Respiration Difficulty

Start mouth-to-mouth artificial respiration immediately. The most important lifesaving action is to get air into the person's lungs quickly.

1. Lay the patient down and quickly loosen clothing about neck and chest.
2. Clear the mouth and throat of foreign objects.
3. Tilt the head back with the jaws jutting out to allow free air passage.
4. Place your mouth directly over the patient's mouth and pinch the patient's nostrils closed to form a seal. Exhale.
5. Timing is important. Breathe steadily at approximately twenty breaths per minute for children and ten to twelve per minute for adults.
6. Always take a deep breath before blowing into a patient's mouth. This act guarantees a greater supply of oxygen.
7. *Do not exhale entire breath* into person's mouth. Blow with a "huff"—just enough to make the chest rise. Do not force air into children's lungs too hard or too fast. *Caution:* If stomach inflates and chest does not rise with each breath, stop and check airway to find out why air is not getting into the lungs.
8. Continue artificial respiration without interruption until person has started breathing naturally or until at least two hours have passed without a sign of life.
9. As soon as possible after the person has started breathing without assistance or when help is available, make the patient comfortable, prevent chilling, and treat for shock.

Priorities in Treatment for Severe Accidents

1. Control bleeding.
2. Restore breathing.
3. Treat for shock.
4. Splint fractured bones.
5. Move the person only when absolutely necessary after performing the preceding steps as required.

ACCIDENT FORMS

It is the principal's responsibility to fill out all school district accident forms in duplicate. One copy should go to the safety office. The other belongs in the school office files.

NOTES

1. Donald B. Stone, Lawrence B. O'Reilly, and James D. Brown, *Elementary School Health Education* (Dubuque, Iowa: Wm. C. Brown Co., 1976), p. 189.
2. The American National Red Cross, *Advanced First Aid and Emergency Care* (Garden City, N.Y.: Doubleday, 1973), pp. 36-37.

CHAPTER 21
School
Health Services

For many years educators have seen that some parents neglect their responsibility to send their children to school healthy. Children do not come to school free of health problems. Minor and major ill health problems can affect students' educations, and therefore, it is necessary for the school to take some responsibility for the main-tenance of their good health.

Teachers have a large influence on the youngsters with whom they come in contact. The primary responsibility for a child's health rests with the parents. The role of the teachers and the schools is to supple-ment parental care. Students who do not receive good health care or instruction at home are dependent on teachers and schools to give them every chance for success in life.

The job of the "health services" part of the school health program includes these responsibilities:

1. Examine each student for health problems.
2. Promote the health of each student.
3. Protect the health of each student.
4. Help each student learn to maintain good health.

The main health-service role of the teacher is to look for health problems and refer or send the information to proper authorities.

Teachers see students every day and therefore should be able to spot changes in appearance, behavior, and emotions that are not normal and may indicate that something is wrong with the student's health. To be sure that students who show signs of illness receive the best care, teachers should advise them and their parents to see a physician or refer the students to the school health nurse or physician. Follow-up procedures will confirm that students who need it receive help for specific health problems.

Health problems of students fall into four main groups:

1. Physiological problems, such as vision, hearing, dental, and postural problems
2. Metabolic problems, such as diabetes and obesity
3. Central nervous system disorders, such as epilepsy
4. Communicable diseases, such as measles and influenza, and allergies, such as plant pollen allergies.

Each type of health problem has characteristic signs and symptoms. Teachers should learn to recognize the signs and symptoms of common health problems and then observe their students closely:

1. At the beginning of the year
2. At different times of the day
3. Under different play and work situations

The clues to existing health problems will come from physical or personal appearance, behavior, and vocalized complaints from the student. If the same clue persists for a period of time, the student may have a health problem. It is wise to get as much help as possible to find any health problems among students. Doctors, nurses, dentists, or other medical helpers will come into the school to do different types of health screening. In some states, general student assessment and health screening programs are mandatory.

A general health assessment usually accompanies entrance into the school system. The children take home a health history sheet for their parents and family physicians to fill out for the information of the school nurse, who reviews it and discusses it with the students and parents if appropriate. Then the school nurse usually checks children's height and weight and notes the status of the skeletal system and the body type; postural deviations sometimes show up as early as kindergarten. Minimal testing for hand-eye coordination, poor nutritional manifestations, speech difficulties, and lateral dominance are all part of the first health examination.

Following this first examination, children undergo routine screening exams, which usually conform to government regulations. Vision testing is required at the first enrollment and at intervals of three or four years thereafter. Hearing screening conventionally takes place at enrollment and then at grades two, five, eight, and ten, although the pattern is not absolute. To enhance communicable disease prevention and control, health services personnel distribute information on prevention and immunizations. At the beginning of each year teachers receive information on the identification of the early symptoms of communicable diseases, and learn the proper procedures for referring students to the school nurse or excluding them from school when they suspect that they have a communicable disease. Some communicable disease tests, such as the Tuberculosis Tine Test, are routine in some schools. Some progressive school districts require cardiac screening with a Phono-Cardio-Scan and stethoscopes. According to several authorities, up to 5 out of every 1000 children may have previously unrecognized heart disease that a heart-sound screening program might detect.

HEALTH SCREENING

Of course, not all school districts have a large professional health screening program. But classroom teachers, using equipment that is usually available, can see that children receive at least minimal examinations.

Hearing Screening

Typically a school classroom has two children with hearing problems in one or both ears. The disability may be complete or partial deafness. Parents cannot always discern hearing problems, especially if their child is in the category called "hard of hearing."

The sound frequencies most commonly affected by otitis media, or middle-ear infections, are within the speech range of 500 to 3000 CPS (cycles per second). This is also the most common test range in screening programs.

The two tests performed with a pure tone audiometer are the *threshold test* and the *sweep test*. The sweep test is usually given first. For this test, the audiometer is preset at an intensity of 25 decibels and frequencies of 250, 500, 1000, 2000, 4000, and 8000 CPS are scanned. Failure to hear two or more tones in either ear warrants another sweep test at a later date, because inflammation from a respiratory infection or another temporary problem may be causing the hearing loss. Children who fail the second screening test undergo the threshold test in which the examiner gradually decreases the volume of a tone in order to measure the lowest volume the individual can hear. A normal threshold score is zero and abnormal thresholds deviate from this standard according to decibels of loss. The threshold test is very accurate for hearing acuity, and is used to diagnose hearing problems as well as to validate screening tests.

Audiologists, nurses, or specially trained technicians, rather than elementary school teachers, usually administer hearing tests, but teachers should understand the procedures. Their observations, together with the nurse's recommendations, complaints by the child, and test results, provide the basis for referring the child to a specialist.

Check your own hearing and use the results as a basis for checking students' hearing. Children who cannot hear at the same distance from a sound as you can may have hearing problems.

Here are some activities that may help to find students with hearing problems.

1. For a few minutes, have the children sit as still as they can. Then have them report every sound they heard during those minutes. Try this procedure inside the building and outside.
2. Bring a bell into the classroom. Ask one child to come to the front of the room and turn away from the class. A second child, who acts as the leader, gives the bell to another child to ring. The child "on stage" must identify the bell's location from the front of the classroom.
3. Ask the class to listen to the trees in the wind and think of words to describe the sounds they make in a gentle breeze, in a steady wind, and in a hurricane. Then have the students write about the experience.
4. Have the children clap their hands or tap their feet in rhythm to the music of a record or use simple percussion instruments.
5. Have a child pop a paper bag at the back of the room when no one expects it. Then ask the class to describe what they were doing at the time and how they felt when they heard the noise.
6. Have the children listen for a certain phonic sound at the beginning, middle, or end of words. Read a series of words and ask them to raise their hands every time they hear that sound.
7. Choose ten "sound makers." Make a screen to conceal the items. Make each sound and instruct the children to identify it on paper.
8. Play several different musical instruments and ask the children if they can distinguish the difference.
9. With a drum, tap out a given number of beats or a particular rhythm. Get a volunteer to reproduce it. (Children must close their eyes for this activity to insure the use of the auditory sense rather than the visual sense.)
10. Tell a story that is familiar to the students, and alter the plot or a particular incident. Ask the students to identify the missing or altered part.

11. Whisper directions: "Anyone who can hear me, sit on the floor." "Anyone who can hear me, clap three times." "Anyone who can hear me, leave for recess."
12. Describe an object or make a statement. If the statement is true, the students raise their hands. If the statement is false, they keep their hands on their desks. For example, fish swim? Frogs jump? Bells run?

VISION SCREENING

Since vision is so vital to the typical education program, teachers should be constantly alert for signs of visual problems (see Table 13-2). Ideally each child should have a complete, competent professional eye examination before entering school and at stated strategic intervals throughout school. Until this goal has become a reality, however, vision screening programs are necessary during the preschool years to identify children who may need professional attention. The National Society for the Prevention of Blindness recommends that in lieu of a professional eye examination, each child should receive an annual test for distance visual acuity. In certain locations, state law requires that teachers "examine every child under his jurisdiction to ascertain if such child has defective sight or hearing" and "notify in writing, the parent or guardian of the child of any such defect and explain to such parent or guardian the necessity of medical attention for such child."[1] Statistical studies show that 25 percent of school-age children may have some eye difficulty that requires professional care. Students who have unknown vision problems not only may experience learning problems but also may have difficulty adjusting to school in general.

As an integral part of the overall school health program, the well-rounded eye health program has three basic elements: direct health services, education of both parents and children, and provision of a healthful environment. The total program includes vision screening and follow-up, instruction in eye health and safety, carefully planned policies to prevent eye accidents, a comfortable and healthful visual environment in which lighting is adequate in quantity and quality, medically approved first aid procedures, and special educational facilities and teaching services for children who have limited vision.

Vision screening in schools should not be considered diagnostic, because screening simply tests a few visual skills. Careful observation both by teachers and by the tester is necessary to detect symptoms of eye trouble. Students whose visual ability is not within the "passing" range of established criteria or who show previously mentioned symptoms need a professional eye examination. Screening does not locate every child who needs eye care, nor does every child who is referred need glasses or treatment. As the term implies, screening merely identifies most of the children who may have eye problems.

Screening Procedures

Authorities agree that a careful, painstaking test for central distance visual acuity is the most important single test of vision. This method identifies more children who require eye care than any other single test. Under proper conditions of illumination, it tests the individual's ability to perceive forms twenty feet away. This distance represents infinity because light rays are almost parallel as they enter the eye from twenty feet or further away.

In the schools the best way to screen vision is to use the Snellen eye chart (see Figures 21-1 and 21-2). Testing may involve exposure of single symbols or exposure of the whole chart. The use of isolated test symbols is recommended with preschool-age children. For kindergarten students, screening by exposure of an entire line of symbols is recommended.

Several research studies have shown that the combination of teacher and tester observation plus the Snellen test has a high correlation with clinical findings by ophthalmologists. This procedure is inexpensive, requires little time per student, and is easy to administer.

Preparation

Hang the Snellen chart on a wall or large portable tackboard covered with white paper. Secure the chart to the board so that it does not swing. Use thumbtacks on the top and bottom of the chart to avoid defacing it. Do not place charts on low or narrow blackboards because the location will make working with them difficult. Replace chart covers when they become soiled or torn or difficult to use.

Elementary students should stand for the screening. Hang the chart so the 30–40 foot lines are at the level of the students' eyes. Intermediate and secondary students may sit on a chair for screening to eliminate having to move the chart up and down.

Measure a distance of 20 feet from the chart and place a piece of masking tape on the floor at that point. To indicate where to stand, the tester may fasten paper footprints to the floor with the heels on the 20-foot line. For seated students, the back of the chair seat should be on the 20-foot line or even with the heel of the footprints.

The light on the chart should have an intensity of 10–30 footcandles with no glare. Approximately 20 footcandles is ideal. Control the light with blinds and drapes and check the intensity periodically with a light meter.

Provide a clean eye cover card for each pupil. A wastebasket placed at the 20-foot line makes disposal of used cards easy.

FIGURE 21-1. *Regular Snellen chart. Charts with different letters are available. (National Society to Prevent Blindness, New York, 1980.)*

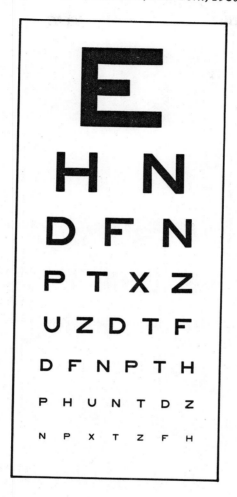

Screening

1. If the examinee has prescription glasses, screen with glasses. Postpone first screening if the child did not bring them. If the pupil forgets them a second time, screen without glasses.
2. Instruct the pupil to keep both eyes open and not to press the occluder (cover card) against the eye.
3. Screen both eyes together, then the right eye and the left. Record the results in the same sequence.
4. Use a cover card to expose four symbols or letters at a time. With a pointer, point to one letter or symbol at a time and move to another one as student responds. Hold the pointer perpendicular

FIGURE 21-2. *Snellen chart for the illiterate child. (National Society to Prevent Blindness, New York, 1980).*

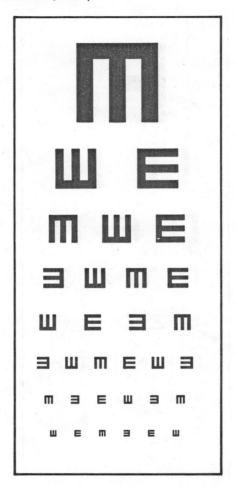

to the chart and one-fourth inch below the symbol. Cover all symbols not in use.
5. Second-grade students and older ones should read the letters aloud as they recognize them.
6. Kindergarten and first-grade pupils can point with the entire arm and hand in the direction in which the legs of the "E" point on the symbol chart.
7. Beginning at the 50-foot line, have the pupil read four symbols on that and each succeeding line. A correct reading of three out of four symbols or letters indicates satisfactory vision. Do not accumulate misses beyond one line. At the 30-foot line, test both eyes and then the left eye and the right eye separately.
8. If the child fails to read the 50-foot line, review your directions

to be sure they are clear. Try the 50-foot line again, and if the student fails again, record appropriately (50–). If the child fails the 30-foot line with both eyes, go to the 40-foot line and examine there. Correct responses at the 40-foot line warrant a second try at the 30-foot line. Record the *last* line on which three out of four replies were correct.

9. To simplify recording, indicate only the number of the last correctly read line.
10. If a student screens 40 or worse wearing glasses, note the date of the last professional eye examination and the doctor's name, if known.

The National Society for the Prevention of Blindness recommends referring children who cannot read the 20/30 line in the third grade and below, and those in the fourth grade and above who cannot read the 20/20 line. The Snellen test, in combination with teacher observation, should identify children who would benefit from a complete eye examination by an ophthalmologist.

Astigmatism Test

Some students may have an irregularly shaped cornea or lens, which causes them to see a blurred image. Commercial astigmatism charts are available or you can make your own (Figure 21–3). Students who report that some lines on the chart look darker than the others ought to receive additional testing.

Referral

Practical criteria for referral based on results of the Snellen test (either isolated symbol or linear method) are as follows:

1. Kindergarten through third grade: Vision of 20/40 or less. The designation 20/40 or less indicates an inability to identify accurately the majority of the letters or symbols on the 30-foot line of the test chart at a distance of 20 feet.
2. Fourth grade and above: Vision of 20/30 or less. This score signifies an inability to identify the majority of the letters or symbols on the 20-foot line of the chart.
3. All grades: A one-line difference between the two eyes.
4. Refer the pupil only after a second screening has been made. Referrals on the basis of one screening are too frequently in error.
5. Rescreen pupils who are unable to follow instructions and any case of questionable findings or significant symptoms on the second screening.
6. Refer all pupils, after a second screening, who do not receive

FIGURE 21-3. *Model for astigmatism chart.*

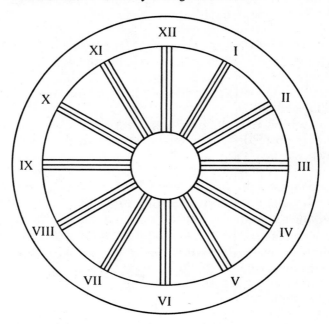

regular eye examinations and who have broken or lost glasses or contact lenses, except:

a. Pupils with 20/40 vision who already wear glasses or contacts, if the correction is recent.

b. Pupils who have had a recent eye examination and correction or whose eyes cannot be helped with glasses or contacts.

In addition to referrals incident to the regular screening program, children who have reading difficulties or other learning problems (among them dyslexia), who experience scholastic failure, who may be mentally retarded, and who have medical problems like cerebral palsy or diabetes should have a thorough, professional eye examination as part of their physical, mental, and emotional evaluation.

Refractive errors can be corrected with glasses. Contact lenses are generally impractical for children because continuing changes in their vision necessitate frequent readjustment of the prescription. Furthermore, proper care and use of contacts usually require a level of responsibility that few elementary schoolchildren display.

Figure 13-2 shows the types of lenses used to correct for myopia and hyperopia. It is desirable for teachers to learn the nature of their students' vision problems early in their association. Generally, looking at their glasses will reveal the handicap. If objects look smaller through the glasses, the child has myopia. On the other hand, lenses for hyperopia cause objects to appear larger. The astigmatic lens distorts objects viewed through it, stretching them in one dimension and shrinking them in the other, an effect that may be exaggerated by looking at objects through the lenses while rotating them. While an inspection of children's glasses may provide a crude assessment of their visual problems, it does not replace the more discriminatory Snellen test. Knowing a child's visual problem early may have considerable value, however. A child whose glasses are borken or who has left them at home may need preferential seating temporarily to obtain the full value of the educational experience.

Other Perceptual Problems

Children who have normal to exceptional intelligence and good hearing and vision may have perceptual problems that cause them to copy symbols in reverse, to print backwards and upside down, or to be unable to spell or read even very simple words. These disorders are usually referred to as *dyslexia, minimal brain damage,* or *minimal brain dysfunction.* Besides the clues that show up in schoolwork, children afflicted with these disorders may also be hyperactive, inattentive, disruptive, awkward, and noisy. Treatment is available for these children but the problem first has to be discovered and referred, usually by teachers.

Handicaps and Chronic Conditions

Teacher observation and classroom tests may lead teachers to suspect and ultimately to find undiagnosed handicaps and chronic health conditions, such as epilepsy, juvenile diabetes, muscle and bone disorders, heart disease, mental and emotional disorders, and numerous other maladies.

One of the first clues that a health problem is developing is a sudden deterioration in schoolwork, such as a change from neat to sloppy writing. Other signs and symptoms include odd behavior; nervous, awkward, or jerky movements; unexplained mood swings; a quick loss of weight, a deterioration in successful social interaction; increased appetite and thirst connected with copious urination and irritability when hungry; and undue fatigue. Many of these signs may point to a developing case of diabetes. Epilepsy may appear for the first time as a grand mal seizure with major convulsions or as a momentary stare, fluttering eyelids, and mild, muscular contractions, including facial twitching, which characterize petit mal.

After a specialist has diagnosed the perceptual problem, teamwork can help the child adjust to the condition and become a successful, functioning adult.

Height-Weight Screening

Growth in height and weight reflects general physical progress in the development process. Students who are big for their age may not necessarily be healthy, however. Increases in height and weight progress at a slow rate from ages six to twelve. Weight increases average four to seven pounds a year and height increases are about two or more inches a year. Usually boys are bigger than girls except between ages ten through fourteen, when most girls are bigger than the boys.

Growth and development are rhythmic, not regular. Humans experience four main periods of growth:

1. Birth to two years: rapid growth
2. Two years to puberty (eight to eleven years): slow growth
3. Eleven to sixteen: rapid growth
4. Sixteen to adult: slow growth

Given this information, teachers may be able to detect a health problem in a student who shows a sudden large change in height and/ or weight.

Have the students keep their own height and weight charts in a log (book) so they can measure themselves once a month and write down the measurements (see Table 21-1). Each student can construct a tape measure out of strong paper. An envelope pasted on the

TABLE 21-1.   Example of Student Log for Height and Weight Measurements

Date	Height	Weight	Waist Size	Arm Circumference	Hand and Foot Measurement
Sept.					
Oct.					
Nov.					
Dec.					
Jan.					
Feb.					
March					
April					
May					
June					

back of the growth record will provide a handy place to store the measurement tape.

Communicable Diseases

Respiratory ailments are the most common communicable disease in children. They commonly begin with watery, puffy eyes, coughing, and "sniffles." Inflamed, watery eyes are also a sign of conjunctivitis (pinkeye). A skin rash, high fever, and a sore throat sometimes herald the coming of other communicable diseases. Listen to children's complaints of headaches, nausea, sore throats, dizziness, and general sickness. A normally outgoing, articulate child who suddenly becomes quiet and uncommunicative may be getting sick.

Skin Conditions

Elementary schoolchildren commonly experience sores, blisters, and rashes. They may be signs of communicable disease or symptoms of an allergy or poor nutrition.

Cold sores, caused by the herpes simplex virus, begin as small, itchy blisters about the nose and mouth. Normally, cold sores are not really something to worry about, but children who get them often should see a physician.

Impetigo, a contagious and potentially serious skin disorder, consists of blisters that become crusty. They appear first on the face, ears, and hands and then spread to other areas of the body. Impetigo usually requires medical treatment.

Eczema is an allergic condition that causes the skin to look constantly chapped, red, and dry. Most often it occurs in patches. The allergic cause (eczema is not contagious) is difficult even for a medical specialist to determine but proper medication can keep it under control.

Ringworm is a highly contagious fungal infection of the skin, scalp, and nails. Beginning as a rounded, puffy, red patch, ringworm spreads outward on the skin. Ringworm in the scalp is characterized by raised, scaly gray patches and loss of hair. Because it is contagious and spreads quickly ringworm should receive prompt diagnosis and treatment.

Another highly infectious disorder is *pediculosis,* or head lice. Children can quickly pick up head lice from each other, regardless of personal hygiene. The eggs the lice lay (nits) are seen as tiny white objects that cling to the hair. The eggs are easier to see than the lice themselves. Other clues include scalp irritation with persistent head scratching and red marks at the hairline.

Scabies, or "the itch," is a contagious and potentially serious skin ailment that can spread throughout the classroom. The cause is a tiny mite (a parasite) that loves to live in the armpits and groin, between fingers, in the hollow of the elbow, and so on. The early signs are small, reddish tracks on the skin. Scratch marks and patches of red skin may be scabies and teachers should refer suspected carriers for examination.

Dental Problems

Dental problems other than tooth decay and severe malocclusion are difficult to spot. Children who have dental problems, however, may be irritable and generally unhappy. Puffy, red gums, foul breath odor, and a complaint of bleeding during toothbrushing are symptoms of gum or gingiva infections. Malocclusion may have a serious negative effect on a child's self-concept. Teachers should refer any child with neglected teeth for examination and treatment. Periodic visits by the school nurse or dental hygienist to the classroom are very helpful and may enhance the teacher's credibility when discussing a child's dental problems with the parents.

Nutrition Problems

Malnutrition can have a serious derogatory effect on the growth, development, and overall success of a child's life. Teachers can build positive nutrition attitudes and knowledge and can influence schools to make good food available. Even so, some children will have nutritional deficiencies and will need help from medical specialists.

The most obvious sign of malnutrition is *obesity,* or overweight. Of course, there are scientific ways to diagnose obesity, but visual judgment is probably sufficient as a screening technique. Children who suffer from undernourishment, on the other hand, may have a short attention span, appear lethargic, and look anemic.

General Health Observation

Normal elementary school students should look healthy. In other words, their hair should be shiny, skin clear, and eyes sparkling, and they should have lots of energy. A teenager in high school may have skin problems (acne, for example), but they should also possess the foregoing characteristics. When something goes wrong in the body, the problem may manifest visible symptoms or the affected student may communicate it verbally.

Imagine you have an old car (motorcycle, boat, etc.) that is not working as it should. If you were a good detective, you would use perceptible signs to identify what was wrong. Then you could find someone who knew about engines (or whatever) to fix it so that it would once again operate efficiently. We can apply this analogy to students. When something is wrong with their health, certain signs and symptoms will become evident. Their health problems will probably hamper their learning. Try to identify their problems and help them to obtain treatment. As a result, they will be better, happier students.

Common danger signals to watch for include the following:

1. *Pain:* Persistent or sharp pain anywhere in the body—head, abdomen, chest, or limbs—particularly if it recurs, is the first danger signal. Pain is a friend, for it often drives us to discover and eradicate its cause before it is too late. Pain is a positive indication that something is wrong. It would be foolish to allow it to continue or to mask its effects with painkilling remedies rather than to seek help.

    Abdominal pain (or bellyache in less elegant language) is a special kind of pain, for sharp abdominal pain heralds a number of serious medical emergencies, including appendicitis. With one very important exception—cancer—most gastrointestinal disorders manifest themselves in abdominal pain. It is very important to remember this rule: *Never administer a laxative in the presence of abdominal pain.* If the pain lasts more than an hour, avoid food and drink also (except for a few small sips of water) and seek medical attention.

    Persistent abdominal pain always demands a medical checkup, but it is not necessary to run to the doctor for every stomach ache. Physicians call the stomach "the greatest liar in the anatomy" because it reflects and reacts to pain stimuli originating far outside its orbit. For example, vomiting may occur as a result of a brain injury. And motion sickness (airsickness, train sickness, car sickness), which really disturbs the balance function of the inner ear, also may produce nausea and vomiting.

2. *Fatigue:* A tired feeling without an immediately obvious cause (such as a late party the night before), a general day-after-day weariness of mind and body, is a second danger signal. Fatigue wears many disguises. Learn to recognize them. Fatigue may cause hesitant and strained speech, emotional outbursts at the slightest provocation, poor posture with head and shoulders bowed forward, red eyelids, dark circles and crow's feet around the eyes, loss of energy by noon, decreased sense of humor, difficulty concentrating on work or play, failure to "catch on" to things ordinarily grasped and a generally tired, listless, and

sluggish demeanor or tension and lack of patience for a considerable period of time.

3. *Weight Change:* Sudden or extreme change in body weight,
whether gain or loss, always needs an explanation.

4. *Headache:* There are hundreds of causes for this common symptom. Recurrent headaches warrant investigation.

5. *Fever:* Fever is practically always a sign of infection. Anything
a degree above normal body temperature (98.6° Fahrenheit by
mouth in adults) suggests a need for prompt medical attention.
Learn the easy technique of reading a clinical thermometer.

6. *Bleeding:* (hemorrhage): From the skin, nose, or any other body
opening.

7. *Indigestion or Malaise:* Especially if it often occurs. Beware
especially of mild but persistent digestive disturbances that
might be ignored.

8. *Insomnia* (sleeplessnes): Often a sign of overfatigue or nervous
disorder. Investigate the cause.

9. *Skin Changes:* Every skin rash, unhealed sore, or unexplained
change in color of the skin or complexion—pale face, ruddy face,
yellow face (yellow is a symptom of jaundice)—demands investigation. Warts and moles require observation to see that they are
not enlarging or changing color.

10. *Personality Changes:* If a lion begins acting like a lamb, or vice
versa, something is wrong. Abnormal restlessness, inattentiveness,
aggressiveness, and shyness all are personality changes that bear
watching.

11. *Vision Changes:* Inattention, eye rubbing, reports of seeing
rainbows around lights, and squinting.

12. *Swelling:* In the abdomen, joints, legs, or any other part of the
body.

13. *Lumps or Growths:* Usually painless—on or under the skin anywhere on the body, especially if they increase in size.

14. *Breathlessness:* After slight exertion.

15. *Coughing and Hoarseness:* If it continues for any period of time.

16. *Sore Throat:* Any that persists for more than a day.

17. *Loss of Appetite:* Or difficulty in swallowing.

18. *Excessive Thirst:* Especially when accompanied by excessive
or painful urination.

19. *Dizziness:* Or giddiness or vertigo.

20. *Bowel-habit Changes:* Notably unaccustomed constipation or
diarrhea.

21. *Changes in Upper Respiratory Function:* Persistent runny nose,
sneezing, and so on.

This list by no means mentions all the signs and symptoms of disease.
Nevertheless, investigation of any one of them decreases greatly the
chances of untimely inconvenience or premature death from disease.

Study the list of common danger signals carefully, but do not overwork it. Do not attempt to interpret the meaning of each symptom; that is the doctor's job. Any one symptom or combination can mean a great many things and can point to a wide range of underlying or incipient diseases.

Health Records

Health records that begin when a child starts school and continue to grow each year are known as *cumulative health records.* They provide information about previous illnesses or medical problems, immunizations, health observations by previous teachers, results of previous screening tests and medical examinations, and any health-related assistance that a child received in the past. Teachers can use cumulative health records to gain a better understanding of the health statuses of their students. It is important for teachers to keep this information confidential to protect students.

Figures 21–4 and 21–5 are examples of school health records. In the absence of a school health-record program, teachers can adapt one of these examples to record all the information that is available to them.

Another important record is the student emergency information card. Figure 21–6 shows an example that school personnel can follow to collect information from students' parents.

Referral and Follow-up Procedures

An efficient health-services program will turn up health problems through student screening and observation. Specific teacher responsibilities for identifying a child with a health problem include the following:

1. Read the family, school, medical, and life history files of each child at the beginning of each school year. If this practice is not possible, scan the medical history of each student for any special needs that you should know about. Observe every child at the beginning of the school year. Observe the children at different times of the day and especially in stressful situations.
2. Observe students carefully for physical, social, and emotional deviations. Ask yourself if each child seems to be progressing academically and maturing personally. Is each child happy and seemingly healthy? Do any of the signs and symptoms listed in a child's school record recur? Create opportunities to visit with each child and record any health complaints.
3. Confirm suspected health problems with further observation in

FIGURE 21-4. *Example of a school health form.*

Pupil's Name_____ Grade_____ Room_____

It is important for the school to have some information about every pupil's health. If possible, please have your family or clinic physician send a report of a recent examination to the schools. Will you ask him to send it on the special forms supplied by the schools?

If a recent health examination has not been performed by a private or clinic physician, please indicate your choice on the form below.

Health clearance is required periodically for participation in swimming classes, ROTC, and certain other school activities. In addition, annual medical appraisals are required for varsity sports.

In order to have health information of value to the school, we would appreciate your responses on the following:

1. Allergies_____   8. Loss of time from school_____

2. Convulsions or seizures_____   9. Serious operations or accidents_____

3. Diabetes_____   10. Known exposure to tuberculosis Yes_____ No_____

4. Frequent colds or sore throats_____   11. Vision_____ Hearing_____

5. Frequent stomach-aches_____   12. Other health problems, such as kidney trouble, ulcers, etc.____

6. Headaches_____   _____

7. Heart trouble_____   _____

HEALTH PRACTICES

1. *Eating*—Breakfast   Yes_____   No_____   Between-meal snacks_____

2. *Rest and sleep*—Average hours_____

3. *Exercise and/or recreation outside of school*—Sports, clubs, music lessons, etc._____

_____

4. *Work activities outside of school*_____

5. *Emotional health*—Assuming responsibilities_____

Getting along with others_____ Liking school_____

IMMUNIZATION RECORD AND TUBERCULIN TESTING (please state year last given)

Smallpox vaccination_____

Diphtheria-Tetanus_____

Polio: Number of Salk (shots) _____

Types of Sabin (oral) doses I_____ II_____ III_____ Trivalent_____

Tuberculin test_____ Negative_____ Positive_____

PLEASE RETURN THIS SHEET PROMPTLY TO THE SCHOOL NURSE AFTER YOU SIGN BELOW

I will have our family or clinic physician give this examination. . . _____
(Sign here)

I wish the school medical appraisal. . . . . _____
(Sign here)

FIGURE 21-5. *Example of a school health form.*

HEALTH APPRAISAL REPORT

SALT LAKE CITY BOARD OF EDUCATION
HEALTH SERVICES DEPARTMENT

THIS INFORMATION IS FOR OFFICIAL USE ONLY AND WILL NOT BE RELEASED TO UNAUTHORIZED PERSONS

NOTE TO PARENT: YOUR CHILD'S SUCCESS IN SCHOOL RESTS TO A VERY GREAT EXTENT ON HIS PHYSICAL WELL BEING. WITH THE CURRENT EMPHASIS ON PHYSICAL FITNESS IT IS EVEN MORE IMPORTANT TO EXCLUDE IN EACH CHILD THE POSSIBILITY OF PHYSICAL HARM FROM ENGAGING IN STRENOUS ACTIVITIES. THE IMPORTANCE OF THESE CONSIDERATIONS DEMANDS YOUR CO-OPERATION SO THAT ANY NECESSARY ADJUSTMENTS CAN BE MADE IN SCHOOL. THE EXAMINATIONS ARE COMPLETED BEFORE THE SCHOOL YEAR STARTS FOR GRADES OF KINDERGARTEN, THIRD, SEVENTH AND TENTH. ALSO ANY NEW STUDENT TO THE DISTRICT AND ON ENTRANCE AND EVERY THREE YEARS FOR STUDENTS IN SPECIAL CLASSES. TAKE YOUR CHILD TO THE MEDICAL DOCTOR OF YOUR CHOICE. YOU SHOULD TAKE WITH YOU A CLEAN FRESHLY VOIDED URINE SAMPLE. LABORATORY TESTS, IMMUNIZATIONS, A SKIN TEST FOR TB OR CHEST X-RAY MAY OR MAY NOT BE INDICATED AND THE SCHOOL RELIES ON YOUR PHYSICIAN'S RECOMMENDATION.

SECTION 1 OF THE FORM SHOULD BE COMPLETED BEFORE YOU REPORT FOR THE DOCTOR'S EXAMINATION. THE BACK OF THE FORM SHOULD THEN BE ADDRESSED TO THE SCHOOL PRINCIPAL AND A STAMP AFFIXED. YOUR DOCTOR WILL MAIL THE FORM DIRECTLY TO THE SCHOOL.

SECTION I

1. Last Name – First Name – Middle Name	2. Date of Birth	3. Age	4. Sex	5. School	6. Grade
7. Home Address	8. Phone	9. Father's Name		10. Mother's Name	

11. FAMILY HISTORY: Has any blood relation of this child ever had any of the following? If yes note relationship at right.

Yes	No		Relationship:	Yes	No		Relationship:	Yes	No		Relationship:	Yes	No		Relationship:
		Tuberculosis				Epilepsy				High Blood Pressure				Cancer	
		Asthma				Hay Fever				Mental Disorder				Rheumatic Fever	
		Hives				Diabetes				Kidney Trouble				Rheumatism	

12. Has child had or does child now have (please check at left of each item.)

YES	NO	(Check each item)	YES	NO	(Check each item)	YES	NO	(Check each item)	YES	NO	(Check each item)
		Scarlet Fever, Erysipelas			Hay Fever			Any Reaction to Serum, Drug or Medicine			Frequent Trouble Sleeping
		Diphtheria			Goiter or Thyroid Trouble			Tumor, Growth, Cyst, Cancer			Frequent or Terrifying Nightmares
		Meningitis			Sugar Diabetes			Rupture			Temper Tantrums
		Rheumatic Fever			Epilepsy or Seizures			Appendicitis			Depression or Excessive Worry
		St. Vitas Dance (chorea)			Tuberculosis			Piles or Rectal Disease			Loss of Memory or Amnesia
		Swollen or Painful Joints			Soaking Sweats			Frequent or Painful Urination			Speech Difficulties
		Mumps			Coughing of Blood			Kidney Stone or Blood in Urine			Bed Wetting
		Whooping Cough			Pneumonia			Kidney or Urinary Disease			Habit Spasm
		Frequent or Severe Headache			Asthma			Boils			Nervous Trouble of Any Sort
		Dizziness or Fainting Spells			Bronchitis or Chronic Cough			Venereal Disease			Poor Eating Habits
		Eye Trouble			Shortness of Breath			Recent Gain or Loss of Weight			Easy Bleeding or Bruising
		Eye Glasses			Pain or Pressure in Chest			Arthritis or Rheumatism			

13. Has Child been immunized for:

	Yes	No	If yes, list most recent year
Tetanus			
Diphtheria			
Small Pox			
Poliomyelitis			

YES	NO	(continued item 12)	YES	NO	(continued)	YES	NO	(continued)
		Ear, Nose, or Throat Trouble			Palpitation or Pounding Heart			Bone, Joint, or Other Deformity
		Mouth Breathing			High or Low Blood Pressure			Lameness
		Running Ears			Cramps in the Legs			Loss of Arm, Leg, Finger or Toe
		Chronic or Frequent Colds			Frequent Indigestion			Foot Trouble
		Severe Tooth or Gum Trouble.			Stomach, Liver or Intestinal Trouble			Paralysis or Poliomyelitis
		Sinusitis			Gall Bladder Trouble			Finger Sucking
		Eczema			Jaundice			Nail Biting

14. Age at Walking	15. Age at Talking	16. Aprox. gain in past 12 months lbs	17. Is child ☐ right handed ☐ left handed	18. Date of Last Dental Check

YES	NO	(Check each item Yes or No. Every item checked "Yes" must be fully explained in the blank space on right.)
		19. Does child take Medication: (If yes, give type, amount and reason)
		20. Is there communicable disease or emotional illness in the home?
		21. Do you know of any reason to limit child's physical activities?
		22. Has child had a chest x-ray? (If yes, why, where, when and result)
		23. Skin Test for Tuberculosis (If yes, give type, data and result)
		24. Has child had difficulty with school studies or teachers? (If yes, give details)
		25. Has child had or been advised to have any operations? (If yes, describe and give age at which occurred)
		26. Has child ever had any illness or injury other than those already noted? (If yes, specify when, where, and give details)

SECTION II

THIS SPACE FOR PHYSICIAN'S ELABORATION OF HISTORICAL DATA:

NOTE TO DOCTOR: WITH THE PRESENT EMPHASIS ON PHYSICAL FITNESS, THE MEDICAL EXAMINATION BECOMES EVEN MORE IMPORTANT. THE TEACHER REQUIRES PRECISE INFORMATION ON EACH PUPIL'S CAPABILITIES OR LIMITATIONS. YOUR SUPPORT IN SUPPLYING COMPLETE INFORMATION IS URGENTLY SOLICITED. KINDLY SEND THE COMPLETED FORM DIRECTLY TO THE SCHOOL.

PHYSICAL ACTIVITY CLASSIFICATION: (Information to be used in determining child's physical education and physical fitness program)

Check One or More (Use space at the right for elaboration)
- ☐ A. Full participation including competitive sports
- ☐ B. Full participation excluding competitive sports
- ☐ C. Restricted participation (Note restrictions)
- ☐ D. No participation in sports
- ☐ E. Limitation of ordinary activity. (Is stair climbing all right?)
- ☐ F. Requires Rest Periods at school
- ☐ G. Special Restrictions only (List)

Comments

FIGURE 21–6. *Example of a form for recording emergency health information.*

EMERGENCY INFORMATION CARD

Name of Pupil _____

Home Address _____ Telephone _____

Name of Father _____ Business Telephone _____

Name of Mother _____ Business Telephone _____

Name of responsible adult who will assume responsibility for the child if parents cannot be reached _____

Address _____ Telephone _____

Physician of choice **(1)** _____ **(2)** _____

                            Telephone _____ Telephone _____

Dentist of choice _____

                            Telephone _____

Hospital of choice _____

                            Telephone _____

Special health condition of child, if any _____

If you and the physician of choice as indicated above cannot be reached in an emergency and if in the judgment of the school authorities immediate medical and/or hospital attention is indicated, do you authorize responsible school authorities to send your child (properly accompanied) to an available hospital or physician?

Yes _____   No _____

                                          _____
                                          Signature of Parent of Guardian
Date _____

---

subsequent weeks. If new behavior patterns appear to relate to the health problem, consider recommending health counseling and referral.

The first of the follow-up procedures is health counseling, which should accomplish the following aims:

1. Give pupils as much information about their health status as they can use to good advantage.
2. Aid in interpreting to parents the significance of health conditions and encourage them to obtain needed care for their children.
3. Motivate pupils and their parents to seek needed treatment and to accept desirable modifications of their school programs.
4. Promote every pupil's acceptance of responsibility for their own health in accordance with their maturity.
5. Contribute to the health education of pupils and parents.
6. Obtain for exceptional pupils educational programs adapted to their individual needs and abilities.

Counseling may involve individual teachers, or it may include the principal and a team of health experts such as a physician, school nurse, health coordinator, counselor, and social worker. This team usually performs follow-up activities in these categories:

1. Detailed examinations to diagnose tuberculosis contacts, fainting spells, heart murmurs, chronic fatigue, and so on
2. Medical correction or treatment of infections (tonsillitis, dental caries, etc.) and allergies
3. Help for parents in meeting parenting responsibilities in regard to malnutrition, insufficient sleep, improved home care, tension and worry in the home, too little play and too much work, and other areas.
4. Mental health problems caused by stress-related factors.

Teachers are in a prime position to observe a health problem and make the first referral. It is important to use the proper channels in the school for referrals. Elementary teachers will logically refer children to the school nurse, who should then assume the referral responsibilities.

A key to the success of follow-up activities is teacher contact with the student's parents. Face-to-face conferences are essential. Notes sent home with the student will not achieve the desired results. It is critical that parents clearly understand a health problem and the part they are to play in the corrective program. Someone must explain it to them in their own language. Potential communication hurdles are poor understanding of English, cultural differences, fears, prejudices, and ignorance. Limited family finances may come to light only after careful sleuthing by teachers, for parents may be too proud to admit their need. Some parents are reluctant to gain medical help as long as their child seems healthy and well. They may not understand the seriousness of a health problem. Some parents accept health problems as a normal part of life. And many other problems may intervene. Teachers must convince the parents that their child's health problem will interfere with success in school and that the situation is urgent in order to guarantee their cooperation. The doctor and nurse can help to accomplish this end.

After referral, the next step is to follow it up. Ask the physician and school nurse for a medical appraisal and an evaluation of the referral. The teacher, school nurse, physician, and parents should then meet together to decide an effective corrective program. Without doubt, teachers are the best people to coordinate the corrective program because of their natural liaison position and daily contact with the student.

After a period of time has passed, an evaluation of a student's progress on the corrective program is essential. This assessment should take place three or four times during the school year.

Although it is easier to ignore health problems, a tremendous amount of professional and human satisfaction comes from helping students overcome health problems. Improved well-being generally leads to improved learning and, later on, to a responsible, well-adjusted, and productive adult. Students who receive this kind of help remember their teachers as successful educators.

UTILIZATION OF COMMUNITY RESOURCES

The health curriculum can reach its full potential only upon identification and use of community resources. Community members can and will work with students and school faculty as a team to promote better community and personal health awareness and more thorough health education.

Each community has a wealth of resources. School personnel must take the initiative to contact and communicate with voluntary community health agencies, public health officials and nurses, physicians, dentists, psychiatrists, other health specialists in private practice, health clinics and hospitals, child guidance clinics, health departments, social service agencies, family service agencies, welfare agencies, and civic and service organizations.

Community health programs can involve elementary students in several ways. For example, they might help the police plan a bicycle safety program or work at a public health department. Visits to water purification plants and fire departments and first aid discussions with paramedics are all very constructive activities. At community-health facilities students can observe firsthand and participate in health careers and services. The schools can also sponsor health fairs and special presentations and invite community and parent participation.

Community health problems in poorer, ghetto areas are more complex and of greater magnitude than in areas where a higher standard of living prevails. Many of the basic health services are not available to insure a high level of wellness among ghetto residents. In these neighborhoods the schools need to take the initiative to stimulate a movement toward better health programs. Mobile units for medical and dental aid, neighborhood nutrition centers and well-baby clinics, community immunization programs, and free treatment centers for venereal disease and drug abuse problems all belong in a comprehensive community "better health program." Informed teachers, in cooperation with the school nurse, can initiate these programs.

NOTE

1. State Law 53-22-1 of Utah Code Annotated 1965.

CHAPTER 22
Principles of Effective Instruction

At one time, teaching involved the cognitive domain almost exclusively. Teachers "told" students what they had to learn, and students memorized facts and information to parrot back at a later date. Today the teaching process is becoming more effective at educating the "whole" student by combining the cognitive (knowledge) and affective (emotional) domains. We now recognize teaching as both an art and a science. We know that children use their body senses to receive messages from their teachers. Learning experiences, then, help them internalize the teacher's message. Teachers can use the scientific approach to formulate realistic behavioral objectives and then select relevant content, materials, and methods to realize the behavioral objectives.

The ultimate goal of today's teachers is to provide learning experiences that will prepare students to become responsible, successful adults (success being determined by the individual). An important part of that preparation is students' involvement in the type of health education and other education that will positively affect their lives.

THE TEACHER'S IMPACT

Individual teachers can have a tremendous personal impact on each student, according to Haim Ginott:

I have come to a frightening conclusion. I am the decisive element in the classroom. It is my personal approach that creates the climate. It is my daily mood that makes the weather. As a teacher, I possess tremendous power to make a child's life miserable or joyous. I can be a tool of torture or an instrument of inspiration. I can humiliate or humor, hurt or heal. In all situations it is my response that decides whether a crisis will be escalated or de-escalated, and a child humanized or de-humanized.[1]

An integral part of being a good educator is giving students room to express feelings, opinions, and values, and cultivating a classroom atmosphere that nurtures expression of those feelings. A true facilitator of learning gives students a voice in planning classroom activities. If students share in the planning, then they feel a sense of responsibility for themselves. The success of this approach requires a non-threatening classroom and lots of resources. Ginott states that teachers should "make it safe for them [the students] to risk failure." He goes on to list some salient points concerning the feeling each student should have about the classroom.

1. In this classroom it is permissible to make mistakes.
2. An error is not a terror.
3. Goofs are lessons.
4. You may err, but don't embrace your error.
5. Mistakes are for correcting.
6. Don't let failure go to your head.[2]

In the last decade, a strong movement in education has been to humanize teaching through the development of a humanistic curriculum. Manning broadly discusses this humanistic curriculum:

This child is a precious thing. Try to know him well. Bring him into your classroom as a loved and esteemed member of the group. Respect him for what he is and guide him to discover what he can do best. Help him to grow in wisdom and skill. Show him that he has within him a capacity for greatness. Give him the will to touch the stars. Protect him, and cherish him, and help him become his finest self.[3]

This philosophy encourages the building of a positive self-concept for each child. The psychologist William Glasser, developer of reality therapy who has also had a great effect on present-day education, likewise emphasizes the development of positive self-concepts. He believes that all students need love and a feeling of self-worth. Glasser says that teachers should care about students as unique individuals and show respect for them as such. Thereby they will help students to respect themselves. This characteristic is essential to a facilitator of learning. Relatedly, Glasser feels that schools should play down two principles:

1. Certainty principle: There is a right and wrong answer to every question.

2. Measurement principle: Nothing is really worthwhile unless it can be measured and assigned a numerical value.[4]

Alschuler helps us understand how to plan a humanistic classroom with the following six-step process:

1. Focus attention on what is happening here and now by creating moderate novelty that is slightly different from what is expected.
2. Provide an intense, integrated experience of the desired new thoughts, actions, and feelings.
3. Help the person make sense out of his experiences by attempting to conceptualize what happened.
4. Relate the experience to the person's values, goals, behavior, and relationships with others.
5. Stabilize the new thoughts, actions, and feelings through practice.
6. Internalize the changes.[5]

Students seem to respond much better to a personal approach than to a fact-oriented approach. Knowledge of subject matter is vital, but it must incorporate the feelings and concerns of students. By combining the cognitive and affective domains, educators can achieve this objective.

THE IMPORTANCE OF HEALTH EDUCATION

We have been discussing education and educators in general. Of all specific subjects, health education demands an affective approach due to its highly personal nature. Health education, therefore, can be much more effective in developing positive health behavior than it has been in the past. According to one survey, American children are deficient in health knowledge. Some of the health problems cited by school administrators who participated in the study are:

1. Failure of the home to encourage the practice of health habits learned in school.
2. Ineffectiveness of instructional methods.
3. Insufficient time in the school day for health education.
4. Inadequate professional preparation of the teaching staff.
5. Lack of interest on the part of some teachers assigned to teach health education.
6. Student indifference to health education.
7. Neglect of health education when combined with the physical education program.[6]

A concluding observation is that teachers may not recognize the real importance of health in the lifeline of their students and, consequently, do not try very hard to involve them in the development of positive health knowledge, attitudes, and behavior. Good health education requires real participation by students.

Additional criteria of effective health education is the projection of a positive health image by teachers and student respect for them. Health education derives as much from teachers' personal health and life-styles as from what comes out of their mouths. Rash addresses this point:

> What you are speaks so loudly I cannot hear what you say! Perhaps it is in patterns of eating, of exercise and sleep, or smoking, of fundamental attitudes and behavior in the realm of personal sex behavior, of integrity, of emotional stability, even of genuine concern for our fellow man that our behavior speaks out so loudly and distinctly.[7]

The goal of health education is to internalize in the student healthy decision making (a process) and positive health behavior. One way to further this goal is through *affective education*. Affective learning involves communication skills, coping skills, creativity, decision-making skills, group interaction, positive self-concept development, and values clarification.

Student involvement stems from reciprocal respect. Mutual respect of teachers and students comes from the expectation of all to impart as well as to receive information, an expectation based on interpersonal relations. Student involvement means integrating their questions, interests, and concerns in the curriculum and strengthening student-teacher relations by attention to learning processes.

THE LEARNING PROCESSES

Communication Skill Building

One of the greatest problems our society has is communicating accurately. When people talk but do not hear, communication breaks down. Strategies and games that stress accurate listening and direction taking help immensely. Risk-taking activities develop trust in oneself and one's peers. Examples are *trust walks* (blind walk) and *trust falls* (a blindfolded student falls backward and is caught from behind by a classmate).

Group Interactions

It is essential to involve students in learning. Asking questions, using lavish praise and encouragement, accepting student ideas and feelings, and using student ideas in teaching all encourage active interest.

Encourage an active learning process. Be cognizant of the kinds of nonverbal communications you are making. Use role-playing and problem-solving techniques. Values-clarification* strategies help students evaluate their own values and discover new ones. It is impossible to teach all the medical knowledge available (the volume of medical knowledge doubles every five years in the United States). Informational knowledge does not always alter behavior anyway. A tragic example of this truth is that people continue to smoke cigarettes even though cigarette smoke is a proven health hazard. Therefore, it is essential for students to develop good health behavior through a learning process. Effective education toward this end involves a combination of the cognitive domain (facts and knowledge), the psychomotor domain (mind-body coordination), and the affective domain (feelings and emotions). Values clarification may involve all three of these domains, but it is primarily the affective domain that handles this task. It takes an excellent teacher to manage feelings and emotion, but that teacher will have more of a positive effect on students' lives.

Decision Making

Today we are witnessing a knowledge explosion. We have more alternatives than ever, especially in the area of life and health. Good decision making is a process of choosing the appropriate alternative. In order to help students understand and use decision-making processes, teachers need to know the three common assumptions for every decision:

1. For every decision there are alternatives.
2. For every decision there are consequences. Consequences are the results, or outcomes, of a decision. The degree of satisfaction with

---

*Values are the standards that we freely choose and hold dear and that determine our behavior. People who are values-clear (know what their values are) are usually more successful and have better mental health than those who are values-confused. Teachers can give students a chance to live healthier lives in all dimensions by helping them to become values-clear. The following references will aid teachers in developing the knowledge, skills, and environment necessary for successful values clarification: Robert C. Hawley and Isabel L. Hawley, *Human Values in the Classroom* (New York: Hart Publishing Co., 1975); Robert C. Hawley, *Value Exploration Through Role Playing* (New York: Hart Publishing Co., 1975); Leland W. Howe and Mary Martha Howe, *Personalizing Education—Values Clarification and Beyond* (New York: Hart Publishing Co., 1975); L. Raths, M. Harmin, and Sidney B. Simon, *Values and Teaching* (Columbus, Ohio: Charles E. Merrill, 1966); Sidney B. Simon, Leland Howe, and Howard Kirschenbaum, *Values Clarification: A Handbook of Practical Strategies for Teachers and Students* (New York: Hart Publishing Co., 1972).

the consequence allows us to distinguish between good and bad decisions.
3. For every decision there is a degree of risk that we will not make the best choice. Skillful decision making reduces the risk or possibility of not making the best choice and increases the chances of choosing satisfying outcomes.

Every decision has three basic components:

1. Personal information: Ideal information is that which is correct, unbiased, complete, and fair. The information used in decision making is seldom ideal, but as personal information approaches the ideal, the amount of risk involved in the decision-making process is reduced.
2. Values. A person's values have a great deal to do with the decision-making process. We prize and cherish our values. Kime et al. state, "A clear picture of personal values allows critical consideration of the information pertaining to all alternatives and the impact of the various alternatives."[8]
3. Style. Kime et al. go on to discuss personal style of living as a somewhat indefinable factor, but as they explain:

Every individual is unique—a character all his own, a direction, a style. Individual style is that uniqueness that results from personal change to deal constructively with environmental limitations. Whether accurate or inaccurate, an individual's impression of his personal style prescribes limits within which choices may be made.[9]

Each component of the decision-making model (see Figure 22-1) may receive more or less emphasis, depending on the nature of the alternatives, but all components are equally important. The degree of risk diminishes as greater consideration is given to each component.

Teachers must help students learn how to make the best decisions. They assist students in reducing the risks of decision making. Because values and value systems come from within, teachers cannot dictate them, but they can facilitate the values clarification process. The day when the effective teacher had only to disseminate information is gone (if it ever existed). Information is only one element of the decision-making process. Kime et al. sum up this idea as follows:

If he understands the components of decision-making, the health educator is equipped to help students face up to and accept decisions and apply their own information, values, and style. By means of such application, the student can reduce his risk when making health decisions.[10]

Behavior Modification

Again, the major goal of health education is to lead the individual to desirable health behavior. One of the basic principles of behavioral

FIGURE 22-1. *The decision-making model. (Redrawn from Kime, Schlaadt, and Tritsch,* Health Instruction, © *1977, p. 128. Reprinted by permission of Prentice-Hall, Inc., Englewood Cliffs, New Jersey.)*

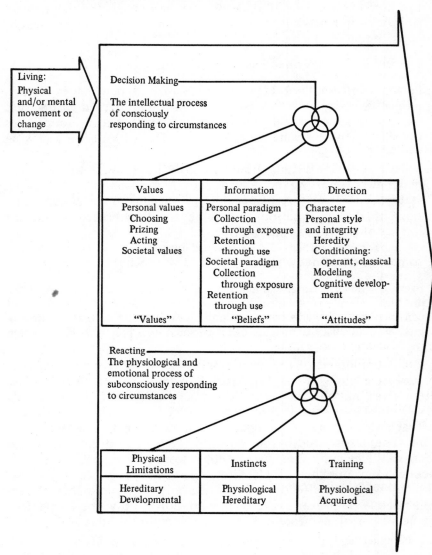

psychology is that rewarded behavior becomes habitual and punished behavior decreases. To achieve behavioral goals, therefore, means strengthening or reinforcing desirable behavior and weakening or removing undesirable behavior. The National Institute of Mental Health lists the following behavior modification principles, which teachers can apply in the classroom:

1. Behavior is learned when it is consistently reinforced.
2. The specific behavior that requires acceleration or deceleration must be identified and the child's strength emphasized.
3. Behavior-modification planning must initially anticipate small gains.
4. The consequences of behavior must be meaningful to the student.
5. Consequences, rewards, or punishments must follow the behavior immediately.
6. Reinforcements may be physical or social.
7. Purposes and goals should be clear.
8. In each instance, the target behavior should be the best one for the particular student. The aim of behavior control should be self control.[11]

Behavior modification techniques are particularly effective in teaching decision making. Specific techniques also can help students to modify health behavior in a positive direction. Through behavior modification, students come to internalize health education to positive effect in their lives. Hochbaum states:

Modification is a process within the individual, not something done to him. . . . It occurs when a person, young or old, has reached an intellectual and emotional state where he is dissatisfied with his present behavior, searches for and discovers a new behavior that promises to be more satisfying to him, and then—if he is able to—modifies behavior accordingly.[12]

Behavior modification offers students the opportunity to choose to modify their behavior or not. A good partner to this method is delegated responsibility, which helps students to develop good habits. Unsatisfactory behavior is amenable to change. The key is to reward appropriate behavior and discourage inappropriate behavior. In addition, encourage discussions about behavior and role models. These methods assist teachers in helping students internalize health education to positively affect behavior.

Affective Films

Educational television now offers some excellent commercial health-education programs for the classroom. The following are two examples of affective film programs:

1. "Inside/Out": Created under the supervision of the Agency for Instructional TV in 1973, this series of thirty fifteen-minute color programs aims at helping eight-to-ten-year-olds achieve and maintain well-being. It covers a broad range of topics involving affective functions such as decision making, interaction and student involvement and acceptance of responsibility. The films are open-ended to encourage discussion. Program subjects include peer-group relationships, prejudice, friendship, and family relationships, in-

cluding divorce and death. The series has been highly successful and is highly recommended. The AIT has also developed a teachers manual, *Inside/Out: A Guide for Teachers,* which explains the purpose of each film and suggests several learning activities.

2. "Self-incorporated." Released in 1975, this program is very similar to the Inside/Out program, but it is for 11-to-13-year-olds. Intended to help this group cope with problems that arise as a result of physical, emotional, and social changes, the fifteen fifteen-minute programs treat the critical issues of boy-girl relationships, peer pressure and sibling rivalry, decision making, and physiological changes. They are open-ended and encourage classroom discussion. Teachers can obtain the useful *Guide to Self-incorporated* from the Agency for Instructional Television, Bloomington, Ind.

HEALTH EDUCATION CURRICULUM PROJECTS

In September 1971, the obvious need for health education prompted the president of the United States to establish the President's Committee on Health Education. The goal of this organization was "raising the level of health consumer citizenship." One of the principal recommendations of this committee was the establishment of a National Center for Health Education, which occurred in 1975. This private, nonprofit organization, in cooperation with the Bureau of Health Education, developed the School Health Education Project (SHEP).

The interest and financial support of the Bureau of Health Education for SHEP derived from its intensive work on the School Health Curriculum Project (SHCP), the Primary Grades Curriculum Project (PGCP), and other school health education projects. The Primary Grades Curriculum Project is for grades K–3, and the School Health Curriculum Project is for grades 2–7. Designed to facilitate individual understanding of and responsibility for the human body and its health, the curricula deal with the biological, cultural, environmental, and social factors that influence the body. They are highly experiential and have been developed and tested in the active classroom setting during the past decade. The School Health Curriculum Project units have been introduced to over 400 school districts in 34 states. The newer Primary Grade Curriculum Project is in 39 school districts in 14 states. The units follow a highly organized, sequential format that integrates completely with the basic curriculum (see Table 22-1).

Anyone in the community can recommend implementation of either curriculum—an educator, a health worker, a parent, a volunteer, or agency. Formal introduction requires three elements: the firm, solid commitment of the school system; funds for training and

TABLE 22-1. Formats of the Primary Grade Curriculum Project and the School Health Curriculum Project

PGCP	SHCP
Kindergarten: Happiness Is Being Healthy Grade 1: Super Me Grade 2: Sights and Sounds Grade 3: Body Framework and Movement	Grade 2: About Our Ears Grade 3: About Our Eyes Grade 4: About Our Digestion Grade 5: About Our Lungs Grade 6: About Our Heart Grade 7: About Our Brain

materials; and training for a team of two classroom teachers at the unit grade level, the principal, and one or two additional curriculum-support personnel.

The K–3 project requires five days of training. The session covers all grade levels simultaneously. The School Health Curriculum Project requires sixty hours training for each grade level unit. Included are periodic monitoring and a nine-month follow-up session. After teaching the unit in the classroom, the experienced team is responsible for training other teams to teach the same grade level.

A film and other information describing the SHCP are available from the National Center for Health Education, School Health Education Project, Suite 215, 901 Sneath Lane, San Bruno, Calif. 94066. Use of the film without attendance of someone who has had experience with the model is not recommended. General brochures are available also from the Bureau of Health Education and the National Center for Health Education.

MEOLOGY[13]

Individual teachers also have developed creative curriculum projects in health education. An example is *meology*, developed by Thomas Okrie of Troy, Mich. This successful program typifies the personal nature of health education and demonstrates how it can very favorably affect students' lives.

Meology includes three operating principles that each student is encouraged to practice:

1. Honesty at all times
2. Mutual respect for each other's opinions and beliefs
3. Trust (what is revealed in class is to stay in the class)

These are the foundation blocks for the philosophy of meology. Spanning from the birth of a person into the world of the future and to old age, death, and dying, this program encourages patient behavior change by focusing on the self-concept as the key ingredient in modification of behavior. The most irreplaceable and delicate feature of meology is the student body. Okrie did not build the program "for" students. Instead he developed it along "with" students. Individual needs dictate the environments and the teaching strategies chosen to meet unique situations. The focal points and structure of the meology program center on six major levels of development:

1. Physical well-being (the body self)
2. Emotional well-being (the feeling self)
3. Mental well-being (the idea self)
4. Interpersonal well-being (the real self)
5. Social well-being (the group self)
6. Spiritual well-being (the value self)

All of these levels are important in the nurturing of human potential. Other sciences take man apart; meology strives to put man together. Meology focuses not on chemicals, neuron responses, or stereotypes but on the unification of all this knowledge into a whole—a whole that works for all people in their particular life situations. Meology is not absorbed or fascinated by the structure and function alone unless these factors strengthen the self-actualization of the individual.[14] Meology puts the parts to work in order to build the whole. Meology is an attempt to synthesize all the knowledge gained and make it work for each child.

Furthermore, every science, well documented and well researched as sciences are, often speaks *about* people and very seldom *to* them. Meology speaks of the information and theories while talking *to* people. The program encourages each participant to value the information by learning to live *through* it. Students share success stories, which are living testimonials that "what I have come to know in theory works in practice." Knowledge is what we possess and living is what we do with what we possess. Knowledge is a necessary part of living, but it is not the sole answer to it. Answers that we find in books do not necessarily provide a formula for living. Living is doing. It is experiencing. Often the experience of living causes the answers to make sense. Meology offers an awareness of what people are—six distinct and complete levels struggling to become a whole. With the help of program, students define the whole of what they have "now." And through the exercise of living what they come to know increases in value everyday and they become all they are meant to be.[15]

This personalized teaching approach is more dependent on style of teaching than on the content. The key is rapport within the classroom, which makes teaching content easier. Okrie strongly believes that teachers should *not* work *for* students but *with* them: "A teacher must become part of the class in order to touch the heart of his class."

For Okrie, every class is a new beginning and therein lies a teacher's central challenge. No two classes are alike. Therefore, Meology uses many different teaching techniques. The most basic teaching tool is called *preping*. "Preping" is a term coined by Okrie to denote the ability to work out the problems in an assignment or lecture before giving it to students. Experienced teachers ought to have a feeling about how students accept their assignments. This knowledge enables a teacher to prepare a prep. Preps can be (and should be) very short, for a prep is no more than an understanding statement explaining why this assignment may be hard and at the same time, why it is necessary. It requires thinking through the problems (and excuses) students are likely to raise and positive reassurance that they can master the task. A prep is empathetic and not a defensive teacher's rationalizing. Assignments become meaningful after teachers have carefully thought through them. Teachers who cannot justify assignment to themselves can expect to face student confrontation.

Sometimes preping, no matter how well a teacher has done it, is not enough. It may be necessary to couple preping with a GAF (glorifying an assignment forever). GAF is an invention of Okrie to characterize an important teaching technique. Anyone can give an assignment, but not everyone can make that assignment seem significant. GAF is a way of making the ordinary assignment significant to the student, making it monumental, lifting it out of the category of classroom work, and giving the assignment value greater than a grade. For example, the traditional way of making an assignment would be to say, "On Friday please hand in ten love thoughts." A GAF approach would have the teacher introduce the assignment this way: "After you have written ten love thoughts, we will try to publish them in a book and sell them in the bookstore. It will also be your job to judge which thoughts are to be considered worthy of merit. A former student who is very good in art can illustrate the book for us." This technique promotes student involvement, preps students for the task, and gives them a reason to work on assignments. With the GAF technique, students learn to value what they do instead of just doing it to get it done. GAF puts students and teachers to work *toward* something and not just *for* something (i.e., letter grades). It elevates assignments to the status of mutual adventures.

Another Meology teaching technique is called the *enshrinement theory*. This theory provides for immortalizing students in Meology, although immortalization is usually not a student goal. It occurs when it seems appropriate at the moment and significant to students' egos. For example, during a discussion on love, one male student remarked: "I do not need love, I can live without it." Rather than writing off the proclamation as a ridiculous statement made by an immature adolescent, the teacher enshrined it as a Meological law. This particular law is called the "McKensie law of affection." There are many of these laws with different philosophical connotations. They serve as a basis for current and future class discussion, during which students analyze, amend, or annotate them. Students seem to find it personally rewarding to be remembered and quoted. It makes them take chances. The enshrinement theory helps teachers to draw students into the class and into the conversation. By taking a stand on something, students begin to build self-concepts.

Two additional techniques that Okrie has used quite frequently in the Meology program are *assimilation* and *weaving*. To effectively use the assimilation technique, teachers must be aware of what is popular on TV or what is currently in vogue in the world. Assimilation is a method in which teachers draw parallels between what is popular and what is happening in Meology. Assimilation serves no educational value other than relieving tension and creating a spirit of competition. For example, Charles Schultz's cartoon character Charlie Brown moralizes as he entertains. Al Capp created Lil' Abner. Meology has a cartoon character called *Meit,* who teaches and moralizes depending on the situation. Similarly, most popular TV shows have theme songs. For "Chico and the Man" and "Welcome Back, Kotter," for example, nationally recognized artists write spirited songs. Meology has a song called "Nobody Spoil Him." Meology assimilates whatever makes life a little less serious and a lot more liveable to keep from becoming too sophisticated and to make it a lot more personable.

Weaving is a technique that ties everything together over and over again through different stories. It uses story pictures, which are diagrams showing where we started, where we are, and where we are headed. They summarize progress and highlight important concepts.

Weaving also provides continuity when conversations seem to sway from the subject under discussion. Students often reveal themselves during moments of conversational drifting. Teachers whose primary concern is content usually do not allow much drifting. By stifling the dialogue, they inevitably limit their effectiveness. No shred of information, memorized fact, or documented statistic can realistically replace the few brief moments of human sharing. It is a firm belief of Meology that a good drift may lead to more meaningful human insights than continued days of drilled content. Drifting is human phenomenon. And at all times, it is absolutely necessary to show interest in students' humanity. Sometimes drifting gives the class a lift. Skilled teachers know how long to pursue a drift and precisely how to weave the pieces together.

A final technique is called *recognition accelerators* (RA). Precise timing is critical to behavior modification. When students are responding to teaching as planned, it is wise to weave an RA into the lecture. Recognition accelerators provide a way to point out progress as soon as a teacher notices it. In other words, recognition accelerators are instant praise. Teachers too often take good behavior for granted. They assume it occurs and fail to realize that it is a goal, not a given fact. Teachers must work *with* students and not take them *for* granted. Harmony is not a continuous part of the classroom environment. It is subject to daily renewal. The seeds teachers plant one day may be ready for harvest the next day. In other words, the recognition of a good day's work today may give the class a head-start tomorrow. Recognition accelerators are signs of appreciation that remind everyone that nothing is owed per se but is earned de facto.

An added value of recognition accelerators is that they stimulate late bloomers. Late bloomers are traditionally called "slow learners," only because they receive no rewards until after the whole task has been finished. Teachers must remember that learning occurs in a stepwise fashion. If teachers reinforce only the end product, then the steps seem to drag on. Teachers must be *with* students on the journey as well as *for* them on arrival. Recognition accelerators are ego building when ego boosts are necessary. And they are necessary *now*. Everything is divisible into parts, and the first important part of teaching the late bloomers is recognition *now* and not the reinforcement of *how well* later.

The ultimate goal of Meology is to bring the student to a reference point of "I am, therefore I can!"

NOTES

1. Haim Ginott, *Teacher and Child* (New York: Macmillan, 1972).
2. Ibid., p. 242.
3. Duane Manning, *Toward a Humanistic Curriculum* (New York: Harper and Row, Publishers, 1971), pp. 3-4.
4. William Glasser, *Schools Without Failure* (New York: Harper and Row, Publishers, 1969), pp. 36-38.
5. Alfred Alschuler, "Humanistic Curriculum," *Education Technology* 10 (May 1970): 58-61.
6. Elena Sliepcevich, *School Health Education Study: A Summary Report* (Washington, D.C.: Samuel Branfman Foundation, 1976).
7. J. Keogh Rash, "An Editorial: The Image of the Health Educator—Are You an Exemplar?" *Journal of School Health* 41 (December 1970), p. 538.
8. Robert E. Kime, Richard G. Schlaadt, and Leonard E. Tritsch, *Health Instruction* (Englewood Cliffs, N.J.: Prentice-Hall, 1977), p. 127.
9. Ibid., p. 129.

10. Ibid., p. 129.
11. Staff of the Center for Studies of Child and Family Mental Health, National Institute of Mental Health, Bethesda, Md., "Behavioral Modification," *Today's Education* 61 (September 1972): 54–55.
12. Godfrey Hochbaum, "Behavior Modification," *School Health Review* 2 (September 1971): 5.
13. Material for this section came from Thomas Okrie, "Meology" (Master's Thesis, Wayne State University, 1977) and from personal correspondence with Okrie.
14. Abraham H. Maslow, *Toward a Psychology of Being* (New York: D. Van Nostrand Co., 1962), p. 135.
15. Thomas Okrie, "Meology" (Master's Thesis, Wayne State University, 1977), p. 43.

RESOURCES

An Introduction to Value Clarification (1972). Educational and Consumer Relations Department, J.C. Penney Company, Inc., 1301 Avenue of the Americas, New York, N.Y. 10019.
Ruth C. Engs, S. Eugene Barnes, and Molly Wantz. *Health Games Students Play.* San Francisco: Kendall Hunt Publishing Co., 1975.
Merill Harmin, Howard Kirschenbaum, and Sidney B. Simon. *Clarifying Values Through Subject Matter.* New York: Hart Publishing Co.
Robert C. Hawley. *Value Exploration Through Role Playing.* New York: Hart Publishing Co., 1975.
Robert A. Hawley and Isabel L. Hawley. *Human Values in the Classroom.* New York: Hart Publishing Co., 1975.
Leland W. Howe and Mary Martha Howe. *Personalizing Education.* New York: Hart Publishing Co., 1975.
Sidney B. Simon and Jay Clark. *Beginning Values Clarification.* New York: Hart Publishing Co.
Sidney B. Simon, Leland W. Howe, and Howard Kirschenbaum. *Values Clarification.* New York: Hart Publishing Co., 1972.
Sidney B. Simon and Howard Kirschenbaum. *Readings in Values Clarification.* New York: Hart Publishing Co., 1975.

CHAPTER 23
Teaching
Health Concepts

The *concept approach* to changing or creating health attitudes and behaviors is the process of piecing together small elements of understanding to form a larger perception of a general principle. A wide variety of learning experiences suggested in this chapter will facilitate children's comprehension of the major concepts in each instructional unit. Our goal here is to summarize teaching ideas that elementary teachers can use to encourage children to think through health learning experiences and form broad concepts or ideas that will fit into their own perpetual plan for healthful living.

Ten principal concepts developed out of the School Health Education Study (SHES). They are:

1. Growth and development influence and are influenced by the structure and functioning of the individual.
2. Growing and developing follow a predictable sequence, yet are unique for each individual.
3. Protection and promotion of health are an individual, community, and international responsibility.
4. The potential for hazards and accidents exists, whatever the environment.
5. There are reciprocal relationships involving man, diseases and environment.
6. The family serves to perpetuate man and to fulfill certain health needs.
7. Personal health practices are affected by a complexity of forces, often conflicting.

8. Utilization of health information, products and services is guided by values and perceptions.
9. Use of substances that modify mood and behavior arises from a variety of motivations.
10. Food selection and eating patterns are determined by physical, social, mental, economic, and cultural factors.[1]

The following presentation focuses on some of these concepts. Resources listed at the ends of the chapters that deal with specific subject areas will help to complete and expand the ten items.

UNIT: GROWTH AND DEVELOPMENT

The family serves to perpetuate humankind and to fulfill certain health needs.

Grade: First and Second

Subconcept

The family is an important part of life for each of us.

1. The family helps us to feel good in many ways
   Learning Activities
   a. Discuss the family members and their roles in the family unit.
   b. Through a puppet show, dramatize how cooperation brings happiness to the family.
   c. Have students draw pictures of what they receive from belonging to a family (food, shelter, love).
   d. Have children list traits they have inherited from their parents.
2. All living things reproduce offspring like themselves.
   Learning Activities
   a. Plant seeds of various types. Show the seeds and allow children to note that:
      1. Seeds produce plants like the parent plants.
      2. Plants produce seeds like the parent seeds.
   b. Have children match pictures of baby animals with pictures of parent animals.

Grade: Third and Fourth

Subconcept

Life produces life through the process of reproduction.

1. Different forms of life have different ways of reproducing themselves.
   Learning Activities
   a. Keep an aquarium with egg-bearing and live-bearing fish.
   b. Use caged mice to show how mammals bear their young.
   c. Prepare an incubator and hatch some eggs.
   d. Show the parts of a plant and how it reproduces itself.
2. Becoming an adult is not the same process for all living things.
   Learning Activities
   a. Develop a chart showing what it takes to make an adult out of:
      1. A marigold seed
      2. A puppy
      3. A monkey
      4. A human
   b. Develop a puppet play to show what would happen if babies received no more from parents than puppies do from dogs.
   c. Discuss how more advanced forms of life have a longer and more involved relationship with parents.
3. Children need help to grow emotionally, mentally, and socially, as well as physically.
   Learning Activities
   a. Role-play how parents help children to mature.
   b. Develop a puppet play about "Growing up is more than getting bigger."
   c. Role-play family situations showing the difference between immature and mature behaviors or reactions.
   d. Have the children tell what the following have to do with growing up:
      1. School
      2. Brothers or sisters
      3. Books and TV
      4. Games and competitive sports.
   e. Keep a record on the wall of each child's physical growth. Ask "What has been the role of your parents in your physical growth?" "What role have you played?"

Grade: Fifth and Sixth

Subconcept

It is a family responsibility to provide experiences that will aid each member in achieving full potential.

1. Each family member should contribute to the growth and happiness of the family unit.

Learning Activities
a. Have students list their talents and indicate how the talents are a benefit to the family.
b. Role-play a family discussion or council meeting ·about a problem typical of the age group. Evaluate autocratic, democratic, and anarchic approaches to solving problems.
c. Discuss the meanings of the following terms and ask what they have to do with family processes:
   1. Patience
   2. Kindness
   3. Courtesy
   4. Respect
   5. Consideration
   6. Self-control
d. Ask how the preceding terms relate to maturity.
2. Many physical changes occur in the body as we grow and mature.
   Learning Activities
   a. Discuss the role of the endocrine glands in maturation.
   b. Develop a mixed-up word puzzle containing the names of glands, hormones, and their functions.
   c. Compare rates of maturation in boys and girls.
   d. Discuss the effects of hormones on secondary sex characteristics.

UNIT: SAFETY

The potential for hazards and accidents exists in every environment.

Grade: First and Second

Subconcept

Rules about safety help us to prevent accidents.

1. Many objects in and around the school are potential safety hazards.
   Learning Activities
   a. Take students on a tour of the school and grounds, and point out or check off safety hazards.
   b. Talk to the principal about playground hazards.
   c. Demonstrate the proper use of playground equipment.
   d. Make bulletin boards showing correct ways to use school equipment and facilities.
   e. Plan activities that would be safe on your school grounds.
   f. Prepare safety rules for various school activities.

2. Accidents happen when we least expect them and fail to follow safety rules.
   Learning Activities
   a. List, demonstrate, or picture safety rules to observe when riding a bicycle, crossing the street, and so on.
   b. Role-play accidents and the rules that would have prevented them.
   c. Have a member of the school safety patrol present and discuss rules for crossing streets.
   d. Let students tell about accidents they have had and what safety violations they involved.
   e. Have students develop a game in which participants earn points for following safety rules on an imaginary trip home.
   f. Demonstrate how courtesy can prevent accidents.
3. Many people help us to be safe.
   Learning Activities
   a. Role-play how mother and father make and keep a safe home.
   b. Tour a fire department and have a fireman discuss fire safety.
   c. Invite a policeman to talk about how police help prevent accidents.
   d. Have students role-play a teacher helping students to learn safety in various school-related activities.
   e. Invite the school nurse to demonstrate how he or she cares for and protects students.
4. Most accidents occur in or around our homes.
   Learning Activities
   a. Have children demonstrate proper care and use of toys.
   b. Have a contest to see who can list the most hazards around the home (i.e., old refrigerators, culverts or canals, cleaning agents, matches, etc.).
   c. Have students draw pictures of hazards discovered on a safety check of their homes.
5. We stay safe by following safety rules.
   Learning Activities
   a. Have students demonstrate:
      1. Safe and unsafe places to play
      2. How to ride a bicycle safely
      3. Proper care and storage of poisonous substances
      4. Proper use of matches
      5. Handling electric appliances safely
      6. Playing safely with rocks and sand
      7. How to react to offers of rides or candy by strangers
      8. Good and bad places to play by drawing maps of their neighborhoods.
      9. Safe and unsafe ways to cross the street by making posters
   b. Have children analyze a personal unsafe behavior and set goals to correct it.

Grade: Third and Fourth

Subconcept

Accidents are a great threat to our health and well-being.

1. Knowledge about the causes of accidents helps us to be more safety-conscious.
   Learning Activities
   a. Prepare a bulletin board showing the causes of several accidents.
   b. Gather news articles about accidents and disease causes and prevention.
   c. Discuss the causes of leading accidents in the home (falls and burns).
   d. Direct the students to detect, correct, and report about a safety hazard at home.
2. We can learn ways to prevent accidents.
   Learning Activities
   a. Prepare a safety checklist to use at home and one to use at school.
   b. Have students review school accident reports (without names) and analyze how the accidents might have been prevented.
   c. Develop a fire-escape plan for home and school and make posters showing safe exit routes.
   d. Organize a "Safety Week," to be officially launched by the principal, and have reports of school accidents, radio announcements, safety drills, poster contests, and so on.
3. Cooperation between parents and children makes a safe home.
   Learning Activities
   a. Report on a home accident telling how parents or children could have prevented it.
   b. Prepare a list of emergency phone numbers to affix to the telephone.
   c. Discuss the roles of parents and children in learning safe use of tools and utensils.
   d. Make a sign or poster warning of a safety hazard for use in the home:
      1. Watch your step.
      2. Don't run in the house
      3. Don't play on the stairs.
4. Many people cooperate in making our environment safe.
   Learning Activities
   a. Write and tell a story about how various people keep us safe:
      1. Firemen
      2. Nurse
      3. Parent

   4. Teacher
   5. Policeman
   6. School lunchroom monitor
b. Have a contest to discover "the safest place in school." Have children list reasons for their choices.

Grade: Fifth and Sixth

Subconcepts

Most accidents are caused by people. They occur because someone or something has failed to function properly under the circumstances.

1. Accidents occur when we begin new activities without learning about them first.
   Learning Activities
   a. Make posters of the risks involved in various activities:
      1. Hiking
      2. Water sports
      3. Hunting and shooting
      4. Camping
   b. Make "expert" badges for learning and reporting on the safety rules for various sports and activities.
   c. Construct a "safe-bicycling" mobile of various road signs.
   d. Develop a play about accidents that occur because people don't know what they are doing (e.g., *The First Day Johnny Tried His Rollerskates*)
2. Safe practices are the key to safe living.
   Learning Activities
   a. Draw posters showing safe practices:
      1. Proper use of matches
      2. Proper use of knives or scissors
   b. Invite a lecturer to speak on safe practices in his or her field:
      1. Police officer
      2. Telephone repair person
      3. Butcher
      4. Factory worker
   c. Draw pictures to illustrate pedestrian safety rules.
3. Safety changes with the seasons.
   Learning Activities
   a. Have children develop stories about what would happen if they tried to do the same things in winter (summer) as they do in summer (winter).
   b. Make posters of seasonal hazards.
   c. Have children prepare reports on weather hazards.

When life-threatening accidents occur, certain procedures are necessary to save lives.

1. Accidents produce emotional as well as physical trauma, which requires proper treatment.
   Learning Activities
   a. Role-play what you would say and do to give emotional and psychological comfort to a victim:
      1. Don't display alarm.
      2. Speak in soft and soothing tones.
      3. Physical contact (i.e., a hand laid gently on forehead, shoulder, or back) is comforting provided you don't touch injured areas.
      4. Don't move the victim, unless it is dangerous to stay put.
   b. Develop posters illustrating "first aid dos and don'ts."
   c. Invite paramedics or other EMT (emergency medical technician) personnel to discuss proper first aid for accident or sudden illness victims.
   d. Demonstrate how to use the phone for emergency dialing.
2. Various types of emergencies may require immediate attention to save life.
   Learning Activities
   a. Discuss these first aid emergencies (see Chapter 20):
      1. Breathing
      2. Bleeding
      3. Poisons
      4. Shock
   b. Demonstrate the proper first aid for the emergencies:
      1. ABC (airway, breathing, circulation)
      2. Hemorrhage
      3. Poisons
      4. Shock
   c. Simulate sudden accident situations and appoint students to respond.
   d. Show Red Cross films of proper first-aid procedures.

Proper care of minor injuries may prevent serious health problems.

1. Wounds are tissue injuries that may lead to infection.
   Learning Activities
   a. Discuss the six types of wounds:
      1. Abrasion (scraping off the top layers of skin)
      2. Incision (sharp, clean cut)
      3. Laceration (jagged, irregular tear of the tissue)
      4. Puncture (small break in skin with shallow to deep penetration by an object)

5. Perforation (penetration by and passage of an object all the way through a body part)
6. Avulsion (tearing away tissue from the body)
   b. Demonstrate proper treatment of wounds (see Chapter 20).

UNIT: COMMUNICABLE DISEASE PROBLEMS

Humans, disease, and the environment have complex interrelationships.

Grade: First and Second

Subconcept

Communicable diseases are microorganism-caused diseases that can spread from one person to another.

1. Microorganisms keep the body from working the way it should.
   Learning Activities
   a. Have the children list some of the diseases they know about.
   b. Have the children role-play what it's like to be sick.
   c. Allow children to look at microorganisms in pond water through a microscope.
   d. Allow children to match pictures and names of some diseases and symptoms.
2. Cleanliness practices help us protect our bodies against disease organisms.
   Learning Activities
   a. Explain the importance of washing hands before eating, after using the bathroom, and so on.
   b. Explain how clean clothes, dishes, and so on protect us against disease.
3. Preventing spread of microorganisms protects others.
   Learning Activities
   a. Describe how microorganisms spread. Demonstrate with a fan and drops of water; blow on a chalk eraser.
   b. Using a feather or cotton ball to represent a microorganism, demonstrate how distance helps prevent giving our diseases to others.
4. When our bodies are strong we can resist microorganisms more effectively.
   Learning Activities
   a. Have students draw pictures of strong bodies fighting disease.
   b. From a group of pictures, let children select the factors that increase resistance (food, immunization, etc.).

5. We can help our bodies overcome sickness.
   Learning Activities
   a. Prepare a bulletin board showing dos and don'ts for someone who is recovering from a disease.
   b. Invite a nurse to talk about care of sick people.
   c. Role-play what parents and children can do in the home to treat disease.

Grade: Third and Fourth

Subconcept

Communicable diseases are caused by specific organisms.

1. Several types of microorganisms are responsible for communicable diseases. (Mention that most microorganisms found in the environment are not harmful and many are very beneficial.)
   Learning Activities
   a. Have the children match pictures of organisms with names of organisms (see Chapter 16).
   b. Have them match types of organisms with the diseases they cause (see Chapter 16).
   c. Expose or touch an agar plate and let children observe the growth of organisms for a few days.
2. Prevention of communicable diseases can take many forms.
   Learning Activities
   a. Discuss factors involved in disease prevention:
      1. Cleanliness
      2. Immunization (see Chapter 16)
      3. Proper food handling (see Chapter 15)
      4. Water purification
      5. Rest and sleep
      6. Immunizations
   b. Have children give reports, draw pictures, or create plays about the preceding disease prevention techniques.
   c. Invite the nurse to discuss and demonstrate immunization.
   d. Have the child establish personal immunization records and evaluate his or her current immunization status.
   e. Have children role-play the ways disease spreads.

Grade: Fifth and Sixth

Subconcept

The infection process passes through a similar sequence in almost everyone (see Chapter 16).

1. Our body defenses have several ways of warding off or healing infections.
   Learning Activities
   a. Discuss skin and membranes as barriers.
   b. Discuss white blood cells, or phagocytes.
   c. Discuss antibodies and immunization (see Chapter 16).
   d. Have students report on scientists who have contributed to our understanding of causes of communicable diseases and their treatment.
   e. Have students pantomime body defenses and disease-causing organisms.
   f. Prepare a bulletin board describing how immunization works.
2. Environmental sanitation is important for communicable disease control and defense.
   a. Have a member of a hospital staff discuss sanitary precautions in a hospital.
   b. Prepare a bulletin board titled "Ways to Kill Germs."
   c. Develop a crossword puzzle containing words related to communicable disease defense.

UNIT: CHRONIC DISEASE PROBLEMS

Grade: Fifth and Sixth

Subconcept

Noncommunicable, chronic diseases are a major health threat in the United States.

1. Chronic diseases are the leading causes of death.
   Learning Activities
   a. List the four leading causes of death in this country;
      1. Heart disease (50 percent of deaths)
      2. Cancer
      3. Stroke
      4. Accidents
   b. Survey the class to find out what caused the deaths of pupils' great grandparents.
2. We can control heart disease by controlling the many factors that contribute to it.
   Learning Activities
   a. Draw posters depicting factors that contribute to heart disease:
      1. Obesity
      2. Smoking
      3. Lack of exercise
      4. High-fat diet

   5. Excess tension
   6. High blood pressure
   7. Infections (rheumatic heart disease)
   b. Develop crossword puzzles containing words related to the heart and heart disease.
   c. Discuss the heart function and parts.
   d. Practice taking pulse:
      1. At rest
      2. During moderate exercise
      3. During heavy exercise
3. Many deaths from cancer are avoidable by intelligent living.
   Learning Activities
   a. Role-play a doctor and patient interview in which the doctor asks the patient about:
      1. Causes of cancer (i.e., smoking, radiation, cancer-causing chemicals)
      2. Danger signs:
         a. Change in bowel or bladder habits
         b. A sore that does not heal
         c. Unusual bleeding or discharge
         d. Thickening or lump in breast or elsewhere
         e. Indigestion or difficulty in swallowing
         f. Obvious change in wart or mole
         g. Nagging cough or hoarseness
   b. Develop a crossword puzzle containing words related to cancer.
   c. Discuss various cancer-producing agents.
   d. Prepare a mobile or bulletin board for the main hall of the school showing the scientific way to treat cancer.

UNIT: DRUG USE AND MISUSE

Use of substances that modify mood and behavior stems from a variety of motivations.

Grade: First and Second

Subconcepts

Maintenance of good health sometimes requires the proper use of drugs or medicines.

1. Drugs are best taken only when a medical doctor or dentist tells us to use them.

Learning Activities
a. Discuss the kind of information a doctor needs to prescribe drugs accurately.
b. Invite the school nurse to talk about the hazards of drugs.
c. Have students draw pictures of people who may legitimately prescribe or sell drugs.
d. Discuss the difference between over-the-counter drugs and prescription drugs.
2. Medicines require careful handling in the home.
Learning Activities
a. Have students draw pictures of places where it is safe to store medicines.
b. Have students clip pictures of bottles of medicine from magazines to make a poster showing where to store medicines.

We should never use some substances because they are always hazardous to our health.

1. Smoking may prevent a person from leading a healthy, active life.
Learning Activities
a. Discuss the effects of smoking on the heart and lungs.
b. Ask students to tell how it feels to inhale smoke or get it in your eyes from a campfire.
c. Make a mobile of disorders caused by or related to smoking:
   1. Lung cancer
   2. Heart disease
   3. Loss of appetite
   4. Irritation to lungs and eyes
d. Have students make up antismoking commercials for TV or radio.
e. Role-play a doctor and patient interview on smoking.
2. Drinks that contain alcohol present some definite risks to health.
Learning Activities
a. Discuss the problems created by misuse of alcohol:
   1. Accidents
   2. Irresponsible behavior
   3. Family problems
   4. Health problems
b. Have students ask their parents about the dangers of alcoholic beverages and report to the class.
c. Invite a police officer to speak about the dangers of alcoholic beverages.
d. Develop a puppet play depicting a doctor and patient discussing problems of alcohol misuse.
e. Prepare a bulletin board depicting some of the problems caused by alcohol.

Grade: Third and Fourth

Subconcept

Whether people use dangerous substances depends on attitudes and motivations.

1. The use of some substances is a habit that is hard to break.
   Learning Activities
   a. Have students describe how they would feel if they could never have ice cream again.
   b. Ask a person who has quit smoking or drinking to talk to the class about:
      1. Reasons for starting
      2. Reasons for stopping
      3. The difficulty of stopping
2. Substance abuse involves many disadvantages and dangers.
   Learning Activities
   a. Have a student panel discuss the advantages and disadvantages of smoking:
      1. Dangers (accidents, disease, etc.)
      2. Expense
      3. Drugs present
   b. Develop a bulletin board illustrating the problems of drinking.
3. People begin to use dangerous substances for a variety of reasons.
   Learning Activities
   a. Develop a puppet play showing ways in which "Smokey" tries to get "No Nonsense Nick" to use cigarettes and how Nick burns Smokey up (makes her mad) by refusing.
   b. Prepare some punch for the class. Give half of the class a note instructing them to refuse the punch at all costs. Give the other half instructions to get the other half to drink some punch.
   c. Role-play the motivations for using drugs and direct a value discussion of these motivations:
      1. Acceptance
      2. Experimentation
      3. Rebellion
      4. Excape
4. The immoderate use of alcohol leads to many personal and family problems.
   Learning Activities
   a. Role-play some of the vices found in alcoholic homes:*
      1. Child abuse
      2. Arguments, fights, and divorce

Caution: Invasion of privacy can become a problem here. Teachers must not draw examples from homes of students.

3. Loss of jobs and money
4. Accidents
5. Loss of friends
   b. Develop a radio or TV spot to educate people about the effects of adult alcoholism on children.
5. Decisions about substance use are based on a variety of factors.
   Learning Activities
   a. Discuss how various factors relate to decisions about substance abuse:
      1. Friends chosen
      2. Family atmosphere
      3. Life experiences and satisfactions
   b. Have students bring advertisements to class and explain how the ads try to get people to drink or smoke:
      1. Artistic beauty
      2. Catchy phrases
      3. Use of movie idols or attractive models.
6. Too large an amount of any substance is unhealthy.
   Learning Activities
   a. Develop a play that shows what happens when people:
      1. Eat too much candy
      2. Breathe too fast
      3. Watch too much TV
      4. Eat too many carrots
   b. Discuss the problems associated with improper use of medicines:
      1. Taking more than prescribed doses
      2. Not heeding warnings (drowsiness)
      3. Taking substances for disorders other than the ones for which they were prescribed:
         a. Have students try to open an empty paint can with a pair of pliers.
         b. Develop a puppet play about using the wrong tools for the job (hammer for watch repairs, etc.)
         c. Invite a law-enforcement officer to talk about the problems associated with unlawful use of drugs.

Grade: Fifth and Sixth

Subconcepts

Use of tobacco products increases chances of coming down with associated diseases.

1. Many serious diseases are related to smoking.
   Learning Activities
   a. Have each student prepare a report on the diseases linked to smoking.

        1. Heart disease
        2. Lung cancer
        3. Ulcers
        4. Emphysema
    b. Prepare a bulletin board showing the relationship of smoking to the foregoing disorders.

2. Concern about the effects of smoking has prompted some government action.

   Learning Activities
    a. Discuss the warnings on cigarette packages.
    b. Have students watch for tobacco ads on radio and TV. They will not find any.
    c. Have students investigate local laws regarding sales of tobacco products to minors and discuss the pros and cons of such laws.

3. Tobacco smoke contains many harmful compounds.

   Learning Activities
    a. Construct a smoking machine and collect the residue from cigarette smoke, which collects in the lungs.
    b. Have students report on the toxins in cigarette smoke and their effects.

4. Smoking has sociological and psychological health implications as well as physical ones.

   Learning Activities
    a. Have students calculate the expense of smoking one pack of cigarettes per day for a year.
    b. Develop a puppet play about the effect of smoke on non-smokers.
    c. Show posters from the American Cancer Society depicting the social implications of smoking.
    d. Assign a panel of "experts" to determine, through questionnaires, why people start smoking.
    e. Have students ask parents how they feel about their children smoking and why.
    f. If you are a smoker, tell the children you plan to quit and why.

Alcohol has the potential for affecting many dimensions of our life.

1. Alcohol modifies behavior through its action on brain centers.

   Learning Activities
    a. Show the parts of the brain and indicate the effects of alcohol on brain functions:
        1. Reflexes
        2. Judgement
        3. Emotions
        4. Reason
        5. Automatic functions

    b. Have students make a bulletin board showing the effects of blood alcohol levels on behavior.

    c. Ask a person from Alcoholics Anonymous to discuss behavior and alcohol with the pupils.

    d. Develop a crossword puzzle about areas of the brain matched with phrases relating the effects of alcohol on behavior.

2. People drink for a variety of reasons.

Learning Activities

    a. Have students ask why people may think that drinking fills different psychological needs.

    b. Invite a lawyer to discuss problems created by drinking.

    c. Construct a bulletin board showing the amount of alcohol in various beverages.

    d. Have a panel discuss the question, "When does drinking become an illness?"

3. Treating alcoholism involves the family as well as the alcoholic.

Learning Activities*

    a. Assign students to extend an invitation to representatives from treatment agencies in the community to discuss how they help alcoholics.

    b. Develop role-playing situations showing how family members should respond to family problems created by an alcoholic family member.

    c. Have students report on their parents' feelings about drinking.

4. The disease of alcoholism produces a considerable drain on society's resources.

Learning Activities

    a. Have students collect news articles relating drinking to accidents.

    b. Invite a police officer to discuss highway accidents and drinking.

    c. Construct a bulletin board comparing the costs of alcoholism to the costs of other diseases to society.

        1. Days work lost

        2. Legal costs

        3. Property losses—accidents

        4. Rehabilitation expenses

        5. Emotional and psychological costs to the family

5. There are many alternatives to the abuse of substances.

Learning Activities

    a. Have the class discuss alternate ways to satisfy needs that lead to substance abuse:

        1. Curiosity

        2. Experimentation

        3. Recognition

**Caution:* Invasion of privacy can become a problem here. Teachers must not draw on examples from homes of students.

     4. Acceptance

     5. Satisfaction

  b. Develop posters illustrating behavioral alternatives.

UNIT: NUTRITION

Food selection and eating patterns are the product of physical, social, mental, economic, and cultural factors.

Grade: First and Second

Subconcept

Proper nutrition is necessary for our bodies to grow strong, healthy, and active.

1. We need food for energy to participate in many activities each day.
   Learning Activities
   a. Have children discuss and demonstrate the many ways we use energy each day.
      1. Walking
      2. Running
      3. Bicycling
      4. Playing
      5. Just being alive
   b. Draw pictures of favorite ways to use energy.
2. We need food for proper growth and development.
   Learning Activities
   a. Relate foods to the health of different body parts (be sure children understand that these are the *best sources* but *not the only sources* of nutrients for the body parts indicated).
      1. Carrots (Vitamin A): vision
      2. Milk and dairy products (calcium): strong bones and teeth
      3. Milk, meat, eggs, beans, peas, nuts (protein): strong muscles.
   b. Have children find names of foods in a mixed-up word puzzle. Place muscle foods across, bone foods down, foods for both diagonal, and so on, and give clues.
3. We need a great variety of foods to ensure proper nutrition and to make eating a pleasant experience.
   Learning Activities
   a. Make a food train showing many different kinds of foods.
   b. Have a food party. Assign different persons to bring favorite salads, soups, meats, casseroles, vegetables, and so on.

c. Have children draw pictures of a good meal.

d. Challenge the children to write the name of a food beginning with each letter in the alphabet.

e. Teach children the concept of the basic four food groups. Have them cut pictures of food from magazines and paste them on a poster listing the basic four.

1. Meat and eggs group
2. Dairy products group
3. Fruits and vegetables group
4. Breads and cereals group

4. We need to make decisions about foods we eat to be healthy.

Learning Activities

a. Give a home assignment to help parents plan meals for a whole day. Ask children to bring the plan to school.

b. Have the children list the foods they ate for lunch in the proper basic four groups.

c. Following the rules of the basic four, have the children select pictures of foods that would make a nutritious breakfast, lunch, and dinner.

Grade: Second and Third

Subconcept

The quality of our nutrition depends directly on our eating habits.

1. We acquire our eating habits early in our lives.

Learning Activities

a. Have children list foods they typically eat at home. Compare lists to show that different families eat different things.

b. Mention certain basic foods (apple, carrots, tuna fish, etc.) and ask the children to describe how it is served in their homes.

c. Have students compare eating habits (food selection) during school lunch.

2. Certain foods are more nutritious than others.

Learning Activities

a. Display pictures of snack foods and ask the children to rank them according to decreasing nutritional value.

b. Have a contest to see who can name the greatest number of high-protein foods (calcium, vitamin, etc.).

c. Make a chart with the basic nutrients listed across the top (fats, carbohydrates, proteins, vitamins, minerals, fiber). From pictures of foods, ask children to select and categorize the ones that are richest in the basic nutrients.

3. How we eat affects our nutrition.
   Learning Activities
   a. Role-play mealtime to show how different emotions and attitudes affect how well we eat.
   b. Develop a puppet show depicting appetizing and unappetizing table habits.
   c. Using puppets as foods, show how foods "feel" when they are left out of a child's eating patterns.
   d. Discuss the nutrients likely to be deficient in a diet when we skip meals (e.g., skipping breakfast may mean we don't eat enough breads and cereals).

Grade: Fifth and Sixth

Subconcepts

Proper nutrition and well-balanced meals require that all nutrients essential for normal health be available most of the time.

1. The diet must contain sufficient calories to meet energy requirements throughout the day.
   Learning Activities
   a. Have students determine their daily energy needs in calories using the approximation formula: $22 \times$ body weight in pounds. (This formula is equal to two times the basal metabolic rate, or BMR, which is given as approximately 11 calories per pound per day. The BMR is the caloric requirement for the body at complete rest.)
   b. Have students calculate their actual intake using the accompanying chart (see Table 23-1).
   c. Have students calculate their caloric intake for one day using the "caloric values of common foods" chart (see Table 23-1).
2. Food selection should emphasize the basic four food groups.
   Learning Activities
   a. Give students a list of common dishes and have them point out how the basic four groups are represented.
   b. Analyze foods from different cultures to find out how other diets fit into the basic four.
   c. Analyze food commercials to determine which food groups are most heavily represented.
   d. Prepare commercials for food establishments that would provide better nutrition than fast-food outlets.

The value of foods lies in the nutrients they provide for optimum growth and development.

TABLE 23-1.   Calories in Some Favorite Foods

Breakfast	Calories	Drinks	Calories
1 Scrambled egg	110	Whole milk, 1 cup	160
2 Slices fried bacon	100	Nonfat milk, 1 cup	90
Ham slice, lean and fat	245	Malted milk, 1 cup	280
1 Wheat pancake	60	Cocoa, 1 cup	235
1 Waffle	210	Orange juice, frozen,	
Grapefruit, ½ whole	55	1 cup diluted	110
Cantaloupe, ½ melon	60	Apple juice, 1 cup	120
Corn flakes, 1 oz.	110	Grape juice, canned, 1 cup	165
Oatmeal, 1 cup	130	Yoghurt, plain, 1 cup	120
White bread, 1 slice	60	Cola drink, 1 cup	95
Butter, 1 pat	50	Ginger ale, 1 cup	70
Jam, 1 tablespoon	55	Beer, 1 cup	100

Lunch or Dinner	Calories	Lunch or Dinner (cont)	Calories
Tomato soup, 1 cup	90	Mashed potatoes, buttered,	
Spaghetti, with meat		1 cup	185
balls and tomato		Pizza, 1 slice	185
sauce, 1 cup	335	Cottage cheese, creamed,	
1 Pork chop, lean	130	1 cup	240
Roast beef, 1 slice lean	125	Custard, 1 cup	285
Hamburger, meat only,		Angelfood cake, 1 slice	110
3 oz.	245	Iced chocolate cake, 1 slice	445
1 Frankfurter, cooked	155	Apple pie, 1 slice	345
Chicken, ½ breast	155	Ice cream, 1 cup	285
Cheddar cheese,		Sherbet, orange, 1 cup	260
1-inch cube	70	Corn starch pudding, 1 cup	275
Bologna, 1 slice	85	Popcorn, 1 cup	65
Peanut butter,		2 Graham crackers	55
1 tablespoon	95	1 Doughnut, cake type	125
Peanuts, roasted, 1 cup	840	Candy, milk chocolate, 1 oz.	150
10 Potato chips	115	Marshmallows, 1 oz.	90
Raisins, dried, 1 cup	460	Pretzels, 5 small sticks	20
1 Apple	70	1 Fig bar	55
1 Banana	85	1 Cookie, 3 inches in diameter	120
1 Navel orange	60		

Source: *Nutritive Value of Foods,* Home and Garden Bulletin No. 72 (Washington, D.C.: U.S. Department of Agriculture, 1977).

1. The nutrients in food meet specific body needs.
   Learning Activities
   a. Have students develop a bulletin board with the seven basic
      nutrients as headings (water, carbohydrates, protein, fats,

vitamins, minerals, fiber). Place pictures of foods under the nutrients that the foods contain in most abundance.

b. Discuss the body needs that each of the basic nutrients meets.

1. Water is the basic medium in which chemical reactions take place. The body requires a constant supply.

2. Carbohydrates supply energy for the body. Primary sources of carbohydrates are breads, cereals, starches, sugars, and so on. Some people consume too much carbohydrate and their bodies convert the excess to fat.

3. Proteins aid in the growth and repair of body cells. They contain amino acids, which are essential to optimum health. Sources of proteins are dairy products, meats, eggs, fish, and legumes (nuts, beans, peas, lentils, etc.).

4. Fats provide large quantities of heat and energy. Many people consume much more fat than is good for optimum health. Diets high in fatty nutrients may lead to obesity complicated by high blood pressure, heart disease, and other health problems. Pastries, meats, and butter are common sources of fat.

5. Vitamins assist in the chemical regulation of the body and are essential in a balanced diet. Recommended amounts of vitamins will also prevent various nutritional-deficiency diseases.

6. Minerals have several purposes in the diet. They aid in regulating the body chemistry, in tooth and bone development, and in the function of heart muscle, skin, and nervous system.

7. Fiber may be an aid to normal digestive-tract function and prevent certain digestive-tract disorders.

c. Construct a vitamins chart telling where we get them and why we need them.

2. Nutritional needs vary from time to time and as circumstances change.

Learning Activities

a. Develop a bulletin board showing how nutritional needs change with:

1. Age (child versus elderly)
2. Season (less active in winter than in summer)
3. Occupation (teacher versus construction worker)

b. Compare two rats—one that is exercised regularly and one that is kept in a small cage—in terms of weight and food consumed.

Diet fads and fallacies are very common and may be harmful.

1. No foods have special powers to provide either physical or mental health.

Learning Activities
a. Invite a nutritionist to speak to the class and answer questions about food fads.
b. Develop a bulletin board comparing the nutrient content of regular and "health" foods:
   1. Yogurt and milk
   2. Honey and sugar
   3. Sprouts and other vegetables
   4. Enriched bread and whole-grain bread
c. Invite a doctor to talk to the class about vitamins and minerals and then prepare a news article about vitamin and mineral risks.
d. Collect notions about the health values of foods from members of another class. Evaluate them—fact and fancy—and make a bulletin board.

UNIT: EVERYDAY PRACTICES IN HEALTH

Protection and promotion of health are an individual, community, and international responsibility.

Grade: First and Second

Subconcepts

Activities that require vigorous physical activity play an important role in our health and well-being.

1. Exercise helps keep our muscles, heart, and lungs healthy.
   Learning Activities
   a. Collect pictures of people performing various types of physical activities.
   b. Develop a puppet play about "Active Happy Healthy Harry" and "Inactive Sad Sickly Sam."
   c. Do a fitness search: Have students tell about someone who is very active from a previous or other class and someone who is inactive, and then compare the fitness of each. *Use no names.* (See Chapter 10 and the Appendix)
2. Group activity helps us be happy and have friends.
   Learning Activities
   a. Have children talk about the activities they like most and why.
   b. Draw pictures of favorite active games.
   c. Explain how sportsmanship is related to friendship:
      1. Fairness
      2. Courtesy

   3. Consideration
   4. Good-natured losing
3. Exercise helps us have good posture.
   Learning Activities
   a. Develop a puppet show called "Miss Stand Tall Helps Sally Slump."
   b. Discuss exercises that aid in the development of good posture.
   c. Develop a fitness demonstration for parents.

Sleep and rest in proper amounts are important for health.

1. Children need sleep for alertness and growth.
   Learning Activities
   a. Have a quiet time each day with appropriate music; talk about how it feels to relax. Teach the children how to relax.
   b. Role-play how it feels to be too tired to do things.
2. When we get too tired we don't feel well.
   Learning Activities
   a. After you have established quiet time, skip it and do regular schoolwork instead. Ask children how they feel.
   b. Have the children ask their parents to keep them up and awake and active very late some night. Let them report in class how it felt.
   c. Have students describe ways of relaxing and resting.
   d. Develop a puppet play showing how adequate sleep and rest produce happiness, activity, and good posture and contrast these results with feelings of tiredness and their effects.
   e. Develop a sleep chart and have the children keep track of the number of hours they sleep every day for a week.

Personal appearance and health benefit from proper oral hygiene.

1. Teeth perform various functions.
   Learning Activities
   a. Help children recognize the letters of the alphabet that require teeth for correct pronunciation (*f, th, v,* etc.). Have them try to say them without using the teeth.
   b. Demonstrate the different chewing functions of the teeth.
      1. Breaking
      2. Biting
      3. Grinding
   c. Help children appreciate the importance of teeth to appearance and personality and how we would look without teeth (show pictures).

2. Regular care of the teeth is necessary to make them last a lifetime.
   Learning Activities
   a. Show a model of the teeth; teach the parts of a tooth.
   b. Have children count their teeth. Tell them which are baby teeth and which are permanent (last molars on each side if there are more than twenty teeth in the mouth).
   c. Invite a dentist or dental hygienist to demonstrate proper care of the teeth to the class.
   d. Discuss dental accidents and appropriate preventive behavior:
      1. Behave appropriately at the water fountain.
      2. Keep hard objects out of the mouth.
      3. Don't use teeth for anything other than chewing food.
   e. Demonstrate ways to clean the teeth when a toothbrush is not available (fibrous foods, swish and swallow).
   f. Show pictures of foods and have the children identify the ones most likely to promote cavities.
   g. Have children note how their teeth feel after eating marshmallows; after eating carrots or celery.
   h. Develop puppet shows about:
      1. Care of teeth and neglect of teeth
      2. A trip to the dentist
      3. Feelings teeth have about sticky, sugary foods

Grade: *Third and Fourth*

Subconcept

Regular, daily health practices will improve health, increase feelings of personal worth, enhance acceptance by others, and promote a better quality of life.

1. Appropriate dress and grooming affects many areas of our lives.
   Learning Activities
   a. Produce a puppet show called "Mergatroid Messy Meets Nelly Neat."
   b. Point out the difference between being badly dressed and being poorly (no money) dressed.
   c. Suggest different occasions, climate, and so on, and ask the children to describe how they should dress.
2. Teeth should last a lifetime with proper care.
   Learning Activities
   a. Tell why straight teeth are healthier.
      1. Better speech

      2. Better appearance
      3. Fewer cavities
      4. Less damage to jaw and mouth structure
   b. Invite an orthodontist to discuss what he or she does and why.
   c. Demonstrate the effect of acid on teeth by placing an egg, shell and all, into a glass of vinegar overnight. Relate the effects to decay produced by acid from bacteria and carbohydrates on the teeth.
   d. Discuss the relationship between eating frequency and bacterial activity:
      1. 30 min. of acid production after breakfast
      2. 30 min. of acid production after lunch
      3. 30 min. of acid production after dinner

Most tooth decay occurs within 30 minutes after sweets enter the mouth. If we eat only three meals per day, we can limit acid production to an hour and a half per day. Contrast:

      1. 30 min.—breakfast
      2. 30 min.—midmorning snack
      3. 30 min.—lunch
      4. 30 min.—midafternoon snack
      5. 30 min.—dinner.
      6. 30 min.—bedtime snack

Eating between meals increases the original 1.5 hours to 3 hours. In addition, if children eat candy or chew gum, the teeth could be in contact with acid-producing materials most of the time.

   e. Conduct a classroom or schoolwide survey to determine:
      1. Number and types of between-meal snacks
      2. Number of visits to the dentist per year
      3. Number of times teeth are brushed each day
      4. Types of toothpaste used
      5. Number of students who floss their teeth

3. Regular exercise makes us feel better.
   Learning Activities
   a. Check the physical fitness of each student (see Appendix B).
   b. Develop exercise routines to music.
   c. Invite an athlete to talk about how regular exercise has influenced his or her life.
   d. Challenge students to promote a family activity and to pursue it regularly one month. Then have them report on the experience.
   e. Develop a bulletin board illustrating the types of exercises that promote:
      1. Strength
      2. Endurance
      3. Agility

TABLE 23-2. Form for Students to Use in Recording Their Pulse Rates During Different Activities

Activity	Pulse Rate at Height of Activity				
	Mon.	Tues.	Wed.	Thurs.	Fri.
Running					
Baseball					
Soccer					
Basketball					
Tag					
Relays					
Football					
Special games					

Grade: Fifth and Sixth

Subconcept

All of us should accept the responsibility for our own health through the regular, daily application of sound health principles.

1. Grooming becomes more important for older students because of their greater social activity and concern.
   Learning Activities
   a. Discuss skin problems such as acne and ringworm. Have students develop posters on the prevention and alleviation of skin problems.
   b. Have students develop a list of likes and dislikes regarding dress and grooming by members of opposite sex.
   c. Develop posters based on slogans to enhance grooming and dress standards in the school.
2. Physical fitness is an essential element to the feeling of well-being.
   Learning Activities
   a. Challenge students to run the distance between San Francisco and Washington, D.C., during the school year. Keep a record of each student's progress.
   b. Develop a bulletin board with these headings: kyphoris, lordo-

sis, prenation. Draw pictures of exercises and activities that prevent and benefit the conditions.

c. Teach students how to check the pulse rate and determine whether an activity enhances cardiovascular fitness.

d. Have each student develop a chart indicating the pulse rate produced by specific types of activities. Have them keep a record of their own pulse rates during different activities for a week (see Table 23-2).

e. Check the fitness of each student (see Appendix).

NOTE

1. *School Health Education Study* (St. Paul, Minn.: Minnesota Mining and Manufacturing Co., 1967).

APPENDIX
Physical Fitness Tests and Norms - Grades 1-6 *

Teachers should frequently have children perform the following calisthenics to insure familiarity with them. Students should achieve a T score of 50 or above. Scores below 50 indicate deficiency and a need for encouragement and correction. Remember that fitness occurs in a context of many factors (nutrition, freedom from diseases, etc.) besides practice in physical education skills.

GRADES 1–4

First Year	Second Year
40-Yard sprint	40-Yard sprint
220-Yard walk and run	220-Yard walk and run
Sit-ups	Sit-ups
Pull-ups	Pull-ups
Standing long jump	Standing long jump

*We gratefully acknowledge the Springfield Public Schools, Springfield, Ore., for providing this material. Norms compare very favorably (in the fifth and sixth grades) with norms established by AAPHER.

Third Year	Fourth Year
40-Yard sprint	40-Yard sprint
440-Yard walk and run	440-Yard walk and run
Sit-ups	Sit-ups
Pull-ups	Pull-ups
Standing long jump	Standing long jump

Sprints

Equipment: Stopwatch.
Starting position: Pupil stands behind the starting line.
Action: The starter takes a position at the finish line with a stopwatch. When he brings his hand down quickly, the pupil leaves her mark. As the pupil crosses the finish line, the starter notes and records the time.
Rules:

1. The score is the lapsed time between when the runner starts and the instant the runner crosses the finish line.
2. Record the time in seconds to the nearest tenth.

Walk and Run

Equipment: Stopwatch.
Starting position: Pupil stands behind the starting line.
Action: On the signal "Ready, go" the pupil starts running the distance (walking only if necessary because the object is to cover the distance in the shortest possible time).
Rules:

1. Record the time in minutes and seconds.

Sit-ups

Starting position: Pupil lies on his back with legs bent, feet about one foot apart. The hands, with fingers interlaced, are grasped behind the neck. Another pupil holds his ankles to keep his feet in contact with the floor and counts each successful sit-up.
Action:

1. Sit up and turn the trunk to the left. Touch the right elbow to the left knee.
2. Return to starting position.

3. Sit up and turn the trunk to the right. Touch the left elbow to the right knee.
4. Return to the starting position.
5. Repeat the required number of times.
6. One complete sit-up is counted each time the pupil returns to the starting position.

Pull-ups

Starting position: Grasp the bar with palms facing forward; hang with arms and legs fully extended, feet free of floor. The partner stands slightly to one side of the pupil being tested and counts each successful pull-up.
Action:

1. Pull body up with the arms until the chin is placed over the bar.
2. Lower body until the elbows are fully extended.
3. Repeat the exercise the required number of times.

Rules:

1. The pull must not be a snap movement.
2. Knees must not be raised.
3. Kicking the legs is not permitted.
4. The body must not swing. If pupil starts to swing, partner stops the motion by holding an extended arm across the front of the pupil's thighs.
5. One complete pull-up is counted each time the pupil's chin goes above the bar.

Standing Long Jump

Starting position: Pupil stands with the feet comfortably apart, toes just behind the takeoff line. Preparatory to jumping, pupil should flex knees and swing arms backward and forward in a rhythmical motion.
Action:

1. Jump, swinging arms forcefully forward and upward, taking off from the balls of the feet.

Rules:

1. Allow three trials.

2. Measure from the takeoff line to the heel of any part of the body that touches the surface nearest the takeoff line.
3. Record best of three trials in feet and inches to the nearest inch.

GRADES 5-6

50-Yard dash
Pull-ups (boys)
Arm-flex (girls)
600-Yard walk and run (boys)
440-Yard walk and run (girls)

50-Yard Dash

Test two students at a time. When they are both in position behind the starting line, give the commands "Get set" and "Go" with downward sweep of the arm. Record the time in seconds to the nearest tenth of a second.

Pull-ups

Raise the horizontal bar high enough for the boy to hang with his legs straight and feet off the floor. Using the overhand grasp, the boy must raise his body by his arms until his chin is over the bar, then lower the body to a full hang. Record the number of pull-ups.

Arm-flex

The girl will stand on a chair or box high enough for her to have her chin at bar height or above. She will grasp the bar with the palms away from the body and hold the chin above the bar while the box or chair is removed. Start the watch when the total weight goes on the arms and stop it when the arms straighten.

600-Yard Walk and Run

Use track or an open marked-off area. The boy uses a standing start and starts running at the signal. Walking is permissible, but the object is to cover distance in the shortest time. Record the time in minutes and seconds.

440-Yard Walk and Run

Use track or an open marked-off area. Girl uses a standing start and starts running at the signal. Walking is permissible, but the object is to cover the distance in the shortest time. Record the time in minutes and seconds.

PHYSICAL FITNESS TEST CONVERSION TABLES

TABLE A–1. First Year, Boys and Girls

40-Yard Sprint			Pull-ups			Sit-ups			220-Yard Walk and Run			Standing Broad Jump		
Test Score Boys	T Score	Test Score Girls	Test Score Boys	T Score	Test Score Girls	Test Score Boys	T Score	Test Score Girls	Test Score Boys	T Score	Test Score Girls	Test Score Boys	T Score	Test Score Girls
6.0	90	7.1	7	90	7	40	90	40	:40	90	:38	5' 6"	90	5' 0"
6.2	76	7.2		76		39	76	39	:41	76	:39	5' 0"	76	4'10"
6.5	72	7.3		72		38	72	38	:43	72	:40	4'10"	72	4' 9"
6.6	70	7.5		70		36	70	36	:45	70	:41	4' 9"	70	4' 8"
6.8	68	7.6		68		32	68	34	:47	68	:42	4' 6"	68	4' 7"
7.0	66	7.7	6	66	6	30	66	32	:48	66	:43	4' 5"	66	4' 6"
7.2	63	7.8	5	63	5	28	63	28	:49	63	:47	4' 4"	63	4' 3"
7.3	61	7.9		61		24	61	24	:50	61	:50	4' 3"	61	4' 0"
7.5	59	8.0	4	59	4	22	59	21	:53	59	:52	4' 2"	59	3'11"
7.6	58	8.1		58		21	58	20	:54	58	:53	4' 1"	58	3'10"
7.7	55	8.3	3	55	3	20	55	18	:55	55	:56	4' 0"	55	3' 9"
7.9	54	8.4		54		19	54	17	:56	54	:57	3'11"	54	3' 8"
8.0	53	8.5	2	53	2	18	53	16	:57	53	:58	3'10"	53	3' 7"
8.1	51	8.6		51		17	51	15	:58	51	:59	3' 9"	51	3' 6"
8.2	50	8.7	1	50	1	16	50	14	:59	50	1:00	3' 8"	50	3' 5"
8.3	49	8.8		49		14	49	13	1:00	49	1:01	3' 7"	49	3' 4"
8.4	48	8.9		48		12	48	12	1:02	48	1:02	3' 6"	48	3' 3"

	T		T		T		T		T		T		T		T
8.5	47	9.0	47	10	47	11	47	1:06	47	1:03	47	3' 5"	47	3' 2"	47
8.6	46	9.1	46	8	46	10	46	1:10	46	1:08	46	3' 4"	46	3' 1"	46
8.7	43	9.2	43	7	43	8	43	1:15	43	1:15	43	3' 3"	43	3' 0"	43
8.8	42	9.3	42	5	42	7	42	1:22	42	1:22	42	3' 2"	42	2'11"	42
9.0	35	9.9	35	4	35	6	35	1:30	35	1:29	35	3' 0"	35	2'10"	35
9.2	28	10.2	28	3	28	4	28	1:42	28	1:38	28	2'11"	28	2' 7"	28
9.8	10	10.5	10	2	10	2	10	1:53	10	1:47	10	2' 9"	10	2' 4"	10
11.0	0	11.0	0	1	0	1	0	1:59	0	1:50	0	2' 0"	0	2' 1"	0

Grades 1–4

Rating	Total T Score
Excellent	296–450
Good	266–295
Fair	241–265
Poor	211–240
Very poor	0–210

TABLE A-2. Second Year, Boys and Girls

40-Yard Sprint			Pull-ups			Sit-ups			440-Yard Run and Walk			Standing Broad Jump		
Test Scores Boys	T Scores	Test Scores Girls	Test Scores Boys	T Scores	Test Scores Girls	Test Scores Boys	T Scores	Test Scores Girls	Test Scores Boys	T Scores	Test Scores Girls	Test Scores Boys	T Scores	Test Scores Girls
5.5	90	6.4	7	90	7	50	90	50	:38	90	:38	5' 7"	90	5' 0"
6.0	76	6.6		76		49	76	49	:39	76	:40	5' 6"	76	4'11"
6.3	72	6.7		72		48	72	48	:40	72	:42	5' 5"	72	4'10"
6.4	70	6.8		70		47	70	47	:41	70	:43	5' 2"	70	4' 9"
6.5	68	6.9		68		45	68	45	:42	68	:45	5' 1"	68	4' 8"
6.6	66	7.0	6	66	6	44	66	44	:43	66	:46	5' 0"	66	4' 7"
6.7	63	7.1	5	63	5	43	63	39	:44	63	:47	4'10"	63	4' 6"
7.0	61	7.3		61		39	61	36	:45	61	:48	4' 7"	61	4' 5"
7.1	59	7.4	4	59	4	31	59	31	:46	59	:49	4' 6"	59	4' 4"
7.2	58	7.5		58		30	58	30	:47	58	:50	4' 5"	58	4' 3"
7.3	55	7.6	3	55	3	27	55	27	:49	55	:51	4' 4"	55	4' 2"
7.4	54	7.7		54		26	54	26	:50	54	:52	4' 3"	54	4' 1"
7.5	53	7.8	2	53	2	25	53	25	:51	53	:53	4' 2"	53	4' 0"
7.7	51	7.9		51		24	51	24	:52	51	:54	4' 1"	51	3'11"
7.8	50	8.0	1	50	1	23	50	23	:53	50	:55	4' 0"	50	3'10"
7.9														
8.0	49	8.1		49		20	49	21	:54	49	:56	3'11"	49	3' 9"
8.1	48	8.2		48		18	48	20	:55	48	:58	3'10"	48	3' 8"
8.2	47	8.3		47		16	47	19	:56	47	:59	3' 9"	47	3' 7"
8.4	46	8.4		46		14	46	18	:58	46	1:00	3' 8"	46	3' 6"
8.5	43	8.5		43		10	43	15	1:02	43	1:02	3' 7"	43	3' 5"

8.9	42		0	8.6	42		9	42	12	1:11	42	1:06	3' 6"	42	3' 4"
9.0	35			8.7	35		8	35	9	1:19	35	1:17	3' 5"	35	3' 3"
9.2	28			8.9	28		6	28	7	1:25	28	1:20	3' 4"	28	3' 1"
9.5	10			9.0	10		4	10	4	1:37	10	1:25	3' 2"	10	2'11"
0.0	0	0		9.6	0		0	0	0	1:43	0	2:02	2' 8"	0	1'10"

Grades 1–4

Rating	Total T Score
Excellent	296–450
Good	266–295
Fair	241–265
Poor	211–240
Very poor	0–210

TABLE A-3. Third Year, Boys and Girls

40-Yard Sprint			Pull-ups			Sit-ups			440-Yard Run and Walk			Standing Broad Jump		
Test Scores Boys	T Scores	Test Scores Girls	Test Scores Boys	T Scores	Test Scores Girls	Test Scores Boys	T Scores	Test Scores Girls	Test Scores Boys	T Scores	Test Scores Girls	Test Scores Boys	T Scores	Test Scores Girls
6.1	90	6.1	8	90	8	60	90	60	1:15	90	1:12	5' 8"	90	5' 6"
6.2	76	6.2		76		59	76	59	1:18	76	1:17	5' 7"	76	5' 5"
6.3	72	6.4		72		58	72	58	1:20	72	1:21	5' 6"	72	5' 4"
6.4	70	6.5		70		57	70	57	1:24	70	1:26	5' 5"	70	5' 3"
6.5	68	6.6		68		56	68	56	1:31	68	1:37	5' 4"	68	5' 2"
6.6	66	6.7	7	66	7	55	66	55	1:35	66	1:38	5' 3"	66	5' 1"
6.7	63	6.8	6	63	6	54	63	50	1:37	63	1:42	5' 2"	63	5' 0"
6.8	61	6.9		61		53	61	46	1:40	61	1:45	5' 1"	61	4'11"
6.9	59	7.0	5	59	5	49	59	42	1:43	59	1:47	4'11"	59	4'10"
7.0	58	7.1		58		47	58	41	1:45	58	1:49	4'10"	58	4' 9"
7.1	55	7.2	4	55	4	42	55	40	1:47	55	1:50	4' 9"	55	4' 8"
7.2	54	7.3		54		39	54	38	1:48	54	1:51	4' 8"	54	4' 7"
7.3	53	7.4	3	53	3	37	53	37	1:49	53	1:53	4' 7"	53	4' 6"
7.4	51	7.5		51		36	51	36	1:52	51	1:55	4' 6"	51	4' 5"
7.5	50	7.6	2	50	2	34	50	34	1:55	50	1:57	4' 5"	50	4' 4"
7.6	49	7.7		49		32	49	32	1:58	49	1:59	4' 4"	49	4' 3"
7.7	48	7.8	1	48	1	30	48	30	1:59	48	2:00	4' 3"	48	4' 2"
7.8	47	7.9		47		28	47	28	2:00	47	2:02	4' 2"	47	4' 1"
7.9	46	8.0		46		26	46	26	2:01	46	2:04	4' 1"	46	4' 0"
8.0	43	8.1		43		23	43	22	2:05	43	2:07	4' 0"	43	3'11"

8.1	42	8.2	42	18	42	2:07	18	42	2:10	3'11"	42	3'10"
8.3	35	8.3	35	13	35	2:10	13	35	2:13	3'10"	35	3' 9"
8.6	28	8.4	28	10	28	2:15	9	28	2:15	3' 8"	28	3' 8"
9.1	10	8.5	10	7	10	2:23	5	10	2:20	3' 6"	10	3' 5"
10.0	0	9.0	0	6	0	3:00	0	0	3:36	2' 5"	0	3' 0"

Grades 1–4

Rating	Total T Score
Excellent	296–450
Good	266–295
Fair	241–265
Poor	211–240
Very poor	0–210

TABLE A-4. Fourth Year, Boys and Girls

40-Yard Sprint			Pull-ups			Sit-ups			440-Yard Walk and Run			Standing Broad Jump		
Test Scores Boys	T Score	Test Scores Girls	Test Scores Boys	T Score	Test Scores Girls	Test Scores Boys	T Score	Test Scores Girls	Test Scores Boys	T Score	Test Scores Girls	Test Scores Boys	T Score	Test Scores Girls
6.0	90	6.0	8	90	8	70	90	70	1:15	90	1:15	6' 6"	90	6' 0"
6.1	76	6.1		76		69	76	65	1:18	76	1:18	6' 0"	76	5' 8"
6.2	72	6.2		72		68	72	64	1:20	72	1:20	5' 9"	72	5' 6"
6.3	70	6.3		70		67	70	63	1:23	70	1:25	5' 8"	70	5' 5"
6.4	68	6.4		68		66	68	61	1:24	68	1:30	5' 7"	68	5' 4"
6.5	66	6.5	7	66	7	65	66	59	1:25	66	1:32	5' 6"	66	5' 3"
6.6	63	6.6	6	63	6	64	63	57	1:27	63	1:35	5' 4"	63	5' 2"
6.7	61	6.7		61		63	61	55	1:30	61	1:37	5' 2"	61	5' 1"
6.8	59	6.8	5	59	5	62	59	53	1:32	59	1:40	5' 0"	59	4'11"
6.9	58	6.9		58		61	58	52	1:34	58	1:43	4'11"	58	4'10"
7.0	55	7.0	4	55	4	60	55	48	1:36	55	1:47	4'10"	55	4' 9"
7.1	54	7.1		54		55	54	47	1:38	54	1:49	4' 9"	54	4' 8"
7.2	53	7.2	3	53	3	53	53	45	1:40	53	1:51	4' 8"	53	4' 7"
7.3	51	7.3		51		52	51	43	1:45	51	1:54	4' 7"	51	4' 6"
7.4	50	7.4	2	50	2	49	50	41	1:48	50	1:56	4' 6"	50	4' 5"
7.5	49	7.5	1	49	1	46	49	40	1:50	49	1:57	4' 5"	49	4' 4"
7.6	48	7.6		48		40	48	37	1:51	48	1:58	4' 4"	48	4' 3"
7.7	47	7.7		47		34	47	35	1:52	47	1:59	4' 3"	47	4' 2"
7.8	46	7.8		46		32	46	29	1:56	46	2:01	4' 2"	46	4' 1"
7.9	43	7.9		43		31	43	25	1:59	43	2:06	4' 1"	43	4' 0"

8.0 42
8.1 35
8.2 28
8.4 10
10.0 0

0

8.0 42
8.1 35
8.2 28
8.3 10
10.0 0

0

30 42
24 35
20 28
15 10
10 0

24 42 2:00 42 2:10 42 4' 0" 42 3'10"
20 35 2:05 35 2:13 35 3'11" 35 3' 8"
18 28 2:07 28 2:18 28 3' 8" 28 3' 5"
10 10 2:10 10 2:21 10 3' 5" 10 3' 2"
 7   0 2:15   0 2:25   0 3' 0"   0 3' 0"

Grades 1–4

Rating	Total T Score
Excellent	296–450
Good	266–295
Fair	241–265
Poor	211–240
Very poor	0–210

TABLE A-5.   Fifth Year, Boys

50-Yard Sprint		Pull-ups		600-Yard Run and Walk	
Test Score	T Score	Test Score	T Score	Test Score	T Score
6.5	90	12	90	1:44	90
6.8	76		76	1:45	76
6.9	72		72	1:46	72
7.1	70		70	1:47	70
7.2	68		68	1:48	68
7.3	66	11	66	1:49	66
7.4	63	10	63	1:50	63
7.5	61	9	61	1:57	61
7.6	59	8	59	2:02	59
7.7	58	7	58	2:06	58
7.8	55	6	55	2:11	55
7.9	54	5	54	2:14	54
8.0	53	4	53	2:17	53
8.1	51	3	51	2:23	51
8.2	50	2	50	2:25	50
8.3	49	1	49	2:27	49
8.4	48		48	2:33	48
8.5	47		47	2:38	47
8.8	46		46	2:41	46
8.9	43		43	2:44	43
9.4	42		42	2:51	42
9.7	35		35	2:56	35
10.1	28		28	2:57	28
10.5	10		10	2:59	10
10.6	0	0	0	3:00	0

Grades 5–6

Rating	Total T Score
Excellent	177–270
Good	159–176
Fair	144–158
Poor	126–143
Very poor	0–125

TABLE A-6.   Fifth Year, Girls

50-Yard Sprint		Arm-flex		440-Yard Run and Walk	
Test Score	T Score	Test Score (seconds)	T Score	Test Score	T Score
6.0	90	65	90	1:14	90
6.3	76	56	76	1:21	76
6.4	72	49	72	1:23	72
6.6	70	44	70	1:25	70
7.0	68	40	68	1:27	68
7.3	66	38	66	1:29	66
7.5	63	35	63	1:31	63
7.8	61	32	61	1:33	61
7.9	59	31	59	1:35	59
8.0	58	30	58	1:37	58
8.1	55	29	55	1:39	55
8.2	54	28	54	1:41	54
8.3	53	27	53	1:43	53
8.4	51	26	51	1:45	51
8.5	50	25	50	1:47	50
8.6	49	24	49	1:49	49
8.7	48	22	48	1:54	48
8.8	47	19	47	2:00	47
8.9	46	17	46	2:07	46
9.0	43	14	43	2:15	43
9.3	42	10	42	2:30	42
9.7	35	7	35	2:45	35
9.9	28	4	28	3:00	28
10.5	10	1	10	3:30	10
11.4	0	0	0	4:00	0

Grades 5–6

Rating	Total T Score
Excellent	177–270
Good	159–176
Fair	144–158
Poor	126–143
Very poor	0–125

TABLE A-7. Sixth Year, Boys

50-Yard Sprint		Pull-ups		600-Yard Run and Walk	
Test Score	T Score	Test Score	T Score	Test Score	T Score
6.0	90	12	90	1:36	90
6.3	76		76	1:37	76
6.5	72		72	1:38	72
6.7	70		70	1:39	70
6.8	68		68	1:43	68
7.0	66	11	66	1:48	66
7.1	63	10	63	1:56	63
7.2	61	9	61	2:02	61
7.3	59	8	59	2:05	59
7.4	58	7	58	2:08	58
7.5	55	6	55	2:11	55
7.6	54	5	54	2:15	54
7.8	53	4	53	2:20	53
7.9	51	3	51	2:21	51
8.0	50	2	50	2:22	50
8.1	49	1	49	2:23	49
8.2	48		48	2:24	48
8.3	47		47	2:27	47
8.4	46		46	2:31	46
8.5	43		43	2:37	43
8.7	42		42	2:40	42
8.9	35		35	2:43	35
9.1	28		28	2:49	28
9.2	10		10	3:05	10
9.3	0	0	0	3:48	0

Grades 5–6

Rating	Total T Score
Excellent	177–270
Good	159–176
Fair	144–158
Poor	126–143
Very poor	0–125

TABLE A–8.   Sixth Year, Girls

50-Yard Sprint		Arm-flex		440-Yard Run and Walk	
Test Score	T Score	Test Score	T Score	Test Score	T Score
6.0	90	75	90	1:12	90
6.3	76	64	76	1:20	76
6.9	72	58	72	1:22	72
7.2	70	53	70	1:24	70
7.3	68	47	68	1:26	68
7.4	66	45	66	1:28	66
7.5	63	41	63	1:30	63
7.6	61	37	61	1:32	61
7.7	59	36	59	1:34	59
7.8	58	35	58	1:36	58
7.9	55	33	55	1:38	55
8.0	54	32	54	1:40	54
8.1	53	31	53	1:42	53
8.2	51	27	51	1:44	51
8.3	50	25	50	1:46	50
8.4	49	24	49	1:48	49
8.5	48	22	48	1:51	48
8.6	47	19	47	1:55	47
8.7	46	17	46	1:59	46
8.9	43	14	43	2:05	43
9.2	42	10	42	2:15	42
9.5	35	7	35	2:30	35
9.7	28	4	28	2:45	28
10.1	10	11	10	3:00	10
10.9	0	0	0	3:30	0

Grades 5–6

Rating	Total T Score
Excellent	177–270
Good	159–176
Fair	144–158
Poor	126–143
Very poor	0–125

Index